# Fetal Neurology

*Guest Editor*

ADRÉ J. DU PLESSIS, MBChB, MPH

# CLINICS IN PERINATOLOGY

www.perinatology.theclinics.com

September 2009 • Volume 36 • Number 3

SAUNDERS an imprint of ELSEVIER, Inc.

**W.B. SAUNDERS COMPANY**
*A Division of Elsevier Inc.*

Elsevier, Inc. ● 1600 John F. Kennedy Blvd. ● Suite 1800 ● Philadelphia, PA 19103-2899

http://www.theclinics.com

**CLINICS IN PERINATOLOGY Volume 36, Number 3**
**September 2009 ISSN 0095-5108, ISBN-10: 1-4377-1259-2, ISBN-13: 978-1-4377-1259-9**

Editor: Carla Holloway
Developmental Editor: Donald Mumford

*Clinics in Perinatology* (ISSN 0095-5108) is published in quarterly by Elsevier Inc., 360 Park Avenue South, New York, NY 10010-1710. Months of issue are March, June, September, and December. Subscription prices are $217.00 per year (US individuals), $321.00 per year (US institutions), $255.00 per year (Canadian individuals), $408.00 per year (Canadian institutions), $314.00 per year (foreign individuals), $408.00 per year (foreign institutions) $105.00 per year (US students), and $153.00 per year (Canadian and foreign students). Foreign air speed delivery is included in all Clinics subscription prices. All prices are subject to change without notice. **POSTMASTER:** Send address changes to *Clinics in Perinatology*, Elsevier Health Sciences Division, Subscription Customer Service, 3251 Riverport Lane, Maryland Heights, MO 63043. **Customer Service: Telephone: 1-800-654-2452** (U.S. and Canada); **1-314-447-8871** (outside U.S. and Canada). **Fax: 1-314-447-8029. E-mail: journalscustomerservice-usa@elsevier.com** (for print support); **journalsonlinesupport-usa@elsevier.com** (for online support).

*Reprints.* For copies of 100 or more, of articles in this publication, please contact the Commercial Reprints Department, Elsevier Inc., 360 Park Avenue South, New York, NY 10010-1710. Tel. (212) 633-3812; Fax: (212) 482-1935; email: reprints@elsevier.com.

*Clinics in Perinatology* is also pubilshed in Spanish by McGraw-Hill Interamericana Editores S.A., P.O. Box 5-237, 06500 Mexico D.F., Mexico.

*Clinics in Perinatology* is covered in *MEDLINE/PubMed (Index Medicus) Current Contents, Excepta Medica, BIOSIS and ISI/BIOMED.*

Printed in the United States of America.

# Contributors

## GUEST EDITOR

**ADRÉ J. DU PLESSIS, MBChB, MPH**
Associate Professor of Neurology, Harvard Medical School; Associate in Neurology and Director, Fetal-Neonatal Neurology Research Group, Children's Hospital Boston; Boston, Massachusetts

## AUTHORS

**JAMES F. BALE, Jr, MD**
Professor and Associate Chair, Division of Pediatric Neurology, Departments of Pediatrics and Neurology, The University of Utah School of Medicine; and Pediatric Residency Office, Primary Children's Medical Center, Salt Lake City, Utah

**LAURA BENNET, PhD**
Professor, Department of Physiology, Faculty of Medical and Health Sciences, University of Auckland, Auckland, New Zealand

**PETER C. BRUGGER, MD, PhD**
Associate Professor, Center of Anatomy and Cell Biology, Medical University of Vienna, Vienna, Austria

**ROMY CHUNG, MD**
Resident, Department of Radiology, University of California, San Diego, School of Medicine, La Jolla, California

**ALEJANDRO L. DIAZ, MD**
Neurogenetics Laboratory, Howard Hughes Medical Institute, Department of Pediatrics and Neurosciences, University of California, San Diego, Leicthag Biomedical Research Building, La Jolla, California

**ADRÉ J. DU PLESSIS, MBChB, MPH**
Associate Professor of Neurology, Harvard Medical School; Associate in Neurology and Director, Fetal-Neonatal Neurology Research Group, Children's Hospital Boston; Boston, Massachusetts

**HARI ESWARAN, PhD**
Associate Professor, SARA Scientific Director, Department of Obstetrics and Gynecology, University of Arkansas for Medical Sciences, Little Rock, Arkansas

**JOSEPH G. GLEESON, MD**
Neurogenetics Laboratory, Howard Hughes Medical Institute, Department of Pediatrics and Neurosciences, University of California, San Diego, Leicthag Biomedical Research Building, La Jolla, California

**RATHINASWAMY B. GOVINDAN, PhD**
Assistant Professor, Department of Obstetrics and Gynecology, University of Arkansas for Medical Sciences, Little Rock, Arkansas

**ALISTAIR JAN GUNN, MBChB, PhD**
Professor of Physiology and Paediatrics, Department of Physiology, Faculty of Medical and Health Sciences, University of Auckland; Department of Paediatrics, Faculty of Medical and Health Sciences, University of Auckland; and Paediatrician, Starship Children's Hospital, Auckland, New Zealand

**GREGOR KASPRIAN, MD**
Fellow, Department of Neuroradiology, Medical University of Vienna, Vienna, Austria

**MARTIN LAMMENS, MD, PhD**
Department of Pathology, Radboud University Nijmegen Medical Center, Nijmegen, The Netherlands

**TALLY LERMAN-SAGIE, MD**, Associate Professor, Pediatric Neurology Unit; and Metabolic Neurogenetic Service, Wolfson Medical Center, Sackler School of Medicine, Tel Aviv University, Tel Aviv, Israel

**BARRY M. LESTER, PhD**
Professor of Psychiatry and Human Behavior, Professor of Pediatrics, Warren Alpert Medical School of Brown University; and Director, Brown Center for the Study of Children, Department of Pediatrics, Women & Infants Hospital of Rhode Island, Providence, Rhode Island

**CATHERINE LIMPEROPOULOS, PhD**
Assistant Professor, Department of Neurology and Neurosurgery, McGill University; Department of Pediatrics, McGill University, Montreal, Quebec; and Fetal-Neonatal Neurology Research Group, Department of Neurology, Children's Hospital Boston and Harvard Medical School, Boston, Massachusetts

**CURTIS L. LOWERY, MD**
Professor, Specialist, Division of Maternal-Fetal Medicine; Chairman, Department of Obstetrics and Gynecology; and Hospital Director of Obstetrics, University of Arkansas for Medical Sciences, Little Rock, Arkansas

**GUSTAVO MALINGER, MD**
Assistant Professor, Prenatal Diagnosis Unit, Department of Obstetrics and Gynecology, Wolfson Medical Center, Sackler School of Medicine, Tel Aviv University, Tel Aviv, Israel

**PAM MURPHY, BSN, RN**
Senior Research Coordinator, Division of Maternal-Fetal Medicine, Department of Obstetrics and Gynecology, University of Arkansas for Medical Sciences, Little Rock, Arkansas

**ERROL R. NORWITZ, MD, PhD**
Professor, Department of Obstetrics, Gynecology and Reproductive Science, Yale University School of Medicine; Co-Director, Division of Maternal-Fetal Medicine, Yale-New Haven Hospital; Director, Maternal-Fetal Medicine Fellowship Program and Director, Obstetrics and Gynecology Residency Program, Yale University School of Medicine; New Haven, Connecticut

**JAMES F. PADBURY, MD**
Oh-Zopfi Professor of Pediatrics and Perinatal Biology, Warren Alpert Medical School
of Brown University; and Pediatrician-in-Chief, Program Director, COBRE for Perinatal
Biology, Department of Pediatrics, Women and Infants Hospital of Rhode Island,
Providence, Rhode Island

**KATHRYN L. PONDER, BS**
Department of Pediatrics, Women and Infants Hospital of Rhode Island; and Department
of Pediatrics, Warren Alpert Medical School of Brown University, Providence,
Rhode Island

**ASURI N. PRASAD, MBBS, FRCPC, FRCPE**
Associate Professor, Section of Clinical Neurosciences, Department of Pediatrics and
Child Health; and Section of Pediatric Neurology, Department of Clinical Neurosciences,
Children's Hospital of Western Ontario, London Health Sciences Centre, University
of Western Ontario, London, Ontario, Canada

**DANIELA PRAYER, MD**
Professor and Director, Department of Neuroradiology, Medical University of Vienna,
Vienna, Austria

**HUBERT PREISSL, PhD**
Research Associate Professor, Department of Obstetrics and Gynecology, University
of Arkansas for Medical Sciences, Little Rock, Arkansas

**RAYMOND W. REDLINE, MD**
Department of Pathology, Case Western Reserve University School of Medicine,
University Hospitals Case Medical Center, Cleveland, Ohio

**AMY L. SALISBURY, PhD**
Assistant Professor of Pediatrics and Psychiatry & Human Behavior, Warren Alpert
Medical School of Brown University; and Brown Center for the Study of Children at Risk,
Department of Pediatrics, Women & Infants Hospital of Rhode Island, Providence, Rhode
Island

**HANS J. TEN DONKELAAR, MD, PhD**
Department of Neurology, Radboud University Nijmegen Medical Center, Nijmegen,
The Netherlands

**ADAM J. WOLFBERG, MD, MPH**
Assistant Professor, Division of Maternal-Fetal Medicine, Department of Obstetrics and
Gynecology, Tufts University School of Medicine, Tufts Medical Center; and Research
Fellow in Neurology, Children's Hospital Boston and Harvard Medical School, Boston,
Massachusetts

# Contents

Alejandro L. Diaz and Joseph G. Gleeson

This article reviews key recent findings in the field of human cortical development. This development is divided into three major time-dependent
phases: neural proliferation of inhibitory and excitatory neurons in spatially
distinct regions, migration through multiple cellular boundaries, and maturation through morphologic changes that result in the elaboration of dendrites and axons and that establish the multitude of cellular contacts
that underlie neuronal processing. Many of the neurocognitive disorders
treated in the clinic can trace their origin to a disorder in one or more of
these key steps. Along with this update, work is highlighted that offers
a glimpse at the future of therapy for developmental brain disorders that
can result from disorders of these cellular events.

Hans J. ten Donkelaar and Martin Lammens

The cerebellum arises from two anatomically and molecularly different proliferative compartments: the cerebellar ventricular zone and the rhombic
lip. The protracted development makes the cerebellum vulnerable to
a broad spectrum of developmental disorders, of which the more frequent
(the Dandy-Walker and related malformations and the pontocerebellar hypoplasias) are discussed in this article. Several genes for congenital malformations of the human cerebellum have recently been identified,
including genes causing Joubert syndrome, the Dandy-Walker malformation, and pontocerebellar hypoplasias.

Adré J. du Plessis

The inaccessibility of the human fetal brain to studies of perfusion and metabolism has impeded progress in the understanding of the normal and abnormal systems of oxygen substrate supply and demand. Consequently,
current understanding is based on studies in fetal animals or in the premature infant (ex utero fetus), neither of which is ideal. Despite promising developments in fetal magnetic resonance imaging (MRI) and Doppler
ultrasound, major advances in fetal neurodiagnostics will be required before rational and truly informed brainoriented care of the fetus becomes
feasible.

a possible common epigenetic mechanism for their potential effects on the developing child. We suggest that exposure to these substances acts as a stressor that affects fetal programming, disrupts fetal placental mono-amine transporter expression and alters neuroendocrine and neurotrans-mitter system development. We also discuss neurobehavioral techniques that may be useful in the early detection of the effects of in utero drug exposure.

There exists a link between the in utero metabolic environment and the de-velopment of the fetal nervous system. Prenatal neurosonography offers a unique, noninvasive tool in the detection of developmental brain malfor-mations and the ability to monitor changes over time. This article explores the association of malformations of cerebral development reported in as-sociation with inborn errors of metabolism, and speculates on potential mechanisms by which such malformations arise. The detection of cerebral malformations prenatally should lead to a search for both genetic etiolo-gies and inborn errors of metabolism in the fetus. Improving the changes of an early diagnosis provides for timely therapeutic interventions and it is hoped a brighter future for affected children and their families.

Current microbial diagnostics enable rapid and specific identification of the agents causing intrauterine and perinatal infections, and CT and MRI allow precise characterization of the central nervous system effects of these pathogens. Although infections with *Toxoplasma gondii*, *Toxo-plasma pallidum*, *Toxoplasma cruzi*, and cytomegalovirus cannot currently be prevented by immunization, postnatal therapy of infected neonates can substantially improve outcome. Therapy with acyclovir should be initiated whenever perinatal herpes simplex virus encephalitis is suspected. De-spite these strategies, intrauterine and perinatal infections remain major causes of permanent deafness, vision loss, cerebral palsy, and epilepsy among children throughout the world.

This article examines recent studies that have systematically dissected features of fetal heart rate responses to labor that may help identify devel-oping fetal compromise, such as the slope of the deceleration, overshoot, and variability. Although repeated deep decelerations are never necessar-ily benign, fetuses with normal placental reserve can fully compensate even for frequent deep but brief decelerations for surprisingly prolonged intervals before developing profound acidosis and hypotension.

> Obstetric care providers and researchers have long relied on analysis of the fetal heart rate tracing for insight into the fetal neurologic status. Although a normal fetal heart rate tracing does provide reassurance of intact neurologic function, an abnormal pattern is a very poor predictor of newborn brain injury. Indeed, if the clinical end point of interest is cerebral palsy, a non-reassuring fetal heart rate tracing has a 99% false positive rate. More recent analyses of fetal heart rate variability and fetal ECG waveforms, however, hold promise for improved diagnostic accuracy.

> Fetal magnetic resonance imaging (MRI) may add important diagnostic information to prenatal sonography and has the power to confirm or change decisions at critical points in clinical care. Recent studies have shown MRI to be a critical clinical adjunct in the evaluation of the developing central nervous system (CNS), especially at early gestational ages, and MRI has been used in three significant ways: (1) for the quantification of brain growth and structural abnormalities using biometry, (2) for the qualitative evaluation of CNS microstructure, and (3) for the qualitative assessment of dynamic fetal movements in utero.

> SQUID Array for Reproductive Assessment is a unique magnetoencephalography device designed for the noninvasive recording of fetal brain activity. In this article, we provide a general overview of the technology and its potential application to fetal medicine. A large number of studies that have been conducted and published describing this device since it was brought into operation are referenced throughout the article.

## GOAL STATEMENT

The goal of *Clinics in Perinatology* is to keep practicing neonatologists and maternal-fetal medicine specialists up to date with current clinical practice in perinatology by providing timely articles reviewing the state of the art in patient care.

## ACCREDITATION

The *Clinics in Perinatology* is planned and implemented in accordance with the Essential Areas and Policies of the Accreditation Council for Continuing Medical Education (ACCME) through the joint sponsorship of the University of Virginia School of Medicine and Elsevier. The University of Virginia School of Medicine is accredited by the ACCME to provide continuing medical education for physicians.

The University of Virginia School of Medicine designates this educational activity for a maximum of 15 *AMA PRA Category 1 Credits*™ for each issue, 60 credits per year. Physicians should only claim credit commensurate with the extent of their participation in the activity.

The American Medical Association has determined that physicians not licensed in the US who participate in this CME activity are eligible for a maximum of 15 *AMA PRA Category 1 Credits*™ for each issue, 60 credits per year.

Credit can be earned by reading the text material, taking the CME examination online at: http://www.theclinics.com/home/cme, and completing the evaluation. After taking the test, you will be required to review any and all incorrect answers. Following completion of the test and evaluation, your credit will be awarded and you may print your certificate.

## FACULTY DISCLOSURE/CONFLICT OF INTEREST

The University of Virginia School of Medicine, as an ACCME accredited provider, endorses and strives to comply with the Accreditation Council for Continuing Medical Education (ACCME) Standards of Commercial Support, Commonwealth of Virginia statutes, University of Virginia policies and procedures, and associated federal and private regulations and guidelines on the need for disclosure and monitoring of proprietary and financial interests that may affect the scientific integrity and balance of content delivered in continuing medical education activities under our auspices.

The University of Virginia School of Medicine requires that all CME activities accredited through this institution be developed independently and be scientifically rigorous, balanced and objective in the presentation/discussion of its content, theories and practices.

All authors/editors participating in an accredited CME activity are expected to disclose to the readers relevant financial relationships with commercial entities occurring within the past 12 months (such as grants or research support, employee, consultant, stock holder, member of speakers bureau, etc.). The University of Virginia School of Medicine will employ appropriate mechanisms to resolve potential conflicts of interest to maintain the standards of fair and balanced education to the reader. Questions about specific strategies can be directed to the Office of Continuing Medical Education, University of Virginia School of Medicine, Charlottesville, Virginia.

The faculty and staff of the University of Virginia Office of Continuing Medical Education have no financial affiliations to disclose.

**The authors/editors listed below have identified no professional or financial affiliations for themselves or their spouse/partner:**
Laura Bennet, PhD; Robert Boyle, MD (Test Author); Peter C. Brugger, MD, PhD; Romy Chung, MD; Alejandro L. Diaz, MD; Adré J. du Plessis, MBChB, MPH (Guest Editor); Hari Eswaran, PhD; Joseph G. Gleeson, MD; Rathinaswamy B. Govindan, PhD; Carla Holloway (Acquisitions Editor); Gregor Kasprian, MD; Martin Lammens, MD, PhD; Tally Lerman-Sagie, MD; Barry M. Lester, PhD; Catherine Limperopoulos, PhD; Curtis L. Lowery, MD; Gustavo Malinger, MD; Pam Murphy, BSN, RN; Errol R. Norwitz, MD, PhD; James F. Padbury, MD; Kathryn L. Ponder, BS; Asuri N. Prasad, MBBS, FRCPC, FRCPE; Daniela Prayer, MD; Hubert Preissl, PhD; Raymond W. Redline, MD; Amy L. Salisbury, PhD; and Hans J. ten Donkelaar, MD; PhD.

**The authors/editors listed below identified the following professional or financial affiliations for themselves or their spouse/partner:**
**James F. Bale, Jr., MD** owns stock in Baxter and Fidelity Healthcare, is employed by the University of Utah, and serves on the Advisory Committee for Primary Children's Medical Center.
**Alistair Jan Gunn, MBChB, PhD** is an unpaid consultant for Brainz Ltd and OlyMed/Natus Ltd.
**Adam J. Wolfberg, MD, MPH** owns stock in and has a patent with MindChild Medical, Inc., and owns stock in Akaza Research, Inc.

*Disclosure of Discussion of Non-FDA Approved Uses for Pharmaceutical Products and/or Medical Devices.*
**The University of Virginia School of Medicine, as an ACCME provider, requires that all faculty presenters identify and disclose any off-label uses for pharmaceutical and medical device products. The University of Virginia School of Medicine recommends that each physician fully review all the available data on new products or procedures prior to clinical use.**

## TO ENROLL

To enroll in the Clinics in Perinatology Continuing Medical Education program, call customer service at 1-800-654-2452 or visit us online at: www.theclinics.com/home/cme. The CME program is available to subscribers for an additional fee of $195.00.

**THE CLINICS ARE NOW AVAILABLE ONLINE!**

Access your subscription at:
**www.theclinics.com**

# Preface

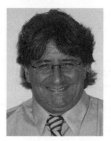

Adré J. du Plessis, MBChB, MPH
*Guest Editor*

That events in the fetal period may be critical determinants of lifelong neuropsycholog-ical function is not a new concept. However, the vast extent and diversity of fetal expe-riences and the broad spectrum of their postnatal impact are rapidly achieving greater recognition. Two apparently parallel avenues begin at this time to intersect in an enticing way. First, the accelerating field of neurogenetics is vitalizing our under-standing of the highly programmed process of brain development and, in cases of brain dysgenesis, its derailment. Second, investigations of internal and external envi-ronmental influences are greatly expanding our understanding of their fundamental role in normal and disrupted fetal brain development. The growing body of data from both these avenues of investigation no longer labels one or the other as primary or secondary but instead highlights their complex interactions. In fact, these discoveries have led to a paradoxic decrease in the distinction between genetic and experiential influences on the developing fetal brain. Increasingly we recognize that the expression of genetic programming may be influenced by environmental factors, even in a trans-generational epigenetic manner. Conversely, genetic predisposition may render some fetuses more vulnerable than others to acquired insults and disrupted brain develop-ment. Advanced fetal neuroimaging suggests that several fetal brain anomalies previ-ously believed to have an as-yet-undiscovered genetic basis may instead result from acquired insults that disrupt the primary developmental program.

With these new intersections in mind, this issue of *Clinics in Perinatology* includes selected topics that highlight areas of major progress in fetal neurology. Inevitably, other very exciting developments could not be included because of limited space. We begin by reviewing recent advances in our understanding of the genetic and envi-ronmental factors involved in normal and abnormal brain development. Areas of focus include fascinating new insights into the development of the cerebral cortex and of the cerebellum. Drs. Diaz and Gleeson offer insights into the role of specific gene products in neuronal migration and organization and the important role of transient structures, such as the subplate zone, during neocortical development. Equally exciting are the significant advances in our understanding of cerebellar development with its complex

Clin Perinatol 36 (2009) xiii–xv
doi:10.1016/j.clp.2009.07.006
0095-5108/09/$ – see front matter © 2009 Elsevier Inc. All rights reserved.          **perinatology.theclinics.com**

patterns of cellular migration, as presented by Drs. ten Donkelaar and Lammens. Few areas of human dysmorphology have been as difficult to categorize in a clinically meaningful manner as anomalies of the posterior fossa. The growing body of genetic and histogenetic information about cerebellar development discussed in their review will hopefully lead to a more rational and prognostically useful template for posterior fossa dysgeneses.

As the discipline of fetal neurology grows and the notion of informed brain-oriented management develops, it will be of critical importance that the normal mechanisms of oxygen/substrate supply to the developing brain be understood and become measurable. In the human fetus, both these challenges remain daunting. My article discusses current concepts of fetal oxygen/substrate supply, largely extrapolated from animal experiments, followed by Dr. Redline's review of placental mechanisms of impaired cerebral oxygen/substrate supply. Dr. Limperopoulos then reviews brain growth impairment in the fetus with congenital heart disease and discusses potential mechanisms by which cardiovascular malformations may disrupt the normal delivery of oxygen/substrate to the fetal brain, impair normal compensatory responses in the fetal circulation, or both. Drs. Gunn and Bennet follow with a discussion of experimental studies into the mechanisms and manifestations of different "doses" of oxygen/substrate deprivation. Their work emphasizes the importance of being able to detect and measure brain insults in the fetus and highlights our current inability to do so reliably.

A multitude of toxic substances and infectious agents are capable of injuring the immature brain and disrupting its developmental program. Here we review two important forms of toxic disruption of normal brain development. Dr. Lester and colleagues first discuss exogenous maternally transmitted substances, prescribed or illicit, capable of disrupting fetal neurotransmitter systems and thereby mediating later neurodevelopmental disturbances, a phenomenon termed "behavioral teratology." Dr. Lerman-Sagie and colleagues review the increasing recognition of an endogenous form of developmental neurotoxicity in fetuses with inherited errors of metabolism; in these cases, the deprivation or excessive accumulation of metabolic substances may disrupt normal structural brain development. The importance of this phenomenon is that clinicians diagnosing a structural brain malformation in infants with neurodevelopmental impairment may assign culpability to a primary (and assumed static) genetic mechanism, whereas progressive neurologic failure may result from ongoing brain toxicity due to the underlying metabolic defect. The role of infection in mediating injury to the immature brain has received widespread attention in recent years; much of it focused on the cytotoxic effects of inflammatory cytokines on the immature oligodendrocyte. However, other infectious agents, particularly viral agents, are capable of disrupting normal brain development and causing encephaloclastic parenchymal injury. Dr. Bale addresses the complex interplay between fetal infection, inflammation, and brain development, wherein the manifestations of fetal infections are determined by the concurrent developmental events in the fetal brain.

The final series of reviews focuses on recent advances in diagnostic techniques for the assessment of fetal well-being. Drs. Bennett and Gunn offer a detailed review of the fetal heart rate response to hypoxia, based on an elegant series of experimental studies in fetal sheep. Drs. Wolfberg and Norwitz discuss a number of innovative attempts not only to extract meaningful quantitative information from the variability patterns in the fetal heart rate (FHR) recording but also to interrogate the fetal electrocardiogram waveform. These techniques are early in development, and extensive validation studies will be necessary before they enter clinical practice. Although the value of FHR monitoring techniques as currently applied has been questioned extensively, ongoing exploration of fetal heart signals remains a very important avenue of research for several reasons. First, the FHR signal is easily accessible, and its measurement widely available. In addition, with the paucity of other promising techniques on the immediate horizon, the FHR signal is likely to remain, at least for the foreseeable future, the only continuous physiologic fetal signal readily available during the intrapartum period.

The successful application of magnetic resonance imaging (MRI) with its vastly superior soft tissue resolution has revolutionized studies of the human fetus, and especially of the fetal brain. Dr. Prayer and colleagues discuss the rapid advances in fetal MRI to date and the anticipated future developments, which promise to open other avenues for fetal brain study. Finally, the lack of established techniques for assessing fetal electrocortical function has confined our assessment of fetal brain function to analysis of fetal movements and behavioral state change. The technique of magnetoencephalography is now firmly established in epilepsy. As presented by Dr. Lowery and colleagues, the successful application of this technique to the noninvasive assessment of fetal electrocortical activity presents a hugely exciting opportunity for more informed fetal neurologic evaluation in future.

In the preface to their book *Fetal Neurology* some 20 years ago, Joseph Volpe and Alan Hill introduced clinicians to the notion of a distinct new discipline focused on "the time of life…that is often the most critical and invariably the most mysterious." Well, certainly the mystery continues! Although their anticipation of a distinct new discipline within a decade of that publication was perhaps optimistic, there can be no denying that a remarkable set of diagnostic instruments has continued to accrue over the intervening period. Given our burgeoning understanding of the immature brain and the hazards confronting it and given the comprehensive battery of diagnostic tools now at our disposal, we have little excuse to further delay in rallying expertise around the critical challenges of ensuring fetal brain well-being.

I am extremely grateful to Elsevier for the opportunity to serve as guest editor for a subject that is very special to me. Also to the collaborating authors, thank you for the uniformly superb reviews of your rapidly evolving fields of expertise. Finally, I owe an enormous debt of gratitude to Shaye Moore and Carla Holloway for their dedicated supervision of all aspects of this project.

Adré J. du Plessis, MBChB, MPH
Department of Neurology, Fegan 11
Children's Hospital Boston
300 Longwood Avenue
Boston, MA 02115, USA

E-mail address:
adre.duplessis@childrens.harvard.edu

# The Molecular and Genetic Mechanisms of Neocortex Development

Alejandro L. Diaz, MD, Joseph G. Gleeson, MD*

**KEYWORDS**

- Neocortex • Development • Neocortical proliferation
- Migration • Cerebral palsy

The mammalian neocortex is a remarkably complex organ. It contains many neuronal cell types, oligodendrocytes, and glia, together accounting for over 10 billion cells in the human brain that form perhaps $10^{13}$ to $10^{15}$ intricate connections (synapses) with other regions of the central nervous system. In its human form, the neocortex exists at its most complex and evolved state. It is the region of our brain responsible for sensation, action, cognition, and consciousness. Despite the seemingly overwhelming complexity of the neocortex, various groups have made significant progress toward unraveling the mystery of how it is formed. This article focuses on the three major processes that give rise to the mature neocortical structure: neurogenesis, neural migration, and maturation or the establishment of functional neocortical connectivity. Definitions of the terms used herein are listed in **Box 1**. In the process of this discussion, we highlight results and ideas that offer a glimpse into the future.

## OVERVIEW OF NEOCORTEX DEVELOPMENT

In humans, as in other vertebrates, the remarkably complex central nervous system begins by the process of neural induction as a relatively simple collection of cells on the dorsal side of the gastrula-stage embryo, the neural plate.[1] The plate eventually expands, its lateral ends fold upward and toward each other at the midline, and the ends fuse into the embryologic neural tube at around embryonic day (E) 30 in humans.[2]

In mammals, the developing neocortex forms in the dorsolateral wall at the rostral end of this neural tube. Here in the embryonic cerebral vesicles, or prosencephalon, the vast majority of neurons that are destined for the neocortex arise in

Neurogenetics Laboratory, Howard Hughes Medical Institute, Department of Pediatrics and Neurosciences, University of California, San Diego, Leichtag Biomedical Research Building, Room 482, 9500 Gilman Drive, La Jolla, CA 92093-0665, USA
* Corresponding author.
*E-mail address:* jogleeson@ucsd.edu (J.G. Gleeson).

Clin Perinatol 36 (2009) 503–512
doi:10.1016/j.clp.2009.06.008
0095-5108/09/$ – see front matter © 2009 Elsevier Inc. All rights reserved.

perinatology.theclinics.com

---

**Box 1**
**Definition of terms relevant to neocortex development**

**Neural induction:** process by which the embryonic chordamesoderm at the three-layer embryo stage coaxes the overlying ectoderm into becoming the neural plate or neuroectoderm

**Neurogenesis:** embryologic process during which neural progenitor cells arise

**Neuronogenesis:** embryologic process during which neural progenitors fully differentiate into neurons as opposed to glia

**Neural progenitors:** pluripotent stem cells that can give rise to either neurons or glia

**Neural migration:** embryologic process by which a neural progenitor travels from its birthplace to a final destination within the nervous system

**Basic helix-loop-helix:** transcription factor protein family (members include MyoD, Beta2/ NeuroD1) named for its structural motif which consists of two alpha helices connected by a short loop

**Long-term depression:** neurophysiologic property characterized by weakened synaptic activity

---

a pseudostratified epithelial cell layer made up of two distinct germinal regions that surround the early ventricular lumen: the ventricular zone (VZ) located immediately adjacent to the ventricle and the subventricular zone (SVZ) which lies superficially on the VZ (**Fig. 1**).[3]

The early cycles of cellular proliferation in the VZ result primarily in the symmetric expansion of cells termed *radial glia*. These radial glia are direct descendants of the neural plate and, as such, have been shown to be pluripotent neural stem cells in nature retaining the capacity for producing multiple neural cell types and for self-renewal.[4–6] This process determines not only the total pool of neural stem cells, or so-called "proliferative units," from which the nascent cortical structure is later derived but also markedly increases the surface area and thickness of the VZ. At around E33 a second phase of proliferation predominates, in which the stem cells begin to divide asymmetrically to produce a single clone and a more committed neural progenitor that temporarily withdraws itself from the cell cycle. This process marks the beginning of neurogenesis.[7]

The next key step in neocortical development following neural progenitor proliferation is migration, which occurs between weeks 10 and 20 in the human.[3] As mentioned earlier, the mature mammalian neocortex contains six layers of neurons. Development of these layers involves both radial and tangential migration routes that are taken by the various neuronal progenitors on their way to their final laminar destination (see **Fig. 1**). Congenital migration disorders may display derangements in either one or both directions.

In the first stage of neural migration, the preplate forms (see **Fig. 1** and **Fig. 2**). It is composed of the first wave of neural progenitors migrating out of the VZ. Concurrently, Cajal-Retzius cells appear at the outermost aspect of the preplate. This specialized population of early neurons secretes reelin, a signaling molecule that helps to attract subsequent waves of migrating neural progenitors.[8] In the next migrational stage, a second wave of postmitotic neural progenitors enters the preplate and splits it into the more superficial marginal zone (MZ) and subplate (SP) below constituting the embryologic cortical plate. Subsequent waves of migrating neuronal progenitors migrate past the subplate, stopping just short of the MZ (or layer I of the mature cortex) and forming the various neocortical lamina in the process. Early birth-dating studies using tritiated thymidine in primates and rodents established that these progenitors

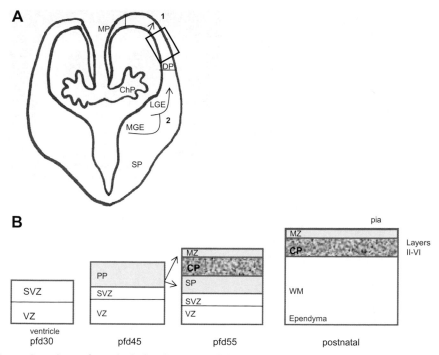

**Fig. 1.** Overview of cortical development. (*A*) Radial (1) and tangential (2) modes of migration. (*B*) Inset from above. Neocortical layering. During early stages (post fertilization day [pfd 30]) the cortex consists of the outer subventricular zone (SVZ) and ventricular zone (VZ). The emergence of the preplate (PP) occurs around pfd 45. Newly generated neurons from the VZ migrate into the cortical plate (CP) and split the PP into the marginal zone (MZ) and subpallium (SP) (*arrows*). The SP has a critical role in establishing the inside-out lamination of cells, as well as the efferent and afferent cortical axonal projections. In the adult, these developmental layers evolve into the white matter (WM). ChP, choroid plexus; DP, dorsal pallium; LGE, lateral ganglionic eminence; MGE, medial ganglionic eminence; MP, medial pallium.

accumulate in their respective layers using a radial, inside-out sequence pattern with the earliest born neurons populating the innermost lamina (or layer VI) and subsequent waves becoming the more superficial layers V, IV, III, and II, respectively.[9,10] Another key recent observation in this field involves cortical neurons that express the neurotransmitter gamma aminobutyric acid (GABA). These neurons appear to derive almost exclusively from the more distant germinal zones of the medial and lateral ganglionic eminences (MGE/LGE). From here they migrate tangentially to their respective laminar destination in the neocortex.[11] Recently, it has also been shown that neurons destined for a specific layer of neocortex are generated closely in time whether they originate in the nearby VZ or the more distant MGE/LGE.[12]

As the development of the brain proceeds, the final process in the formation of the fully mature mammalian neocortex is the establishment of functional connections between the various brain regions. One of the more fascinating stories to have developed in recent years involves the role of transient laminar zones within the developing neocortex known as the SP (see **Fig. 2**), which act as "waiting rooms" where axons

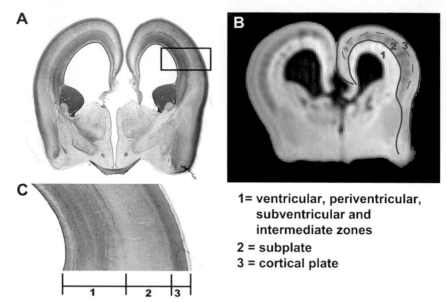

1= ventricular, periventricular,
   subventricular and
   intermediate zones
2 = subplate
3 = cortical plate

Fig. 2. Layers of the developing cerebral cortex from humans. (A–C) Coronal histologic slides of a 17-week fetal brain, similar to a coronal slice taken by diffusion tensor imaging of a 17-week fetal brain, and an enlarged region corresponding to the boxed area. The red contour establishes the boundary of the cortical plate and subplate (CP+SP). The dashed red curve separates the cortical plate and subplate. The annotation of each boundary is shown at bottom right. (*From* Huan H, Xue R, Zhang J, et al. Anatomical characterization of human fetal brain development with diffusion tensor magnetic resonance imaging. J Neurosci 2009;29:4263; with permission.)

making their way to the cortex temporarily arrest before continuing on toward their respective targets. The SP is easily visible as a major structure in the fetal brain on pathology or brain MRI but after development is largely replaced by white matter in the adult.

## ADVANCES IN NEOCORTICAL NEUROGENESIS

Much of our understanding of the generation of cell type diversity found in the mature neocortex is based on studies primarily in chicks and mice. In particular, the results from work on spinal cord and retina development in these animals have revealed that, across the entire central nervous system, various compartments share common developmental strategies. One such strategy involves the specification (around the time of neural tube formation) or patterning of the early neocortical primordium in response to extracellular (often secreted) morphogen gradients, such as sonic hedgehog (Shh), bone morphogenetic protein (Bmp), and fibroblast growth factor (Fgf).[13–15] A number of transcription factor genes, most notably of the homeodomain and basic helix-loop-helix (bHLH) class, are resultantly expressed and inform their respective progenitor "pools" to commit to a particular cellular fate.[16,17] This process has been deemed the transcriptional factor "combinatorial code." It allows an exponential number of cellular fates to be generated by a relatively modest amount of transcription factor gene products. In theory, a code based on only two homeodomain and three bHLH genes can result in as many as 25 different specific neocortical cell types.

Besides the laminar organization that the developing neocortex takes on, the mature neocortex also subdivides in a tangential fashion. Two main mechanisms appear to take hold of the development of the neocortex along this axis. The first holds that the tangential subdivisions of the early neocortex are prespecified into a sort of "protomap" by gradients and countergradients of molecules during neurogenesis.[18–20] The second mechanism or "protocortex hypothesis" holds that a particular neuron's fate is determined by its attachment to thalamocortical afferents that made their way into the developing neocortex.[21,22] Recent molecular evidence strongly supports both of these mechanisms as fundamental in establishing the final elements of mature neocortical differentiation and functional connectivity.

Primary microcephaly (MCPH) is the clinical finding of a reduced fronto-occipital head circumference of greater than 3 standard deviations below age- and sex-matched controls, reflecting a reduced brain volume[23] in the absence of other causes or physical findings. It has been hypothesized that the reduced size of the brain in MCPH patients is due to premature asymmetric division of neural stem cells in proliferative zones such as the VZ, resulting in a reduced number of postmitotic neural progenitors. Microcephalic individuals generally have a small cerebral cortex; hence, the majority are mentally retarded. MCPH in particular is typically an autosomal recessive disorder resulting directly from hypoplasia of the cerebral cortex with a generalized reduction in the overall size of the brain. Occipital-frontal circumferences are typically 4 to 12 standard deviations below normal, and patients have mild-to-severe mental retardation as a result. Surprisingly these patients tend to lack any other predominant neurologic features such as spasticity or epilepsy.

MCPH is genetically heterogeneous, mapping thus far to six known loci, four of which have been identified.[24] Immunofluorescence studies reveal that these loci encode proteins that localize to the cellular centrosome, suggesting a mitotic yet brain-specific mechanism responsible for limiting the number of neural progenitors produced. Further insights into the role of MCPH gene products will no doubt be of therapeutic significance in the future, in particular toward identifying or establishing clinically beneficial neural stem cell lines for transplant.

## ADVANCES IN NEURAL MIGRATION

Despite its similarity with the spinal cord and retina, there exists an important added complexity with respect to the generation of the cell diversity found within the mature neocortex. There are two broad classes of neocortical neurons: (1) interneurons that express the neurotransmitter GABA and make relatively local connections, and (2) projection neurons that express glutamate and extend axons to both local intracortical and distant subcortical and subcerebral targets. During development, projection neurons are generated primarily in the dorsolateral (or pallial) wall of the telencephalon in the germinal VZ and SVZ zones previously mentioned.[25] From there they migrate relatively locally in a radial inside-out fashion to their respective lamina. This development is in contrast to that of GABA-containing interneurons which are generated in the ganglionic eminences of the ventral (or subpallial) telencephalon and migrate relatively long distances to their final neocortical destination.

Compelling evidence suggests that these cells find their final destination within the developing neocortex specifically through a rearrangement of cytoskeletal components in response to extracellular cues mediated by various intracellular signaling pathways.[26] Thought of in this way, three large classes of genes underlie the vast majority of neural migration disorders that are seen clinically: (1) those involving the formation of the extracellular environment encountered by migrating neurons and axons, (2) those encoding for intracellular signaling mechanisms, and (3) those encoding the intracellular machinery that mediates cellular and axonal physical movement.[27] One such family of genes involved in the extracellular environment encodes for the enzymatic regulators of glycosylation, which, in turn, control the appearance of a specific extracellular cue that is encountered by migrating cells. Mutations in this group appear to delineate boundaries along a particular pathway where a cell may arrest during migration. An example in humans are the genes involved in the brain phenotype known as cobblestone lissencephaly, in which the surface of the brain has a disorganized bumpy exterior lacking both gyri and sulci. Microscopically, these bumps consist of collections of neurons that abnormally migrated past the pial layers and into the meninges. In some instances, the abnormally migrating neurons have been thought of as having crossed from one side of the cerebral hemisphere to the other, fusing the two together at the midline. Cobblestone lissencephaly is only one feature in a group of conditions known as the congenital muscular dystrophies. These disorders, which are characterized by the features of muscular dystrophy, developmental eye abnormalities, and cobblestone lissencephaly, include Fukuyama congenital myotonic dystrophy, muscle eye-brain disorder, and Walker-Warburg syndrome. Recent work involving the genetic background of these disorders reveals that the mutated genes in this group encode actual or putative glycosyltransferases that detrimentally affect the dystrophin-glycoprotein complex.[28–31] Cobblestone lissencephaly itself appears to be the result of loss of the integrity of the limiting glial membrane, loss of the "stop signal" found there, or the dissociation of migrating neurons from the otherwise intact migrational scaffold.

## ADVANCES IN NEURAL CONNECTIVITY

When neurons near their final laminar destination, they send and receive axons and form dendrites and synapses with local and distant cerebral structures. This process begins in the second half of gestation and extends into the postnatal period. An interesting feature is the role of transient layers of cells from the earliest migrations that seem to behave as a "waiting room" for the axons of distant afferents making their way into the neocortex. One example of these layers is the SP that forms when the early preplate is split by a second wave of early neocortical progenitors.

When the SP was initially characterized, first in the human and then in the monkey in mid-1970s, few prominent neuroscientists recognized the significance of its existence.[32–34] This fact is not surprising given that the earliest reports essentially argued for a reinterpretation of neocortical laminar development. Another reason for missing the significance of the SP had to do with its seemingly underdeveloped state and relatively small size in experimental rodents in comparison with humans and monkeys where it had initially been characterized.[35] It was not until 1991 that Rakic first demonstrated in the rhesus monkey that thalamocortical axons destined for the visual cortex in fact wait in the SP just before migrating into and past the cortical plate.[36] Work by Shatz and colleagues provided conclusive evidence of the role of the SP in establishing not only functional thalamocortical connections but development of the neocortex's functional columnar architecture.[37,38] Although several genes are known to be expressed in SP neurons, there is as yet no evidence for specific genetic derangements leading to absence or prolonged existence of the SP.

The SP is present in all mammals, but its morphologic characteristics and persistence in adulthood vary among species. In the human, the SP exists during the period from 13 weeks post fertilization through 6 to 9 months' postnatal. In fact, SP neurons and the afferent synaptic connections that meet them essentially represent the most significant reservoir of functional connectivity in the preterm infant. Thought of in this way, the SP exists at a time when neocortical synaptic architecture is still relatively immature or even absent, and more importantly coincides with the age of peak vulnerability to perinatal brain injury.[39,40] Blindness due to impairment of visual cortex formation ("cortical blindness") is particularly common in infants with perinatal white matter injury. Much of this association may be directly attributed to the vulnerability of the SP and its relative importance to the development of normal visual cortex.[41] Some encouraging results in the field of neuroimaging demonstrate that thalamocortical fibers residing in the SP and designated for the somatosensory cortex may, in fact, detour around a particular lesion.[42]

## LOOKING INTO THE FUTURE

The study of human fragile X syndrome provides a hopeful glimpse into the possibility not only of better treatment but ultimately of prevention of the most common type of congenital mental retardation and autism. In humans, fragile X syndrome is caused by transcriptional silencing of the Fmr1 gene that normally encodes the fragile X mental retardation protein (FMRP). This silencing is specifically caused by expansion of a CGG repeat sequence in the Fmr1 promoter region that disrupts the formation of a functional RNA polymerase complex. FMRP normally regulates the translation of mRNA by inhibitory binding. One way FMRP accomplishes this binding is by inhibiting translation of certain proteins at the synapse.[43] The resultant effect is increased dendritic arborization leading to hyperconnectivity or the retainment of too many functional synapses.[44]

In addition, the protein metabotropic glutamate receptor 5 (mGluR5) appears to be involved in local protein synthesis at the synapse in response to glutaminergic activity. In particular, it appears to establish a "lasting effect" as seen in a model for long-term depression, which may have a role in the impaired brain activity seen in patients who have fragile X syndrome.[45–47] Taken together, these findings have led to the mGluR theory of fragile X syndrome. A particularly exciting prospect of this theory has been the development of potentially disease-modifying agents acting through mGluR5.[48–50] Human trials of mGluR5 antagonists have begun for fragile X syndrome and a broad range of other neuropsychiatric conditions.

A causal connection has also been established concerning neuronal migration during development and altered neocortical excitability. The brains of individuals presenting with pharmacologically intractable epilepsy frequently contain foci of abnormally migrated neurons. Until the development of more effective anti-epileptic medications, surgical resection may be the best alternative for reducing the number of seizures in refractory cases. For individuals whose defects are more widespread, the risks of surgery actually offer a worse prognosis. In subcortical band heterotopia, a strip of heterotopic gray matter largely composed of abnormally migrated neurons can be found between the ventricular wall and the cortical mantle separated by a band of white matter. Subcortical band heterotopia is most often caused in females by mutations in the X-linked gene for doublecortin (Dcx), a microtubule-binding protein found to be essential for normal migration. A rat model for subcortical band heterotopia showed that delayed expression of Dcx rescued the formation of this condition while also reducing seizure risk.[51]

## SUMMARY

Congenital brain malformations are a significant cause of morbidity and mortality. In recent years, significant advances in basic neuroscience research have improved our understanding of the molecular and genetic underpinnings of neocortical development. Continued advances in genomics and proteomics research will no doubt move us toward an even better understanding of these and other developmental processes, with the hope of one day being able to provide parents and clinicians with the information they so desperately need to make informed decisions. To say that a leap from these basic laboratory studies into the clinical realm will occur in the next few years is probably naïve at best. Instead, we hope to convey that while the basic mechanisms of neocortical development continue to be worked out along with overcoming the proper technical hurdles, we will begin to enter a new age of research, diagnosis, and treatment of congenital brain malformations and their associated disorders.

## REFERENCES

1. Chitnis AB. Control of neurogenesis–lessons from frogs, fish and flies. Curr Opin Neurobiol 1999;9:18–25.
2. O'Rahilly R, Müller F. The embryonic human brain: an atlas of developmental stages. 3rd edition. Hoboken (NJ): Wiley-Liss; 2006.
3. Bystron I, Blakemore C, Rakic P. Development of the human cerebral cortex: Boulder Committee revisited. Nat Rev Neurosci 2008;9:110–22.
4. Haubensak W, Attardo A, Denk W, et al. Neurons arise in the basal neuroepithelium of the early mammalian telencephalon: a major site of neurogenesis. Proc Natl Acad Sci U S A 2004;101:3196–201.
5. Anthony TE, Klein C, Fishell G, et al. Radial glia serve as neuronal progenitors in all regions of the central nervous system. Neuron 2004;41:881–90.
6. Noctor SC, Martinez-Cerdeno V, Kriegstein AR. Neural stem and progenitor cells in cortical development. Novartis Found Symp 2007;288:59–73 [discussion: 73–8, 96–8].
7. Bystron I, Rakic P, Molnar Z, et al. The first neurons of the human cerebral cortex. Nat Neurosci 2006;9:880–6.
8. Ogawa M, Miyata T, Nakajima K, et al. The reeler gene-associated antigen on Cajal-Retzius neurons is a crucial molecule for laminar organization of cortical neurons. Neuron 1995;14:899–912.
9. Rakic P. Neurons in rhesus monkey visual cortex: systematic relation between time of origin and eventual disposition. Science 1974;183:425–47.
10. Angevine JB Jr, Sidman RL. Autoradiographic study of cell migration during histogenesis of cerebral cortex in the mouse. Nature 1961;192:766–78.
11. Anderson SA, Marin O, Horn C, et al. Distinct cortical migrations from the medial and lateral ganglionic eminences. Development 2001;128:353–63.
12. Valcanis H, Tan SS. Layer specification of transplanted interneurons in developing mouse neocortex. J Neurosci 2003;23:5113–22.
13. Placzek M, Briscoe J. The floor plate: multiple cells, multiple signals. Nat Rev Neurosci 2005;6:230–40.
14. Aboitiz F, Montiel J. Origin and evolution of the vertebrate telencephalon, with special reference to the mammalian neocortex. Adv Anat Embryol Cell Biol 2007;193:1–112.
15. Fuccillo M, Joyner AL, Fishell G. Morphogen to mitogen: the multiple roles of hedgehog signalling in vertebrate neural development. Nat Rev Neurosci 2006; 7:772–83.
16. Molyneaux BJ, Arlotta P, Menezes JR, et al. Neuronal subtype specification in the cerebral cortex. Nat Rev Neurosci 2007;8:427–37.

17. Rallu M, Corbin JG, Fishell G. Parsing the prosencephalon. Nat Rev Neurosci 2002;3:943–51.
18. O'Leary DD. Do cortical areas emerge from a protocortex? Trends Neurosci 1989; 12:400–46.
19. Mallamaci A, Stoykova A. Gene networks controlling early cerebral cortex areal-ization. Eur J Neurosci 2006;23:847–56.
20. Rakic P. Specification of cerebral cortical areas. Science 1988;241:170–6.
21. Sur M, Rubenstein JL. Patterning and plasticity of the cerebral cortex. Science 2005;310:805–10.
22. Price DJ, Kennedy H, Dehay C, et al. The development of cortical connections. Eur J Neurosci 2006;23:910–20.
23. Woods CG. Human microcephaly. Curr Opin Neurobiol 2004;14:112–7.
24. Cox J, Jackson AP, Bond J, et al. What primary microcephaly can tell us about brain growth. Trends Mol Med 2006;12:358–66.
25. Anderson SA, Kaznowski CE, Horn C, et al. Distinct origins of neocortical projec-tion neurons and interneurons in vivo. Cereb Cortex 2002;12:702–79.
26. Ayala R, Shu T, Tsai LH. Trekking across the brain: the journey of neuronal migra-tion. Cell 2007;128:29–43.
27. Bielas S, Higginbotham H, Koizumi H, et al. Cortical neuronal migration mutants suggest separate but intersecting pathways. Annu Rev Cell Dev Biol 2004;20: 593–618.
28. Winder SJ. The complexities of dystroglycan. Trends Biochem Sci 2001;26: 118–24.
29. Beltran-Valero de Bernabe D, Currier S, Steinbrecher A, et al. Mutations in the O-mannosyltransferase gene POMT1 give rise to the severe neuronal migration disorder Walker-Warburg syndrome. Am J Hum Genet 2002;71:1033–43.
30. Yoshida A, Kobayashi K, Manya H, et al. Muscular dystrophy and neuronal migra-tion disorder caused by mutations in a glycosyltransferase, POMGnT1. Dev Cell 2001;1:717–24.
31. Kobayashi K, Nakahori Y, Miyake M, et al. An ancient retrotransposal insertion causes Fukuyama-type congenital muscular dystrophy. Nature 1998;394:388–92.
32. Kostovic I, Molliver ME. A new interpretation of the laminar development of cere-bral cortex: synaptogenesis in different layers of neopallium in the human fetus. Anat Rec 1974;178:395.
33. Kostovic I, Rakic P. Developmental history of the transient subplate zone in the visual and somatosensory cortex of the macaque monkey and human brain. J Comp Neurol 1990;297:441–70.
34. Rakic P. Prenatal development of the visual system in rhesus monkey. Philos Trans R Soc Lond B Biol Sci 1977;278:245–60.
35. Kostovic I, Jovanov-Milosevic N. Subplate zone of the human brain: historical perspective and new concepts. Coll Antropol 2008;32(Suppl 1):3–8.
36. Rakic P. Experimental manipulation of cerebral cortical areas in primates. Philos Trans R Soc Lond B Biol Sci 1991;331:291–4.
37. Ghosh A, Shatz CJ. A role for subplate neurons in the patterning of connections from thalamus to neocortex. Development 1993;117:1031–47.
38. Kanold PO, Kara P, Reid RC, et al. Role of subplate neurons in functional matu-ration of visual cortical columns. Science 2003;301:521–55.
39. Volpe JJ. Encephalopathy of prematurity includes neuronal abnormalities. Pediat-rics 2005;116:221–5.
40. McQuillen PS, Sheldon RA, Shatz CJ, et al. Selective vulnerability of subplate neurons after early neonatal hypoxia-ischemia. J Neurosci 2003;23:3308–15.

41. McQuillen PS, Ferriero DM. Perinatal subplate neuron injury: implications for cortical development and plasticity. Brain Pathol 2005;15:250–60.
42. Staudt M, Grodd W, Gerloff C, et al. Two types of ipsilateral reorganization in congenital hemiparesis: a TMS and fMRI study. Brain 2002;125:2222–37.
43. Vanderklish PW, Edelman GM. Differential translation and fragile X syndrome. Genes Brain Behav 2005;4:360–84.
44. McKinney BC, Grossman AW, Elisseou NM, et al. Dendritic spine abnormalities in the occipital cortex of C57BL/6 Fmr1 knockout mice. Am J Med Genet B Neuropsychiatr Genet 2005;136B:98–102.
45. Huber KM, Kayser MS, Bear MF. Role for rapid dendritic protein synthesis in hippocampal mGluR-dependent long-term depression. Science 2000;288:1254–7.
46. Grossman AW, Aldridge GM, Weiler IJ, et al. Local protein synthesis and spine morphogenesis: fragile X syndrome and beyond. J Neurosci 2006;26:7151–5.
47. Huber KM, Gallagher SM, Warren ST, et al. Altered synaptic plasticity in a mouse model of fragile X mental retardation. Proc Natl Acad Sci U S A 2002;99:7746–50.
48. Bear MF. Therapeutic implications of the mGluR theory of fragile X mental retardation. Genes Brain Behav 2005;4:393–8.
49. Aschrafi A, Cunningham BA, Edelman GM, et al. The fragile X mental retardation protein and group I metabotropic glutamate receptors regulate levels of mRNA granules in brain. Proc Natl Acad Sci U S A 2005;102:2180–5.
50. Yan QJ, Rammal M, Tranfaglia M, et al. Suppression of two major fragile X syndrome mouse model phenotypes by the mGluR5 antagonist MPEP. Neuropharmacology 2005;49:1053–66.
51. Manent JB, Wang Y, Chang Y, et al. Dcx reexpression reduces subcortical band heterotopia and seizure threshold in an animal model of neuronal migration disorder. Nat Med 2009;15:84–90.

# Development of the Human Cerebellum and Its Disorders

Hans J. ten Donkelaar, MD, PhD[a],*, Martin Lammens, MD, PhD[b]

**KEYWORDS**

- Cerebellar development • Pontocerebellar hypoplasia
- Joubert syndrome • Dandy-Walker malformation
- Congenital disorders of glycosylation
- Rhombencephalosynapsis

The cerebellum is one of the best studied parts of the brain. Its three-layered cortex and well-defined afferent and efferent fiber connections make the cerebellum a favorite field for research on development and fiber connections of the central nervous system.[1,2] The cerebellum plays a role not only in motor control but also in motor learning and cognition.[3,4] The cerebellum develops over a long period of time, extending from the early embryonic period until the first postnatal years. This protracted development makes the cerebellum vulnerable to a broad spectrum of developmental disorders, ranging from the Dandy-Walker and related malformations to medulloblastoma, a neoplasia of granule cell precursors.[2,5–8] Ultrasonography and MRI make it possible to detect cerebellar malformations at an early stage of development.[9–12] In mice, the molecular mechanisms of cerebellar development are rapidly being unraveled.[13–18] Similar mechanisms are likely to be involved in the development of the human cerebellum. This article reviews the morphogenesis and histogenesis of the cerebellum, the mechanisms involved, and its more frequent developmental disorders, such as the Dandy-Walker and related malformations and the pontocerebellar hypoplasias.

## MORPHOGENESIS OF THE CEREBELLUM

The cerebellum arises bilaterally from the alar (dorsal) layers of the first rhombomere.[19,20] The two cerebellar primordia are generally considered to unite dorsally to form the vermis, early in the fetal period. Rostrally, the paired cerebellar anlagen

[a] Department of Neurology, 935, Radboud University Nijmegen Medical Center, Reinier Postlaan 4, 6525 GC, PO Box 9101, 6500 HB Nijmegen, The Netherlands
[b] Department of Pathology, 825, Radboud University Nijmegen Medical Center, Geert Grooteplein Zuid 10, PO Box 9101, 6500 HB Nijmegen, The Netherlands
* Corresponding author.
*E-mail address:* h.tendonkelaar@neuro.umcn.nl (H. ten Donkelaar).

Clin Perinatol 36 (2009) 513–530
doi:10.1016/j.clp.2009.06.001
0095-5108/09/$ – see front matter © 2009 Elsevier Inc. All rights reserved.

are not completely separated. Sidman and Rakic[21] advocated Hochstetter's[22] view that such a fusion does not take place, and suggested one cerebellar primordium (the tuberculum cerebelli) in the form of an inverted V (**Fig. 1A**). Recent genetic fate mapping studies of *Engrailed1* and *Engrailed2* in mice corroborate this view.[23] The arms of the tuberculum cerebelli are directed caudally and laterally, and thicken enormously, whereas its rostral, midline part remains small and inconspicuous. During the sixth week of development, the limbs of the cerebellar tubercle thicken rapidly and bulge downward into the fourth ventricle on each side giving rise to the internal cerebellar bulge, which together form the corpus cerebelli (see **Fig. 1B**). One week later, the rapidly growing cerebellum bulges outward as the external cerebellar bulges; these represent the flocculi, delineated by the posterolateral fissures. In the early fetal period, growth of the midline component accelerates and begins to fill the gap between the limbs of the tuberculum cerebelli, thereby forming the vermis. By the twelfth to thirteenth weeks of development, lateral and rostral growth have reshaped the cerebellum to a transversely oriented bar of tissue overriding the fourth ventricle (see **Fig. 1C**). Then, fissures begin to form transverse to the longitudinal axis of the brain, first on the vermis and then spreading laterally into the hemispheres. The first fissure to appear (ie, the posterolateral fissure) separates the main body of the cerebellum from the flocculonodular lobe.

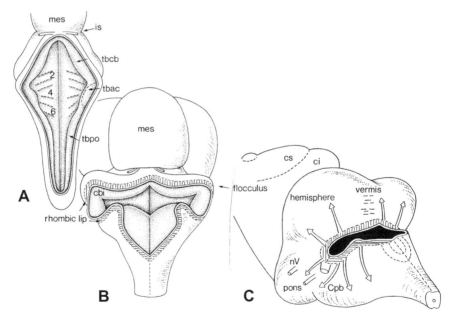

**Fig. 1.** Embryonic development of the human cerebellum. (*A*) At approximately 4 weeks of development. (*B*) At the end of the embryonic period. (*C*) At 13 weeks of development. The V-shaped cerebellar tubercle surrounds the rostral part of the fourth ventricle. The upper and lower rhombic lips are indicated by vertical and horizontal hatching, respectively. cbi, internal cerebellar bulge; ci, colliculus inferior; Cpb, corpus pontobulbare; cs, colliculus superior; is, isthmus; mes, mesencephalon; nV, trigeminal nerve; tbac, tuberculum acusticum; tbcb, tuberculum cerebelli; tbpo, tuberculum ponto-olivare; 2, 4, 6, rhombomeres. (*Data from* references[8,21,22]).

## FOUR BASIC STEPS IN THE DEVELOPMENT OF THE CEREBELLUM

The histogenesis of the cerebellum occurs in four basic steps:[2,8,14,15,17,19,24] (1) characterization of the cerebellar territory in the hindbrain; (2) formation of two compartments of cell proliferation, giving rise to the Purkinje cells and the granule cells, respectively; (3) inward migration of the granule cells; and (4) differentiation of cerebellar neurons. A large number of genes are involved in the formation of the cerebellum.[13–15,17,18,25] More than 20 spontaneous mice mutations are known that affect the cerebellum.[14,26,27]

### Characteristics of the Cerebellar Territory

Transplantation and gene expression studies in avian and murine embryos have shown that a transverse patterning center at the midbrain-hindbrain boundary, also known as the "isthmus organizer," regulates the early development of the mesencephalon and the rostral part of the rhombencephalon.[28–30] In avian embryos, Louvi and coworkers[31] found that a restricted medial domain located at the midbrain-hindbrain boundary produces the local roof plate. Cells migrating rostrally from this region populate the caudal midbrain roof plate, whereas cells migrating caudal populate the cerebellar roof plate. The adjacent paramedian isthmic neuroepithelium also migrates caudal and participates in the formation of cerebellar midline structures. These data and data from mutant mice[23,31] suggest that isthmus-derived cells are essential for the cerebellar fusion process.

Midbrain-hindbrain boundary cells secrete fibroblast growth factors and Wnt proteins, which are required for the differentiation and patterning of the hindbrain and midbrain.[29,32] In *Wnt* knockout mice, the mesencephalon is malformed and a cerebellum is hardly present.[33] A number of homeobox-containing transcription factors are expressed across the isthmus, such as homologues of the *Drosophila* genes *En1* and *En2*. Mutations in these genes cause deletions of mesencephalic and cerebellar structures.[34–37] Sarnat and coworkers[38] described two neonates with congenital absence of the midbrain and hypoplasia of the cerebellum and rostral pons, showing a striking resemblance to the phenotype of the *En2* knockout mice. Cerebellar agenesis is extremely rare.[2,5,6,39] Gardner and colleagues[40] proposed the term "near-total absence of the cerebellum" as a distinct entity, associated with pontine hypoplasia and relatively mild clinical affection.

Less is known about the dorsoventral patterning of the cerebellar territory. Rhombencephalosynapsis (**Fig. 2**), a rare cerebellar malformation characterized by vermian agenesis or hypogenesis and dorsal fusion of the cerebellar hemispheres and dentate nuclei,[41–44] may be explained by an embryologic defect of dorsal patterning at the midbrain-hindbrain boundary,[43] possibly by underexpression of a dorsalizing gene.[45] A candidate molecule may be *Lmx1a*, identified in the neurologic mutant *dreher*, which lacks a vermis, resulting in apparent fusion of the cerebellar hemispheres and the inferior colliculi.[46,47] In rhombencephalosynapsis, clinical findings range from mild truncal ataxia and normal cognitive abilities to severe cerebral palsy and mental retardation.[42] Most cases are sporadic, and most patients die early in life.

### Formation of Two Proliferative Compartments

The histogenesis of the cerebellum comprises the three further steps of cerebellar development: (1) formation of two proliferative compartments, (2) inward migration of granule cells, and (3) formation of cerebellar circuitry and further differentiation (**Fig. 3**). The main cell types of the cerebellum arise from two anatomically and molecularly different progenitor zones: the cerebellar ventricular zone, expressing the bHLH

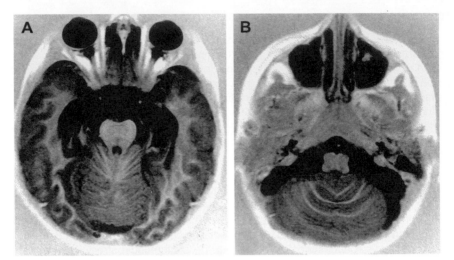

**Fig. 2.** A case of rhombencephalosynapsis. (*Courtesy of* Dr. Berit Verbist, Department of Radiology, Leiden University Medical Center, Leiden, the Netherlands.)

factor Ptf1a; and the rhombic lip, expressing the bHLH factor Math1.[18,24,48–50] GABAergic cerebellar neurons, including the Purkinje cells, the stellate and basket cells, and a subset of deep cerebellar neurons, forming the main outflow tracts of the cerebellum, arise from the ventricular zone of the metencephalic alar plates. All glutamatergic neurons are generated by the rhombic lip. In mice, in the absence of Ptf1a, the cerebellar ventricular zone fails to generate all GABAergic cerebellar neurons.[51]

Purkinje cells migrate along radial glial cells to their future position, making use of a Reelin-dependent pathway. *Reeler* mice show severe malformations of the cerebellum, caused by mutations of the *Reelin (Reln)* gene.[27] Most of the Purkinje cells fail to migrate, and they reside in an ectopic position. Granule cells reach the internal granular layer but are greatly reduced in number. Malformations in the inferior olivary nucleus are also present.[52,53] The human *REELIN (RELN)* gene is localized on chromosome 7q22. *RELN* mutations cause autosomal-recessive lissencephaly with cerebellar hypoplasia.[54] Two other genes, *LIS1* and *DCX/XLIS*, are responsible for the autosomal-dominant and X-linked forms of lissencephaly with cerebellar hypoplasia, respectively.[55]

Toward the end of the embryonic period, granule cell precursors are added from the rhombic lip (see **Fig. 3**B). The rhombic lip is the dorsolateral part of the alar plate, and it forms a proliferative zone along the length of the hindbrain. Cells from its rostral part (the upper rhombic lip) reach the superficial part of the cerebellum, and form the external germinal or granular layer at the end of the embryonic period. The rhombic lip expresses the bHLH factor Math1.[48,49] The upper rhombic lip gives rise not only to the glutamatergic granule cells, but also to all known glutamatergic neurons of the cerebellum, including unipolar brush cells and the glutamatergic subset of deep cerebellar nuclei neurons.[56–59] In *Math1* knockout mice, no granular layer is formed. Granule cell precursors express the netrin receptors DCC, Unc5H2 and Unc5H3.[60,61] Disruption of *Unc5H3* signaling leads to the rostral cerebellar malformation in which granule and Purkinje cells spread ectopically into the caudal mesencephalon.[60,62] Netrin has a general role in guiding ventral migration of rhombic lip derivatives,[61,63] but its role in the migration of granule cell precursors to the external granular layer is not entirely clear. Cerebellar development is undisturbed in *Netrin1*

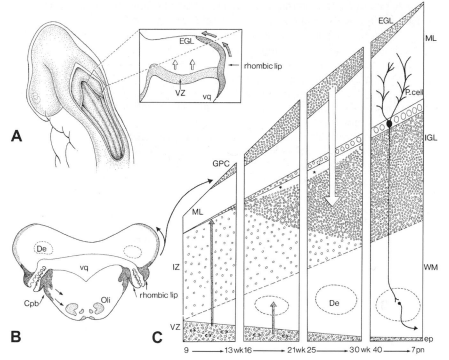

**Fig. 3.** Overview of the histogenesis of the human cerebellum. (*A*) Dorsolateral view of an human embryo is shown and part of the cerebellar tubercle is enlarged, showing the two proliferative compartments: the ventricular zone, giving rise to all GABAergic neurons, including the Purkinje cells and the deep cerebellar nuclei; and the external germinal or granular layer, generating the glutamatergic granule cells. (*B*) The position of the rhombic lip is shown in a transverse section of the brainstem at the level of the lateral recess of the fourth ventricle. The upper rhombic lip is found lateral to the lateral recess, and the lower rhombic lip medial to that recess. (*C*) Formation of the several layers of the cerebellum is shown in four periods from the early fetal period until 7 weeks postnatally. With asterisks the transient lamina dissecans is indicated. The arrows in *A* to *C* show the migration paths. Cpb, corpus pontobulbare; De, dentate nucleus; EGL, external granular layer; ep, ependyma; GPC, granule precursor cells; IGL, internal granular layer; IZ, intermediate zone; ML, molecular layer; Oli, oliva inferior; P-cell, Purkinje cell; vq, ventriculus quartus; VZ, ventricular zone; WM, white matter. (*Data from* references[13,20,21]).

knockout mice.[63] In the mouse mutant *weaver*, the granule cells degenerate after their first cell division.[27,64] *Weaver* mice have a near-total loss of granule cells in the cerebellar vermis that accounts for a diminutive cerebellum and an ataxic gait. *Staggerer* mice also show a near-total absence of granule cells.[65]

### Inward Migration of Granule Cells

Granule cells are formed in the external granular layer, which persists for up to 1 to 2 years after birth.[66] The granule cells form axons, the parallel fibers, and migrate along the processes of Bergmann glia cells to their deeper, definitive site, the internal granular layer (see **Fig. 3**C). In the fetal period, the internal granular layer is formed by further proliferation and migration of the external germinal cells, and constitutes the definitive granular layer of the cerebellar cortex. A transient layer, the lamina dissecans, separates the internal granular layer from the Purkinje cell layer. Ultimately, this layer is filled by migrating granule cells and disappears.[21]

Sonic hedgehog (Shh), a member of the hedgehog family of secreted signaling proteins, is expressed in migrating and settled Purkinje cells, and acts as a potent mitogenic signal to expand the granule cell progenitor population.[67,68] Medulloblastoma, a brainstem tumor of childhood, may originate from granule cell precursor cells that become transformed and fail to undergo normal differentiation. Mutations in the *PATCHED1* (*PTCH1*) gene that is activated by SHH, may give rise to medulloblastoma.[68]

Disturbed proliferation and differentiation of granule cell precursors may give rise to diffuse hypertrophy of the cerebellar cortex,[69] known as "Lhermitte-Duclos" disease.[70] The gene involved, *PTEN*, is a tumor-suppressor gene playing roles in cell cycle control, apoptosis, and mediation of adhesion and migration signaling. *PTEN* germline mutations have been described in various familial tumor syndromes, including Cowden disease and Bannayan-Zonana syndrome.

Primary degeneration of the granular layer of the cerebellum (granular layer aplasia) occurs as an autosomal-recessive disorder.[71,72] All of the pathologically documented granular layer aplasia cases showed aplasia or severe hypoplasia of the cerebellar granular layer accompanied by widespread architectonic disturbances of the Purkinje cell layer.[72] Pascual-Castroviejo[73] described seven cases with features consistent with granular layer aplasia and heterozygous deficiency of phosphomannomutase type 2.

### Differentiation of Cerebellar Neurons

Granule cell differentiation is characterized by a prolonged period of clonal expansion that occurs after progenitors have been specified. In contrast, Purkinje cells cease proliferation within the ventricular zone and rapidly express numerous differentiation markers.[17,24,25] *Math1* is expressed in the rhombic lip and, subsequently, in the external granular layer, but its expression is downregulated at later stages of granule cell development.[48] The interaction of Purkinje and granule cells is clearly demonstrated in *PTF1A* mutations. Mutations in the *PTF1A* gene were first identified in a large family with both cerebellar agenesis and neonatal diabetes.[74] This gene is well-known for its role in pancreas development.[75] Studies in mice showed the crucial role of *Ptf1a* in the specification of cerebellar GABAergic neurons and, moreover, revealed that the complete cerebellar agenesis phenotype seen at birth in both humans and mice is a secondary phenotype.[50] In the absence of *Ptf1a*, the failure to generate GABAergic neurons leads to massive prenatal death of all cerebellar glutamatergic neurons because their GABAergic targets are not present.[50]

### DEVELOPMENT OF PRECEREBELLAR NUCLEI

The precerebellar nuclei form a group of brainstem nuclei with efferent projections largely or exclusively to the cerebellum. They all arise from the lower rhombic lip.[16,19,76] The pontine nuclei and the pontine reticular tegmental nucleus form the upper precerebellar neurons, whereas the inferior olivary nucleus with its accessory olivary nuclei, the external cuneate nucleus, and the lateral reticular nucleus form the lower precerebellar nuclei.[19] Neurons of these upper and lower precerebellar systems migrate along various pathways, the corpus pontobulbare in particular, to their ultimate position in the brainstem (see **Figs. 1** and **3B**). Netrin has a general role in guiding ventral migration of precerebellar neurons.[61,63,77] Neurons migrating toward the pontine nuclei express the netrin receptor DCC[60,61,77] and upregulate a second receptor, Unc5H3, at their target.[60] Cells migrating to the inferior olive also express *Dcc* and *Unc5H* homologues. *Netrin1* knockout mice show a reduced inferior olive and ectopic neurons expressing inferior olive markers.[63]

Inferior olive malformations are found as heterotopia and as dysplasias.[2,5,6] Heterotopia of the inferior olivary nuclei are typically associated with lissencephalies. They are also found in the Dandy-Walker malformation (DWM) and other vermis malformations. They consist of single or multiple irregularly shaped islands of gray matter dispersed along a line extending from its normal position to the lateral floor of the fourth ventricle near the corpus restiforme. Olivary heterotopia mimic the characteristic convoluted shape of the inferior olive. Dysplasias of the shape of the inferior olivary nucleus occur with cerebellar malformations, trisomies 13 and 18, Zellweger syndrome, and holoprosencephaly. Segments of the nucleus are thickened with obliteration of the normal undulating profile. In more severe lesions, the inferior olive has a greatly simplified C-shape.

## DEVELOPMENTAL DISORDERS OF THE CEREBELLUM

Anatomically, cerebellar malformations may be classified into unilateral and bilateral abnormalities. Unilateral cerebellar malformations are most likely caused by acquired insults, such as intracerebellar bleeding associated with prematurity.[78,79] Depending on the part of the cerebellum involved, bilateral cerebellar malformations may be further classified into midline or vermis malformations, and malformations affecting both the vermis and the cerebellar hemispheres.[2,7–9,12] The combination of pontine hypoplasia with cerebellar malformation is considered as a separate group (ie, the pontocerebellar hypoplasias).[7,12,80] Many of the newly identified genes, including genes causing DWM, Joubert syndrome, and pontocerebellar hypoplasia, have not been previously implicated in cerebellar development.[18] Global cerebellar hypoplasia may result from a variety of exogenous or endogenous factors.[5–7,71] Global cerebellar hypoplasia is found as a result of intrauterine exposure to drugs (eg, phenytoin) or irradiation, and as an autosomal-recessive trait in a variety of chromosomal disorders, such as trisomies 13, 18, and 21.

### Midline or Vermis Malformations

Agenesis or hypoplasia of the vermis may be found in a large number of malformations of the brain,[2,5–7,9,10,12,81,82] including (1) the DWM and syndromes with agenesis of the vermis as a constant feature, such as the Joubert and Walker-Warburg syndromes; (2) a large group of syndromes in which absence of the vermis may occur, such as the Meckel-Gruber and Smith-Lemli-Opitz syndromes; and (3) dysgenesis of the vermis in rare disorders, such as rhombencephalosynapsis, tectocerebellar dysraphia, and Lhermitte-Duclos disease. Major malformations of cerebellar midline structures are also found in the Chiari malformations, the most common of which, type II, is almost always associated with a myelomeningocele, and forms part of the neural tube spectrum defect.[83,84] Vermal malformations have also been noted in idiopathic autism[85] and in dyslexic children.[86,87]

DWM, a relatively common malformation occurring in at least 1 in 5000 liveborn infants,[12] is characterized by the following triad:[5,6,9,10,12,81,82] (1) cystic dilatation of the fourth ventricle and an enlarged posterior fossa with upward displacement of the lateral sinuses, confluens sinuum, and tentorium cerebelli; (2) varying degrees of vermian aplasia and hypoplasia; and (3) hydrocephalus (**Fig. 4**A). Hydrocephalus, associated with a bulging occiput, is unusual at birth but is present by 3 months of age in about 75% of patients.[10] Early shunting of the cyst and hydrocephalus is

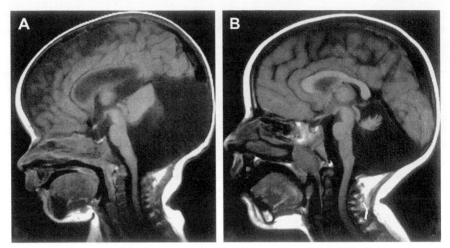

**Fig. 4.** The Dandy-Walker malformation (*A*) and the Dandy-Walker variant (*B*). Note in *A* the large cyst in the posterior fossa, the hydrocephalus, elevation of the structures, forming the roof of the posterior fossa, and hypoplasia of the corpus callosum. In the Dandy-Walker variant (*B*), no hydrocephalus and a normal corpus callosum can be seen. (*Courtesy of* Dr. Henk O.M. Thijssen, Department of Radiology, Radboud University Nijmegen Medical Center, Nijmegen, the Netherlands.)

advocated because early management may give mental development a better chance and improve prognosis.[12,82,88] Most cases are sporadic with a low recurrence risk. Associated central nervous system malformations are present in two thirds of the cases, the most common of which is agenesis or hypogenesis of the corpus callosum (see **Fig. 4**A). The etiology of DWM remains unknown. Probably, the malformation arises late in the embryonic period. Hypotheses include developmental arrest in the formation of the hindbrain, atresia of the fourth ventricular outlet foramina, and delayed opening of the aperture of Magendie. The *ZIC1* and *ZIC4* genes on chromosome 3q24 may be involved in DWM.[89] The *del3q24* DWM phenotype is extremely variable, ranging from classic DWM to only mild vermis hypoplasia.

Barkovich and others[10,82,90] advocated the Dandy-Walker complex as a continuum of posterior fossa anomalies, comprising DWM, the Dandy-Walker variant, and the mega cisterna magna. In the Dandy-Walker variant, the posterior fossa is hardly enlarged; there is hypoplasia of the vermis and communication between the fourth ventricle and arachnoid space, and hydrocephalus is absent (see **Fig. 4**B). The mega cisterna magna consists of an enlarged posterior fossa, secondary to an enlarged cisterna magna, but a normal vermis and fourth ventricle are found. Kollias and Ball[9] suggested the broad term "vermian-cerebellar hypoplasia" for malformations of the posterior fossa with prominent cystlike cerebrospinal fluid–containing spaces that fail to fulfill all the criteria for the diagnosis DWM. Parisi and Dobyns[12] introduced the term "cerebellar vermis hypoplasia-dysplasia" as an alternative for many cases of the Dandy-Walker variant and mega cisterna magna. Several families with cerebellar vermis hypoplasia-dysplasia follow X-linked inheritance.[91] Mutations of the *oligophrenin-1* gene (*OPHN1*) at Xq12, previously associated with X-linked mental retardation, have been identified in affected males from several clinically rather heterogeneous families with mental retardation and vermis hypoplasia with a 50% overall recurrence risk.[92,93] The prognosis for individuals with this and related conditions is often worse than for classic DWM.[93]

The prenatal diagnosis of DWM remains problematic.[12] Prenatal imaging cannot reliably differentiate between true DWM and cerebellar vermis hypoplasia-dysplasia. Although the cisterna magna can be visualized in approximately 95% of fetuses between 15 and 25 weeks of gestation, determination of pathology can be difficult in cases with mild dilatation. Moreover, false appearance of an enlarged cisterna magna may occur because of an improper transducer angle.[11,94] Nyberg and coworkers[94] studied 33 fetuses with an enlarged cisterna magna, 55% of which were found to have a chromosomal abnormality associated with a poor prognosis. They were either electively terminated or died at birth or soon thereafter. Fetuses with a more dramatic ventricular enlargement were less likely to have a chromosomal abnormality and more likely to have classic DWM with a reasonable good prognosis.

Joubert syndrome is a relatively rare, autosomal-recessive disorder with an estimated prevalence of approximately 1 in 100,000.[12] It is defined by vermis hypoplasia (**Figs. 5** and **6**); hypotonia; developmental delay; typical facial features (prominent forehead, upturned nose, open mouth); and at least one of two additional manifestations (abnormal breathing pattern [hyperpnea intermixed with central apnea in the neonatal period] or abnormal eye movements).[95–100] On imaging, the significant feature of Joubert syndrome and related disorders, such as Dekaban-Arima, COACH, Senior-Loken, and OFD VI syndromes, is the "molar tooth" sign. This sign depends on a specific malformation of the brainstem and cerebellum in axial MRIs at the isthmus level,[101] characterized by a deepened interpeduncular fossa, hypoplasia of the vermis, and elongated superior cerebellar peduncles. In the ophthalmologic literature, Joubert syndrome is known as a condition with a variable combination of central nervous system defects together with a distinctive congenital retinal dystrophy and oculomotor abnormalities in early infancy.[102] Many patients with Joubert syndrome have, apart from retinal dystrophy, also renal fibrocystic disease (nephronophthisis), two conditions related to defective function of cilia. Ataxia, mental retardation, and behavioral

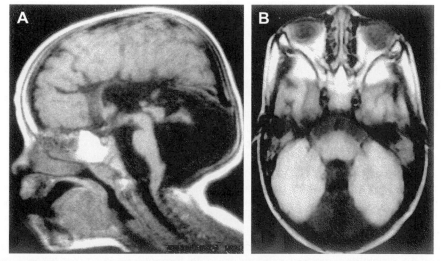

**Fig. 5.** The Joubert syndrome. MRI data in a girl at the age of 1 year and 4 months. Note in (A) and (B) a large fluid-filled cyst in the posterior fossa and the absence of the vermis. (B) The molar-tooth sign is not clear, possibly because of the complete absence of the vermis. (*From* ten Donkelaar HJ, Hoevenaars F, Wesseling P. A case of Joubert's syndrome with extensive cerebral malformations. Clin Neuropathol 2000;19:85–93; with permission.)

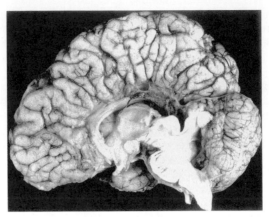

**Fig. 6.** Medial view of the brain of the girl in **Fig. 5** with Joubert syndrome; macrophoto taken at autopsy at 3 years of age. Note the complete absence of the vermis, the malformed roof of the midbrain, a rather wide aqueduct, well-developed fornices, and absence of the corpus callosum.

disorders become manifest in late infancy and childhood, at a time when the respiratory anomalies decrease and become undetectable.[103] The prognosis for Joubert syndrome is poor. There is severe mental and motor retardation and the 5-year survival is about 50%.[97] At least eight genetic loci have been mapped for various subtypes of Joubert syndrome, and seven genes have been identified: (1) *AHI1*; (2) *nephrocystin-1 (NPHP1)*; (3) *CEP290*; (4) *TMEM67*; (5) *ARLI3B*, a retinitis pigmentosa gene; (6) *RPGRIP1L*; and (7) *CC2D2A*.[104–111] These genes encode mediators of signal transduction pathways at the primary cilium. In the cerebellum, primary cilia have been identified in both Purkinje cell and granule cell progenitors.[112,113] The primary defect in Joubert syndrome may be compromised granule cell proliferation, resulting in cerebellar hypoplasia.[17,18]

### Pontocerebellar Hypoplasias

The pontocerebellar hypoplasias form a large group of disorders, characterized by a smaller volume of the pons and varying degrees of cerebellar hypoplasia up to near-total absence of the cerebellum.[7,12,40,80] Most types of pontocerebellar hypoplasias arise in the fetal period, suggesting a rhombic lip defect and the *MATH1* gene as a candidate for this disorder. Most pontocerebellar hypoplasias are autosomal-recessive disorders with a recurrence risk of 25%; for most of these, the responsible gene defect has not yet been identified. Two cases of pontocerebellar hypoplasia are shown in **Fig. 7**. Pontocerebellar hypoplasias may be classified into congenital olivopontocerebellar atrophy,[114,115] and the type 1 and 2 pontocerebellar hypoplasias with spinal muscular atrophy[116–118] and extrapyramidal dysfunction,[119–122] respectively. There are other less defined forms of pontocerebellar hypoplasia that have already been classified as type 3, with linkage to chromosome 7,[123,124] and type 5, an intrauterine variant.[125] Several reports suggest that what was originally categorized as type 4[125] might be a more severe fatal neonatal form of type 2, so that types 2 and 4 may represent a continuum of increasingly severe pathology.[121,126,127]

The congenital disorders of glycosylation are autosomal-recessive, multisystemic disorders characterized by glycosylation defects of glycoproteins, which are involved in many different metabolic functions.[128] *CDG1a* presents clinically with a congenital

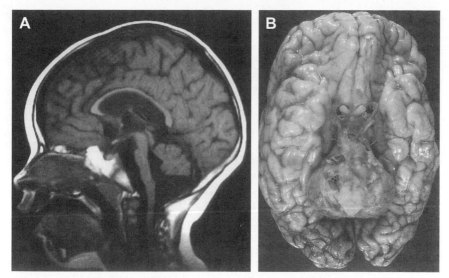

**Fig. 7.** (*A, B*) Two examples of pontocerebellar hypoplasias. Note that in the basal view of the brain with pontocerebellar hypoplasia caused by carbohydrate-deficient glycoprotein type 1a (*B*) the width of the pons does not exceed that of the medulla. (*From* ten Donkelaar HJ, Lammens M, Wesseling P, et al. Development and developmental disorders of the human cerebellum. In: ten Donkelaar HJ, Lammens M, Hori A. Clinical neuroembryology: development and developmental disorders of the human central nervous system. Berlin-Heidelberg-New York: Springer; 2006. p. 309–44; with permission.)

pontocerebellar hypoplasia, which is an early progressive cerebellar atrophy.[129–131] The type 1a carbohydrate-deficient glycoprotein syndrome (Jaeken syndrome) is a multisystem disorder with major neurologic involvement. The major manifestations are dysmorphic features (convergent strabismus, large dysplastic ears, subcutaneous fat deposits with lipodystrophy at the lower part of the back, and orange-peel skin); mental retardation; retinopathy; hyporeflexia; trunk ataxia; and hypogonadism. The basic biochemical defect is deficient transformation of mannose-6-phosphate into mannose-1-phosphate because of deficiency of the enzyme phosphomannomutase. Matthijs and coworkers[132] identified 11 different missense mutations at the phosphomannomutase gene *PMM2*. In carbohydrate-deficient glycoprotein type 2d, Peters and coworkers[133] found DWM and myopathy. Carbohydrate-deficient glycoprotein can be demonstrated by isoelectric focusing of the serum transferrin pattern, which should be routinely performed in neonates presenting with congenital cerebellar hypoplasia.

Mitochondrial disease[134] and congenital muscular dystrophies[135] may also present with congenital pontocerebellar hypoplasia. Recent studies showed that several forms of cerebellar malformation (cerebellar hypoplasia, vermian hypoplasia, cerebellar dysplasia, and cerebellar cysts) are present in different forms of muscular dystrophy with defective dystroglycan glycosylation caused by mutations in *POMT1*, *POMT2*, *POMGnT1*, or *LARGE*.[136]

**REFERENCES**

1. Voogd J. Cerebellum and precerebellar nuclei. In: Paxinos G, Mai JK, editors. The human nervous system. 2nd edition. Amsterdam: Elsevier; 2004. p. 321–92.

2. ten Donkelaar HJ, Lammens M, Wesseling P, et al. Development and developmental disorders of the human cerebellum. In: ten Donkelaar HJ, Lammens M, Hori A, editors. Clinical neuroembryology: development and developmental disorders of the human central nervous system. Berlin-Heidelberg-New York: Springer; 2006. p. 309–44.
3. Middleton FL, Strick PL, editors. Special issue: cerebellum. Trends Neurosci 1998;21:367–419, Trends Cogn Sci 1998;2:313–71.
4. Schmahmann JD. Disorders of the cerebellum: ataxia, dysmetria of thought, and the cerebellar cognitive affective syndrome. J Neuropsychiatry Clin Neurosci 2004;16:367–78.
5. Friede RL. Developmental neuropathology. 2nd edition. Berlin-Heidelberg-New York: Springer; 1989.
6. Norman MG, McGillivray BC, Kalousek DK, et al. Congenital malformations of the brain. pathological, embryological, clinical, radiological and genetic aspects. New York: Oxford University Press; 1995.
7. Ramaeckers VT, Heimann G, Reul J, et al. Genetic disorders and cerebellar structural abnormalities in childhood. Brain 1997;120:1739–51.
8. ten Donkelaar HJ, Lammens M, Wesseling P, et al. Development and developmental disorders of the human cerebellum. J Neurol 2003;250:1025–36.
9. Kollias SS, Ball WS. Congenital malformations of the brain. In: Ball WS, editor. Pediatric neuroradiology. Philadelphia: Lippincott-Raven; 1997. p. 91–174.
10. Barkovich AJ. Pediatric neuroimaging. 3rd edition. Philadelphia: Lippincott; 2000.
11. Pilu G, Visentin B, Valeri B. The Dandy-Walker complex and fetal sonography. Ultrasound Obstet Gynecol 2000;16:115–7.
12. Parisi MA, Dobyns WB. Human malformations of the midbrain and hindbrain: review and proposed classification scheme. Mol Genet Metab 2003;80:36–53.
13. Hatten ME, Alder J, Zimmerman K, et al. Genes involved in cerebellar specification and differentiation. Curr Opin Neurobiol 1997;7:40–7.
14. Millen KJ, Millonig JH, Wingate RJT, et al. Neurogenetics of the cerebellar system. J Child Neurol 1999;14:574–82.
15. Wang VY, Zoghbi HY. Genetic regulation of cerebellar development. Nat Rev Neurosci 2001;2:484–91.
16. Wingate RJT. The rhombic lip and early cerebellar development. Curr Opin Neurobiol 2001;11:82–8.
17. Chizhikov V, Millen KJ. Development and malformations of the cerebellum in mice. Mol Genet Metab 2003;80:54–65.
18. Millen KJ, Gleeson JG. Cerebellar development and disease. Curr Opin Neurobiol 2008;18:12–9.
19. Altman J, Bayer SA. Development of the cerebellar system: in relation to its evolution, structure and functions. Boca Raton (FL): CRC Press; 1997.
20. O'Rahilly R, Müller F. Human embryology and teratology. 3rd edition. New York: Wiley-Liss; 2001.
21. Sidman RL, Rakic P. Development of the human central nervous system. In: Haymaker W, Adams RD, editors. Histology and histopathology of the nervous system. Springfield (MA): Thomas; 1982. p. 3–145.
22. Hochstetter F. Contributions to the developmental history of the human brain, Vol. II, Part 3: The development of the mid- and hindbrain. Vienna: Deuticke; 1929 [German].
23. Sgaier SK, Millet S, Villanueva MP, et al. Morphogenetic and cellular movements that shape the mouse cerebellum; insights from genetic fate mapping. Neuron 2005;45:27–40.

24. Hatten ME, Heintz N. Mechanisms of neural patterning and specification in the developing cerebellum. Annu Rev Neurosci 1995;18:385–408.
25. Goldewitz D, Hamre K. The cells and molecules that make the cerebellum. Trends Neurosci 1998;21:375–82.
26. Caviness VS Jr, Rakic P. Mechanisms of cortical development: a view from mutations in mice. Annu Rev Neurosci 1978;1:297–326.
27. Mullen RJ, Hamre KM, Goldowitz D. Cerebellar mutant mice and chimeras revisited. Perspect Dev Neurobiol 1997;5:43–55.
28. Wassef M, Joyner AL. Early mesencephalon/metencephalon patterning and development of the cerebellum. Perspect Dev Neurobiol 1997;5:3–16.
29. Rhinn M, Brand M. The midbrain-hindbrain boundary organizer. Curr Opin Neurobiol 2001;11:34–42.
30. Wurst W, Bally-Cuif L. Neural plate patterning: upstream and downstream of the isthmic organizer. Nat Rev Neurosci 2001;2:99–108.
31. Louvi A, Alexandre P, Métin C, et al. The isthmic neuroepithelium is essential for cerebellar midline fusion. Development 2003;130:5319–30.
32. Sato T, Joyner AL, Nakamura H. How does Fgf signaling from the isthmic organizer induce midbrain and cerebellum development? Dev Growth Differ 2004; 46:487–94.
33. Mastick GS, Fan C-M, Tessier-Lavigne M, et al. Early detection of neuromeres in *Wnt-1-/-* mutant mice: evaluation by morphological and molecular markers. J Comp Neurol 1996;374:246–58.
34. Millen KJ, Wurst W, Herrup K, et al. Abnormal embryonic cerebellar development and patterning of postnatal foliation in two mouse Engrailed-2 mutants. Development 1994;120:695–706.
35. Millen KJ, Hui CC, Joyner AL. A role for En-2 and other murine homologues of *Drosophila* segment polarity genes in regulating positional information in the developing cerebellum. Development 1995;121:3935–45.
36. Wurst W, Auerbach AB, Joyner AL. Multiple developmental defects in Engrailed-1 mutant mice: an early midbrain-hindbrain deletion and patterning defects in forelimbs and sternum. Development 1994;120:2065–75.
37. Kuemerle B, Zanjani H, Joyner A, et al. Pattern deformities and cell loss in *Engrailed-2* mutant mice suggest two separate patterning events during cerebellar development. J Neurosci 1997;17:7881–9.
38. Sarnat HB, Benjamin DR, Siebert JR, et al. Agenesis of the mesencephalon and metencephalon with cerebellar hypoplasia: putative mutation in the *EN2* gene – report of two cases in early infancy. Pediatr Dev Pathol 2002;5:54–68.
39. Glickstein M. Cerebellar agenesis. Brain 1994;117:1209–12.
40. Gardner RJM, Coleman LT, Mitchell LA, et al. Near-total absence of the cerebellum. Neuropediatrics 2001;32:62–8.
41. Obersteiner H. A cerebellum without vermis. Arb Neurol Inst (Wien) 1914;21: 124–36 [German].
42. Toelle SP, Yalcinkaya C, Kocer N, et al. Rhombencephalosynapsis: clinical findings and neuroimaging in 9 children. Neuropediatrics 2002;33:209–14.
43. Yachnis AT. Rhombencephalosynapsis with massive hydrocephalus: case report and pathogenetic considerations. Acta Neuropathol (Berl) 2002;103:301–4.
44. Pasquier L, Marcorelles P, Loget P, et al. Rhombencephalosynapsis and related anomalies: a neuropathological study of 40 fetal cases. Acta Neuropathol (Berl) 2009;117:185–200.
45. Sarnat HB. Molecular genetic classification of central nervous system malformations. J Child Neurol 2000;15:675–87.

46. Manzanares M, Trainor PA, Ariza-McNaughton L, et al. Dorsal patterning defects in the hindbrain, roof plate and skeleton in the dreher [dr(J)] mouse mutant. Mech Dev 2000;94:147–56.

47. Millonig JH, Millen JK, Hatten ME. The mouse Dreher gene Lmx1a controls formation of the roof plate in the vertebrate CNS. Nature 2000;403:764–9.

48. Ben-Arie N, Bellen HJ, Armstrong DL, et al. *Math1* is essential for genesis of cerebellar granule neurons. Nature 1997;390:169–72.

49. Jensen P, Smeyne R, Goldowitz D. Analysis of cerebellar development in *Math1* null embryos and chimeras. J Neurosci 2004;24:2202–11.

50. Hoshino M, Nakamura S, Mori K, et al. Ptf1a, a bHLH transcriptional gene, defines GABAergic neuronal fates in cerebellum. Neuron 2005;47:201–13.

51. Pascual M, Abasolo I, Mingorance-Le Meur A, et al. Cerebellar GABAergic progenitors adopt an external granule cell-like phenotype in the absence of Ptf1a transcription factor expression. Proc Natl Acad Sci U S A 2007;104: 5193–8.

52. Goffinet A. The embryonic development of the inferior olivary complex in normal and reeler mutant mice. J Comp Neurol 1983;219:10–24.

53. Goffinet A, So K-F, Yamamoto M, et al. Architectonic and hodological organization of the cerebellum in *reeler* mutant mice. Brain Res 1984;16:263–76.

54. Hong SE, Shugari YY, Huang DT, et al. Autosomal recessive lissencephaly with cerebellar hypoplasia is associated with human *RELN* mutations. Nat Genet 2000;26:93–6.

55. Ross ME, Swanson K, Dobyns WB. Lissencephaly with cerebellar hypoplasia (LCH): a heterogeneous group of cortical malformations. Neuropediatrics 2001;32:256–61.

56. Machold R, Fishell G. Math1 is expressed in temporally discrete pools of cerebellar rhombic-lip neural progenitors. Neuron 2005;48:17–24.

57. Wang VY, Rose MF, Zoghbi HY. Math1 expression redefines the rhombic lip derivatives and reveals novel lineages within the brainstem and cerebellum. Neuron 2005;48:31–43.

58. England C, Kowalczyk T, Daza RA, et al. Unipolar brush cells of the cerebellum are produced in the rhombic lip and migrate through developing white matter. J Neurosci 2006;26:9184–95.

59. Fink AJ, Englund C, Daza RA, et al. Development of the deep cerebellar nuclei: transcription factors and cell migration from the rhombic lip. J Neurosci 2006;26: 3066–76.

60. Engelkamp D, Rashbass P, Seawright A, et al. Role of Pax6 in development of the cerebellar system. Development 1999;126:3585–96.

61. Alcantara S, Ruiz M, De Castro F, et al. Netrin 1 acts as an attractive or as a repulsive cue for distinct migrating neurons during the development of the cerebellar system. Development 2000;127:1359–72.

62. Ackermann SL, Kozak LP, Przyborski SA, et al. The mouse rostral cerebellar mutation gene encodes an UNC-5-like protein. Nature 1997;386:838–42.

63. Bloch-Gallego E, Ezan F, Tessier-Lavigne M, et al. Floor plate and netrin-1 are involved in the migration and survival of inferior olivary neurons. J Neurosci 1999;19:4407–20.

64. Rakic P, Sidman RL. Sequence of developmental abnormalities leading to granule cell deficits in cerebellar cortex of *weaver* mutant mice. J Comp Neurol 1973;152:103–32.

65. Sidman RL, Lane PW, Dickie MM. *Staggerer,* a new mutation in the mouse affecting the cerebellum. Science 1962;137:610–2.

66. Lemire RJ, Loeser JD, Leech RW, et al. Development of the human nervous system. Hagerstown (MD): Harper & Row; 1975.

67. Dahmane N, Sanchez P, Gitton Y, et al. The Sonic hedgehog-Gli pathway regulates dorsal brain growth and tumorigenesis. Development 2001;128:5201–12.

68. Wechsler-Reya R, Scott MP. The developmental biology of brain tumors. Annu Rev Neurosci 2001;24:385–428.

69. Beuche W, Wickboldt J, Friede RL. Lhermitte-Duclos disease: its minimal lesions in electron microscope data and CT findings. Clin Neuropathol 1983;2:163–70.

70. Lhermitte J, Duclos P. On a diffuse ganglioneuroma of the cerebellar cortex. Bull Assoc Fr Etud Cancer 1920;9:99–107 [French].

71. Sarnat HB, Alcalá H. Human cerebellar hypoplasia: a syndrome of diverse causes. Arch Neurol (Chic) 1980;37:300–5.

72. Pascual-Castroviejo I, Gutierrez M, Morales C, et al. Primary degeneration of the granular layer of the cerebellum: a study of 14 patients and review of the literature. Neuropediatrics 1994;25:183–90.

73. Pascual-Castroviejo I. Congenital disorders of glycosylation syndromes. Dev Med Child Neurol 2002;44:357–8.

74. Sellick GS, Barker KT, Stolte-Dijkstra I, et al. Mutations in PTF1A cause pancreatic and cerebellar agenesis. Nat Genet 2004;36:1301–5.

75. Kumar M, Melton D. Pancreas specification: a budding question. Curr Opin Genet Dev 2003;13:401–7.

76. Essick CR. The development of the nuclei pontis and the nucleus arcuatus in man. Am J Anat 1912;13:25–54.

77. Yee KT, Simon HH, Tessier-Lavigne M, et al. Extension of long leading processes and neuronalmigration in the mammalian brain directed by the chemoattractant netrin-1. Neuron 1999;24:607–22.

78. Grunnet ML, Shields WD. Cerebellar hemorrhage in the premature infant. J Pediatr 1976;88:605–8.

79. Volpe JJ. Neurology of the newborn. 5th edition. Philadelphia: Elsevier; 2008.

80. Barth PG. Pontocerebellar hypoplasias: an overview of a group of inherited neurodegenerative disorders with fetal onset. Brain Dev 1993;15:411–22.

81. Hart HH, Malamud N, Ellis WG. The Dandy-Walker syndrome: a clinicopathological study based on 28 cases. Neurology 1972;22:771–80.

82. Bordarier C, Aicardi J. Dandy-Walker syndrome and agenesis of the cerebellar vermis: diagnostic problems and genetic counseling. Dev Med Child Neurol 1990;32:285–94.

83. Cai C, Oakes WJ. Hindbrain herniation syndromes: the Chiari malformations (I and II). Semin Pediatr Neurol 1997;4:179–91.

84. ten Donkelaar HJ, Mullaart RA, Hori A, et al. Neurulation and neural tube defects. In: ten Donkelaar HJ, Lammens M, Hori A, editors. Clinical neuroembryology: development and developmental disorders of the human central nervous system. Berlin-Heidelberg-New York: Springer; 2006. p. 145–90.

85. Kaufmann WE, Cooper KI, Mostofski SH, et al. Specificity of cerebellar vermian abnormalities in autism: a quantitative magnetic resonance imaging study. J Child Neurol 2003;18:463–70.

86. Habib M. The neurological basis of developmental dyslexia: an overview and working hypothesis. Brain 2000;123:2373–99.

87. Voeller KKS. Dyslexia. J Child Neurol 2004;19:740–4.

88. Pascual-Castroviejo I, Velez A, Pascual-Pascual S-I, et al. Dandy-Walker malformation: an analysis of 38 cases. Childs Nerv Syst 1991;7:88–97.

89. Grinberg J, Northrup H, Ardinger H, et al. Heterozygous deletion of the linked genes ZIC1 and ZIC4 is involved in Dandy-Walker malformation. Nat Genet 2004;36:1053–5.

90. Barkovich A, Kjos BO, Norman D, et al. Revised classification of posterior fossa cysts and cyst-like malformations based on the results of multiplanar MR imaging. AJNR Am J Neuroradiol 1989;10:977–88.

91. Wakeling EL, Jolly M, Fisk NM, et al. X-linked inheritance of Dandy-Walker variant. Clin Dysmorphol 2002;11:15–8.

92. Bergmann C, Zerres K, Senderek J, et al. Oligophrenin 1 (OPHN1) gene mutation causes syndromic X-linked mental retardation with epilepsy, rostral ventricular enlargement and cerebellar hypoplasia. Brain 2003;126:1537–44.

93. Philip N, Chabrol B, Lossi AM, et al. Mutations in the oligophrenin-1 gene (OPHN1) cause X-linked congenital cerebellar hypoplasia. J Med Genet 2003; 40:441–6.

94. Nyberg DA, Mahony BS, Hegge FN, et al. Enlarged cisterna magna and the Dandy-Walker malformation: factors associated with chromosome abnormalities. Obstet Gynecol 1991;436–42.

95. Joubert M, Eisenring J-J, Robb JP, et al. Familial agenesis of the cerebellar vermis: a syndrome of episodic hyperpnea, abnormal eye movements, ataxia, and retardation. Neurology 1969;19:813–25.

96. Kendall B, Kingsley D, Lambert SR, et al. Joubert syndrome: a clinico-radiological study. Neuroradiology 1990;31:502–6.

97. Saraiva JM, Baraitser M. Joubert syndrome: a review. Am J Med Genet 1992;43: 726–31.

98. Maria BL, Boltshauser E, Palmer SC, et al. Clinical features and revised diagnostic criteria in Joubert syndrome. J Child Neurol 1992;14:583–91.

99. Yachnis AT, Rorke LB. Neuropathology of Joubert syndrome. J Child Neurol 1999;14:655–9.

100. ten Donkelaar HJ, Hoevenaars F, Wesseling P. A case of Joubert's syndrome with extensive cerebral malformations. Clin Neuropathol 2000;19:85–93.

101. Maria BL, Quisling RG, Rosainz LC, et al. Molar tooth sign in Joubert syndrome: clinical, radiologic, and pathologic significance. J Child Neurol 1999;14:368–76.

102. Lambert SR, Kriss A, Gresty M, et al. Joubert syndrome. Arch Ophthalmol 1989; 107:709–13.

103. Aicardi J. Diseases of the nervous system in childhood. 2nd edition. Cambridge, UK: Cambridge University Press; 1998.

104. Dixon-Salazar T, Silhavy JL, Marsh SE, et al. Mutations in the AHI1 gene, encoding Jouberin, cause Joubert syndrome with cortical polymicrogyria. Am J Hum Genet 2004;75:979–87.

105. Ferland RJ, Eyaid W, Collura RV, et al. Abnormal cerebellar development and axonal decussation due to mutations in AHI1 in Joubert syndrome. Nat Genet 2004;36:1008–13.

106. Valente EM, Silhavy JL, Brancati F, et al. Mutations in CEP290, which encodes a centrosomal protein, cause pleitropic forms of Joubet syndrome. Nat Genet 2006;38:623–5.

107. Sayer JA, Otto EA, O'Toole JF, et al. The centrosomal protein nephrocystin-6 is mutated in Joubert syndrome and activates a transcription factor ATF4. Nat Genet 2006;38:674–81.

108. Arts HH, Doherty D, van Beersum SE, et al. Mutations in the gene encoding the basal body protein RGPRIP1L, a nephrocystin-4 interactor, cause Joubert syndrome. Nat Genet 2007;39:882–8.

109. Delous M, Baala L, Salomon R, et al. The ciliary gene RGRPIP1L is mutated in cerebello-oculo-renal syndrome (Joubert syndrome type B) and Meckel syndrome. Nat Genet 2007;39:875–81.
110. Cantagrel V, Silhavy JL, Bielas SL, et al. Mutations in the cilia gene ARL13B lead to the classical form of Joubert syndrome. Am J Hum Genet 2008;83:170–9.
111. Gorden NT, Arts HH, Parisi MA, et al. *CCD2A* is mutated in Joubert syndrome and interacts with the ciliopathy-associated basal body protein CEP290. Am J Hum Genet 2008;83:559–71.
112. Del Cerro MP, Snider RS. The Purkinje cell cilium. Anat Rec 1969;165:127–30.
113. Del Cerro MP, Snider RS. Studies on the developing cerebellum. II. The ultra-structure of the external granular layer. J Comp Neurol 1972;144:131–64.
114. Young IS, McKeever PA, Squier MV, et al. Lethal olivopontocerebellar hypo-plasia with dysmorphic features in sibs. J Med Genet 1992;29:733–5.
115. Park S-H, Becker-Catania S, Gatti RA, et al. Congenital olivopontocerebellar atrophy: report of two siblings with paleo- and neocerebellar atrophy. Acta Neuropathol 1998;96:315–21.
116. Goutières F, Aicardi J, Farkas E. Anterior horn cell disease associated with pontocerebellar hypoplasia in infants. J Neurol Neurosurg Psychiatr 1977;40:370–8.
117. Weinberg AG, Kirkpatrick JB. Cerebellar hypoplasia in Werdnig-Hoffmann disease. Dev Med Child Neurol 1995;17:511–6.
118. Muntoni F, Goodwin F, Sewry C, et al. Clinical spectrum and diagnostic difficul-ties of infantile ponto-cerebellar hypoplasia type 1. Neuropediatrics 1999;30:243–8.
119. Peiffer J, Pfeiffer RA. Hypoplasia ponto-neocerebellaris. J Neurol 1977;215:241–51.
120. Barth PG, Vrensen GFJM, Uylings HBM, et al. Inherited syndrome of micro-cephaly, dyskinesia and pontocerebellar hypoplasia: a systemic atrophy with early onset. J Neurol Sci 1990;97:25–42.
121. Barth PG, Aronica E, de Vries L, et al. Pontocerebellar hypoplasia type 2: a neuropathological update. Acta Neuropathol (Berl) 2007;114:373–86.
122. Steinlin M, Klein A, Haas-Lude K, et al. Pontocerebellar hypoplasia type 2: vari-ability in clinical and imaging findings. Eur J Paediatr Neurol 2007;11:146–52.
123. Rajab A, Mochida GH, Hill A, et al. A novel form of pontocerebellar hypoplasia maps to chromosome 7q11-21. Neurology 60:1664–7.
124. Durmaz B, Wollnik B, Cogulu O, et al. Pontocerebellar hypoplasia type III (CLAM): extended phenotype and novel molecular findings. J Neurol, in press.
125. Patel MS, Becker JE, Toi A, et al. Severe, fetal-onset form of olivopontocerebellar hypoplasia in three sibs: PCH type 5? Am J Med Genet A 2006;140:594–603.
126. Hevner RF. Progress on pontocerebellar hypoplasia. Acta Neuropathol (Berl) 2007;114:401–2.
127. Leroy JG, Lyon G, Fallet C, et al. Congenital pontocerebellar atrophy and telen-cephalic defects in three siblings: a new subtype. Acta Neuropathol (Berl) 2007;114:387–99.
128. Jaeken J, Carchon H. What's new in congenital disorders of glycosylation? Eur J Paediatr Neurol 2000;4:163–7.
129. Stibler H, Jaeken J. Carbohydrate-deficient serum transferrin in a new systemic hereditary syndrome. Arch Dis Child 1990;65:107–11.
130. Stibler H, Westerberg B, Hanefeld F, et al. Carbohydrate-deficient glycoprotein (CDG) syndrome: a new variant, type III. Neuropediatrics 1993;24:51–2.
131. Jaeken J, Casaer P. Carbohydrate-deficient glycoconjugate (CDG) syndromes: a new chapter of neuropediatrics. Eur J Paediatr Neurol 1997;1:61–6.

132. Matthijs G, Schollen E, Pardon E, et al. Mutations in PMM2, a phosphomannomutase gene on chromosome 16p13, in carbohydrate-deficient glycoprotein type I syndrome (Jaeken syndrome). Nat Genet 1997;16:88–92.

133. Peters V, Penzien JM, Reiter G, et al. Congenital disorder of glycosylation IId – a new entity: clinical presentation with Dandy-Walker malformation nd myopathy. Neuropediatrics 2002;33:27–32.

134. de Koning TJ, de Vries LS, Groenendaal F, et al. Pontocerebellar hypoplasia associated with respiratory chain defects. Neuropediatrics 1999;30:93–5.

135. Voit T, Cohn RD, Sperner J, et al. Merosin-positive congenital muscular dystrophy with transient brain dysmyelination, pontocerebellar hypoplasia and mental retardation. Neuromuscul Disord 1999;9:95–101.

136. Clement E, Merculi E, Godfrey C, et al. Brain involvement in muscular dystrophies with defective dystroglycan glycosylation. Ann Neurol 2008;64:573–82.

# Cerebral Blood Flow and Metabolism in the Developing Fetus

Adré J. du Plessis, MBChB, MPH[a,b,*]

**KEYWORDS**

• Fetal brain • Fetal circulation • Brain development
• Fetal hypoxia • Fetal energy metabolism

Acute and long-term oxygen substrate deprivation is a major cause of disrupted fetal brain development and long-term neurologic morbidity. Before truly informed and meaningful brain-oriented fetal care can become a clinical reality, major advances will be required in the understanding of fetal brain hazards and the mechanisms by which normal brain development is derailed. Although a myriad of potential insults may disturb brain development, this article focuses primarily on those intrinsic systems that reduce the risk of fetal cerebral energy deprivation by maintaining a positive balance in cerebral oxygen–energy substrate demand and supply. Because of the inability of the human fetal brain to direct measurements of hemodynamics and metabolism, current understanding is based in large part on data from experimental animal models and from studies of the premature infant, or ex utero fetus. Although both models have provided important insights, neither is ideal, and the understanding of the primary and compensatory support systems for in vivo brain metabolism in the human fetus remains poor. This article reviews the current status of this understanding.

## ENERGY SUBSTRATE DEMANDS FOR NORMAL FETAL BRAIN DEVELOPMENT

The energy demands of the developing brain can be classified broadly as those required for its structural growth (accretion) and maintenance and those required for the functional activation of neuro-axonal and glial populations of the brain. These two sources of energy demand are of course wholly interdependent, and particularly

This work was supported by grants from the National Institute of Child Health and Human Development (R21HD056009), National Institute of Neurologic Disorders and Stroke (K24NS057568), the LifeBridge Fund, and the Trust Family Foundation.

[a] Harvard Medical School, Boston, MA, USA
[b] Department of Neurology, Fegan 11, Fetal-Neonatal Neurology Research Group, Children's Hospital Boston, 300 Longwood Avenue, Boston, MA 02115, USA
* Corresponding author. Department of Neurology, Fegan 11, Fetal-Neonatal Neurology Research Group, Children's Hospital Boston, Boston, MA.
*E-mail address:* duplessis@childrens.harvard.edu

during the later stages of development, the microstructural development of the imma-ture brain depends heavily on activation-related trophic stimulation.[1–3] Given the rapid increase in brain mass, which is caused by explosive development of synaptic, dendritic, and axonal elements in the cortical and subcortical gray matter, the cerebral oxygen substrate demands increase exponentially during the later stages of pregnancy.

### Structural Brain Development

Anatomic events in early brain development provide the structural substrate upon which later functionally driven changes in microstructural development are imposed. The critical events in brain development of the human fetus are reviewed in more detail in other articles in this issue; however, the broad stages of brain development may be summarized as follows. Primary neurulation leading to formation of the neural tube occurs before 4 weeks of gestation, and by 5 weeks, the neural tube has a well-defined rostral–caudal and dorsoventral organization. Development of the prosencephalon commences between 8 and 12 weeks of gestation, with neuronal proliferation and migration occurring between 8 and 20 weeks of gestation. These phases are followed by major events in cortical organization starting around 20 weeks of gestation and persisting well into postnatal development. Although myelination of the posterior fossa structures occurs during the fetal period, that of the supratentorial tissues occurs primarily after term gestational age.

Around the 11th week of gestation, formation begins of the transient subplate layer, which serves as a relay holding area for thalamocortical projections; this is the site of the first synapses, the activity of which is critical for developing cortical and thalamic projections.[4] Between 24 and 28 weeks of gestation, there is a period of major refine-ment of cortical connections with an explosive increase in cortical synapse formation and remodeling, and the development of functionally coordinated outputs from the cerebral cortex.[5–7] In fact, the developing cortex has about 40% more synapses than the mature brain, with the excess synapses being trimmed back by active remod-eling. These cortical activities coincide with a phase of major disassembly of subplate synapses and the energy-dependent programmed death of subplate neurons.

Between 28 weeks of gestation and term, these cortical events are largely respon-sible for an almost threefold increase in brain weight.[8] The features of this period of accelerated brain growth have been described by quantitative in vivo magnetic reso-nance imaging (MRI) studies in premature infants[9] and more recently in the fetus (see the article by Limperopoulos elsewhere in this issue). Such studies have shown that over the course of the third trimester, the cerebral cortex volume increases four-fold,[9,10] as does the volume of the cerebellar hemispheres.[10] This phase of rapid cortical development demands a major increase in energy supply, because cerebral microstructural development depends on functional activation of neuroaxonal units, which in turn depends upon repeated restoration of transmembrane ionic gradients by energy-dependent enzymes (such as Na-K/adenosine triphosphatase [ATPase]).

### Functional Brain Development

The functional development of the fetal brain can be viewed from both electrochemical and behavioral perspectives. The accelerated electrochemical maturation of the brain during the latter half of gestation is associated with an increasingly complex repertoire of fetal movement patterns and the emergence of behavioral states. The onset of spontaneous electrocortical activity in the developing human brain remains unclear. Scalp electroencephalography (EEG) recordings in premature infants, however, show bursts of activity alternating with periods of quiescence as early as 24 weeks of gestation.[11,12] These discontinuous patterns of electrocortical activity evolve with gestational age, becoming increasingly more continuous.[13,14] Although the energy requirements of these EEG patterns have not been defined clearly, the bursts of EEG activity have been associated with concurrent changes in cerebral oxygenation.[15] the apparent coupling between these EEG bursts and cerebral hemodynamics suggests that the bursts are energy-dependent. Of note, in the mature brain, electrocortical activity consumes about 60% of all cerebral oxygen delivered to maintain the neuronal ionic gradients required for synaptic and neural activation.

The functional activation of the fetal brain is a critical stimulus for the development of brain structure, especially during the third trimester. Cortical development depends on early neuronal activation patterns, because these guide critical processes of neuronal differentiation, neuronal migration, synaptogenesis, and formation of neuronal networks.[16] One proposed model for somatosensory cortex development is that spontaneous spinal and subcortical discharges elicit motor activity in the periphery, where sensory events associated with these movements then activate afferent signals back to the sensory cortex; in this manner, topographic representation of afferent input to the sensory cortex becomes established.[17] This paradigm is supported by data showing that spindle-burst EEG oscillations (delta brushes) are triggered by sensory feedback from movements in the periphery activated by subcortical discharges.[16–18] Another example of the complexity of these developmental electrobehavioral phenomena relates to fetal heart rate changes coupled to fetal movements. These heart rate accelerations initially were thought to reflect an increase in cardiac output in response to the energy demands of the motor activity. Both the frequency and amplitude of these heart rate changes, however, persist even in paralyzed fetal animals, suggesting that both the movements and heart rate changes are mediated by concurrent central efferent discharges.[19] Although much about these processes is not understood, it is likely that they are energy-dependent neural discharges that will be impaired by cerebral energy deprivation. Whether the time course and development of these EEG patterns in the preterm infant are similar to those in the gestational age-equivalent fetus remains unclear. The exciting novel techniques for assessing electrocortical development in the human fetus discussed by Lowery colleagues elsewhere in this issue may provide important insights into these complex developmental events.[20]

Characterization of the development of fetal movement patterns and behavioral states has been advanced by fetal ultrasound studies, particularly the advent of four-dimensional ultrasound and the more recent development of fetal MRI (see the article by Prayer and colleagues elsewhere in this issue). These techniques have shown the evolution of fetal behavior patterns, which include an increasingly complex array of spontaneous and reflex movements of varying speed and amplitude, and the development of fetal state changes.[21] Fetal movements start in the late first trimester and expand in repertoire and frequency throughout pregnancy. During the second and third trimesters, these movements become organized into increasingly complex and clearly distinct behavioral patterns. After midgestation, human fetal behaviors develop a periodic nature, in which movements alternate with periods of quiescence.[22,23] The initial simple movement patterns originate from spontaneous discharges in the spinal and brainstem circuitries; the subsequent emergence of complex and variable movements denotes modulation of these spinal–brainstem activities by descending input from higher brain centers. From around 28 weeks of gestation, the topographic organization of neural connections reaches a level that allows goal-directed behaviors to emerge.[24] Fetal sensorimotor reflex systems may be tested using vibroacoustic stimuli to elicit fetal startle responses.[25] Because such responses may originate at a brainstem–spinal level, however, a more reliable test for cerebral modulation of these behaviors is development of habituation to repeated stimuli.[26] From around 36 weeks of gestation, fetal behavioral states emerge, characterized by combinations of behavioral conditions that remain stable for periods of time.

## DEVELOPMENTAL CONSEQUENCES OF IMPAIRED CEREBRAL ENERGY SUPPLY IN THE FETUS

The precise metabolic needs of the developing brain, especially in early pregnancy, remain poorly understood. Oxygen substrate deprivation, however, has been implicated in various developmental lesions in the fetal brain. More detailed discussion of these issues appears elsewhere in this issue. It suffices to say that oxygen substrate deprivation may cause long-term effects through disturbances in fetal programming, selective cell-specific injury, disruption of programmed brain development, or frank encephaloclastic lesions, depending on the nature and timing of the insult. The specific effects on brain development triggered by these disturbances in oxygen substrate supply depend on several factors, including the nature of the insult and the specific developmental events at the time of the insult.

In addition to oxygen–energy substrate deprivation, specific nutritional deficiencies have been implicated in specific developmental anomalies of the nervous system. For example, dietary folate deficiency has been associated with early first trimester disruption of neural tube development.[27] During later first trimester prosencephalic development, maternal diabetes and disturbed fetal cholesterol metabolism have been associated with malformations in the holoprosencephaly spectrum.[28,29] Later in gestation, interruptions in oxygen–energy substrate supply have been implicated in neuronal migration defects, such as lissencephaly and the more localized schizencephaly lesion and postmigrational disturbances such as layered polymicrogyria.[30,31] Disturbances in brain growth have been described by quantitative MRI studies in premature infants with intrauterine growth restriction (IUGR).[32,33] Furthermore, IUGR has been associated with impaired neuropsychological outcome.[34–36] Delayed brain development with structural immaturity recently was described in populations at risk for cerebral oxygen–glucose deprivation, such as fetuses with certain congenital heart lesions (see the article by Limperopoulos, elsewhere in this issue).[37] The relationship between hypoxia and the developmental stage is also evident on a cellular level. For example, recent studies suggest that hypoxia has different effects on the oligodendrocyte lineage at different stages of development. Akundi and colleagues[38] have suggested that very early oligodendrocyte precursors exposed to hypoxia undergo accelerated maturation, while hypoxia later in oligodendrocyte development triggers either degeneration or maturational arrest.[39] These are some examples of the interaction between cerebral energy deprivation and adverse fetal brain development. It is likely that a far wider range of cellular and subcellular disturbances will be elucidated in the future with more advanced research techniques.

## SYSTEMS THAT SUPPORT OXYGEN SUBSTRATE SUPPLY TO THE DEVELOPING FETAL BRAIN

Normal fetal growth and development depend upon a supply system that keeps pace with the escalating oxygen substrate demands. From the perspective of brain development, such a supply system involves multiple complex arrangements along the path from the placental circulation (both maternal and fetal components) to the fetal systemic and cerebral circulations. Disturbances at any point along this path will jeopardize normal fetal brain development.

## Development of the Placental Circulation

The placenta plays a complex and active role in fetal development, as discussed elsewhere in this issue in the article by Redline. Disturbances in placental function may cause a spectrum of sequelae, from fetal demise to cerebral developmental disruption, to the adverse effects of fetal programming, a mechanism whereby an insult at a critical period of fetal development exerts remote effects in later years.[40] Placental function evolves in a developmentally programmed sequence of steps across gestation, allowing it to support the 40-fold increase in the fetal/placental weight ratio between 6 and 40 weeks of gestation.[40] Insults such as hypoxia during this process may disturb future placental function, including disturbances in nutrient transfer and transporter protein expression.[40–42]

The placenta is perfused by two circulations (ie, the maternal uteroplacental circulation and the fetal umbilicoplacental circulation). Although these two circulations share a close anatomic relationship, being separated by only a single tissue layer several cells thick, these two circulations are for the most part functionally distinct.[43] However, as the only sources of fetal oxygen substrate supply, alterations in either circulation may have important consequences for fetal growth and development. There is an exponential increase in placental perfusion during the second half of pregnancy, mediated by different mechanisms in the two circulations. Normally, the volume of uteroplacental blood flow far exceeds that required for fetal growth, creating a buffer zone or safety margin.[43] The uteroplacental blood flow increases by four- to fivefold without significant increases in arterial number. Instead, this uteroplacental blood flow occurs primarily because of vasodilation of uterine resistance vessels (spiral and more proximal arteries) during the later stages of pregnancy. Concurrently, there is an exponential volumetric increase in umbilicoplacental blood flow during the last trimester that primarily is caused by increased growth of the placental vascular bed and, to a lesser extent, vasodilation. Consequently, with advancing gestation, there is a progressive decrease in umbilicoplacental resistance as detected by Doppler ultrasound.[44,45]

Umbilical and placental vessels lack autonomic innervation, and regulation of placental perfusion depends upon local or circulating vasoactive substances.[46–50] There are important functional changes in the placental response to endogenous vasoactive agents, with certain notable differences in the reactivity of the two circulations. During normal pregnancies, women develop changes in reactivity of their systemic and placental circulations that favor enhanced placental perfusion. For example, there is a decreased response of the systemic vasculature overall to the vasoconstrictor angiotensin-II; however, this effect is most striking in the umbilicoplacental circulation,[51] creating a relative perfusion steal toward the placenta.[51] Of note, this response does not occur in women who develop pregnancy-associated hypertension,[52] in whom relative placental hypoperfusion may develop.[53] A similar attenuation in systemic vasoreactivity to the vasoconstrictor effects of the catecholamines develops in pregnant women. This attenuated vasoreactivity, however, is less prominent in the uteroplacental circulation compared with the systemic circulation; as a result, during periods of endogenous catecholamines, the uteroplacental circulation is not protected, and placental hypoperfusion may develop. The umbilicoplacental circulation differs from the uteroplacental circulation in that angiotensin-II is a potent vasoconstrictor,[54] while catecholamines at physiologic doses have minimal effect on umbilicoplacental blood flow. As a result, the increase in catecholamines during fetal hypoxemia causes significant vasoconstriction in the fetal peripheral circulation but not in the umbilicoplacental, myocardial, or cerebral circulations.

The placenta also plays a pivotal role in regulating the fetal endocrine and metabolic physiology. For example, glucocorticoids are important for the growth and development of fetal organ systems through several different pathways. Excess glucocorticoid exposure, however, may affect fetal development adversely, for example by decreasing the expression and function of glucose transporters.[55] The placenta regulates fetal glucocorticoid exposure by, for example, the placental enzyme 11β-hydroxysteroid dehydrogenase (11β-HSD), which converts active cortisol to inactive cortisone, protecting the fetus from excessive maternal cortisol production.[56] The levels of placental 11β-HSD production increase with fetal maturation,[57] but its expression and activity are decreased by hypoxia.[58]

### Development of the Fetal Systemic Circulation

Given the dependence of the fetus on the placenta rather than the lungs and Intestine for oxygen and nutrient supply, there are of necessity major differences between the fetal and postnatal circulatory systems. The fetus has two arterial circulations operating in parallel and connected by intra- and extracardiac shunts, whose patency is critical for normal fetal development. The primary communication between these arterial systems is at the aortic isthmus, which is the watershed between the circulation to the brain and upper body on one side, and between the subdiaphragmatic and placental tissues on the other side.[59] Two special features of the fetal systemic circulation are important for the normal development of the fetal brain. First, under normal conditions, there is preferential oxygen substrate delivery to the aorta and cerebral circulation. Second, the fetal central circulation is very flexible, with adaptive mechanisms capable of maintaining preferential oxygen substrate supply to the developing fetal brain during periods of fetal hypoxia. Specifically, this is achieved by changes in regional vascular resistance in the two circulations, which in conjunction with fetal shunts (discussed later in this article) provide preferential oxygen substrate supply to the developing brain by changes in both the volume and oxygen substrate composition of regional tissue.[60,61]

The highest fetal oxyhemoglobin saturations (85% to 90%) are in the umbilical vein as it enters the fetal abdomen. About half of this umbilical venous return enters the ductus venosus, bypassing the liver and thereby minimizing oxygen extraction. The oxygen substrate rich blood in the ductus venosus enters the inferior vena cava just proximal to the right atrium, from where it is diverted across the foramen ovale into the left heart and ascending aorta. In this manner, blood perfusing the coronary arteries and cerebral circulation has an oxyhemoglobin saturation significantly higher (65%) than that passing through the pulmonary artery (50% to 55%), ductus arteriosus, and into the descending aorta. These preferential streaming patterns have been demonstrated in the human fetus and in animals.[62] Under normal circumstances, the vascular resistance of the placental circulation is significantly lower than that of the pulmonary circulation, enabling the right ventricle to drive systemic perfusion through the ductus arteriosus.[63] In fact, the low placental vascular resistance allows half the combined ventricular output to pass into the umbilical circulation. When placental resistance increases in pathologic conditions, however, the upstream effects may increase the amount of deoxygenated blood from the vena cavae that is diverted across the foramen ovale and into the ascending aorta.

The fetal cardiovascular system differs in other important ways from that of the term newborn infant. The fetal myocardium generates lower active tension to myocardial stretch but has a higher resting tension, which limits diastolic performance.[64,65] Earlier studies suggested that the immature fetal myocardium was limited in its ability to increase stroke volume, leaving it dependent on increasing heart rate to increase cardiac output.[66] Subsequent studies showed that the fetal myocardium follows the basic Frank-Starling model, and that fetal cardiac output can increase by mechanisms other than heart rate.[63] Autonomic, and particularly sympathetic, innervation of the fetal heart is immature and incomplete. The expression of myocardial β-adrenergic receptors is initially low and increases with gestation, while α-adrenergic receptor expression is initially higher and decreases with maturation. Although myocardial norepinephrine stores are low in the fetus,[67] the immature myocardium has an increased sensitivity to circulating norepinephrine,[68] which is important during labor and the early newborn period, particularly in the stressed newborn, when circulating catecholamine levels increase.

### Development of the Fetal Brain Circulation

By the end of the first month of development, soon after closure of the neural tube, a primordial system of endothelium-lined vascular channels is present in the developing nervous system. By the end of the embryonic period, an extensive mesh of leptomeningeal arteries covers the cerebral hemispheres. Subsequent development of the brain vasculature is coupled tightly to the structural development of the brain. Arterial development of earlier developing structures proceeds more rapidly and is completed in the brainstem and cerebellum between 20 and 24 weeks of gestation, and in the basal ganglia and diencephalon by 24 to 28 weeks of gestation. The phase of accelerated third trimester cerebral hemispheric development is accompanied by rapid development of the hemispheric vasculature. Initially, a single vascular plexus covers the cerebral surface with extensive anastomoses between the major arteries of supply. From this surface network, superficial vessels begin to penetrate the brain parenchyma around 7 weeks of gestation, starting with large caliber basal penetrators that supply the basal ganglia and diencephalon and the germinal matrix in the subependymal periventricular zones. Thinner penetrating vessels descend from the cerebral surface; by 24 weeks of gestation, when the major phase of cerebral neuronal migration has been completed, these long penetrating vessels extend from the pial surface into the periventricular regions. The period between 24 and 28 weeks of gestation is one of particularly rapid cortical organization, axonal outgrowth, and synapse formation, and it is accompanied by rapid ingrowth of short penetrators between the earlier long penetrators.

Functional development of cerebral vasoreactivity follows a similar pattern. Specifically, the muscularis layer responsible for regulating cerebral vascular resistance initially is confined to the pial vessels and superficial penetrators, descending with maturation into the cerebral parenchyma.[69] Consequently, cerebral vasoregulation in the earlier fetal brain occurs largely in the superficial regions more remote from distal vascular beds than the precapillary arterioles of the mature brain. This fact may be of relevance to the vasoregulatory mechanisms that will be discussed.

### Cerebral Metabolism in the Immature Brain

Very little is known about the specific energy requirements of the immature brain in the human fetus, particularly during the first half of gestation. This lack of knowledge is largely because of the inaccessibility of the fetal brain to currently available measurement techniques. In fact, current understanding is based largely on data extrapolated from animal studies, and studies in the premature infant (ex utero fetus).[70–73] Besides postconceptional age equivalency, however, the major differences in internal and external environment of the fetus and premature newborn seriously limit the applicability of data from premature infants to the fetus.

For several reasons, anaerobic glycolysis has been considered an important energy source for fetal cerebral metabolism. First, the partial pressure of oxygen in the umbilical vein is significantly lower than in the normal postnatal circulation. Second, earlier studies had demonstrated an inefficient coupling between oxygen availability and energy production in the immature brain, limiting its capacity for mitochondrial oxidative phosphorylation and making it less efficient at energy synthesis.[74] Third, the immature fetal brain is uniquely capable of using alternative energy substrates such as lactate and ketones during periods of glucose limitation.[75] The ability of the immature brain to metabolize alternative substrates relates to the maturational arrangement of cerebral membrane proteins that mediate transport of organic substrates into the developing brain. Specifically, the two distinct types of transporter proteins, namely glucose transporters (GLUT)[76,77] and monocarboxylic acid transporters (MCT), have opposite trajectories of developmentally regulated expression. In early gestation, GLUT expression in the immature brain is low but increases with brain development.[78,79] Conversely, MCT expression, which facilitates transport of lactate and ketones into the immature brain, decreases with brain maturation.[79,80]

Although the immature brain is capable of using these alternative energy substrates, which in animal models may support up to 60% of cerebral energy demand,[81] the principal substrate supporting normal fetal cerebral metabolism throughout all phases of development is glucose, and most of it is consumed aerobically, with little or no production of lactic acid. At no point in development is anaerobic glycolysis solely capable of supporting the energy requirements of the developing brain. Fetal tissue oxygen delivery, on the other hand, depends only on the partial pressure of oxygen but also upon the circulating oxygen content and blood flow. When considered in these terms, there is little difference in oxygen delivery between the fetus and ex utero animal. Several facts support the notion that the umbilical venous oxygen supply is sufficient to support aerobic metabolism in fetal tissues. First, during fetal hypoxemia, the umbilical venous–arterial oxygen extraction fraction increases from around 40% up to 50% to 60%. Conversely, under normal baseline conditions, supplemental maternal oxygen with fetal hyperoxia does not increase fetal oxygen extraction. Finally, under normal circumstances, the umbilical venous–arterial lactic is not increased; in fact, umbilical venous lactate may be higher, suggesting fetal lactate uptake. The notion that oxygen delivery to the normal fetal brain is adequate to support cerebral energy metabolism is supported further by the fact that energy use is substantially lower in the immature animal brain.[82] For example, cerebral energy use in the newborn rat is 20 times lower than in the adult rat brain.[83] For these reasons, it has been argued that although immature animals are capable of using alternative energy sources, their ability to survive significantly longer periods of hypoxia than adult animals is largely because of their decreased cerebral energy requirements.[82] Although cerebral energy demand starts off low in early fetal life, it escalates rapidly during the third trimester to support the function of enzymes, such as Na/K-ATPase, which are critical for maintaining electrocortical activity and the propagation of action potentials. With these escalating cerebral energy demands, there is a concurrent increase in the number and functional capacity of cerebral mitochondria, with increasingly efficient energy production.[74]

Studies of cerebral metabolism in the immature human brain are confined to the ex utero premature infant. Positron emission tomography (PET) has been used to study in vivo oxygen and glucose metabolism in premature and term infants. Altman and colleagues[72] studied the cerebral metabolic rate of oxygen (CMRO2) in third trimester newborns ranging between 26 to 40 weeks of gestation. The CMRO2 was reduced in all infants, but particularly in the smallest, presumably reflecting the functional immaturity of the brain.[84] In the fetal brain, both oxygen and glucose metabolism are highest in the brainstem and deep gray matter and decrease in a rostral direction, being lowest in the subcortical and other white matter structures. In premature infants between 25 and 37 weeks of gestation, cerebral glucose metabolism as measured by PET was lower than in full-term infants.[70,71] As with oxygen metabolism, glucose metabolism was highest in the brainstem and cerebellar structures.

## COMPENSATORY SYSTEMS THAT PRESERVE OXYGEN SUBSTRATE AVAILABILITY IN THE FETAL BRAIN

Restriction in fetal oxygen substrate supply triggers several endogenous fetal compensatory responses at both systemic and cerebral levels, aimed at preserving a positive energy balance by decreasing energy demand and by increasing substrate supply.[85-89] The efficiency of these adaptive responses decreases as the insult dose (duration and severity) increases. In fetal sheep, these adaptive circulatory responses can be maintained for prolonged periods of moderate hypoxemia as long as metabolic acidosis does not develop.[90-93] In fact, in these animals, global and cerebral oxygen metabolism fails only when the circulating pH falls below 7.0.[91,93]

### Fetal Responses that Decrease Energy Utilization

Several physiologic responses triggered by hypoxemia aim to restrict fetal energy expenditure, both in the systemic and cerebral tissues.[94-98] For example, myocardial energy consumption is decreased by means of a neural reflex through which hypoxemia activates chemoreceptors, which in turn elicit a vagally mediated bradycardia[99-103] with an initial fall in blood pressure. This response is followed by a marked vasoconstriction in the peripheral circulation and an increase in blood pressure, a sympathetic response likely triggered in part by the hypoxemic stimulation of the chemoreceptors. With increased sustained hypoxemia, this bradycardia cannot be reversed by atropine, indicating that it no longer is mediated vagally but likely caused by hypoxic myocardial suppression.[103] At the level of the nervous system, the powering down of neuronal activity manifests as a decrease in fetal movements. This decrease in movement is accompanied by changes in the fetal EEG background to a high-voltage slow-wave pattern, which is less energy-demanding. In turn, it is likely that these EEG changes result from neuronal suppression. Adenosine is a breakdown product of adenosine triphosphate (ATP), which accumulates during failure of ATP resynthesis. Through actions at inhibitory presynaptic receptors and dilating vascular receptors, adenosine suppresses neuronal activation and increases perfusion.[89] These responses differ to some extent depending on the mechanism of fetal hypoxemia and level of fetal maturation. If hypoxemia develops very slowly, fetal behavior may not decrease until acidosis develops.[98] Severe cerebral hypoxia will limit cerebral oxygen metabolism directly during the terminal phases, leading to irreversible cellular injury.[104] When hypoxemia develops as a result of umbilical cord compression, the pattern of responses may be different. Specifically, umbilical arterial compression triggers an immediate increase in blood pressure with marked bradycardia, caused in this case by an early baroreceptor rather than chemoreceptor response.[102] In the preterm sheep fetus, hypoxemia fails to trigger bradycardia or an increase in blood pressure, possibly because of a lack of chemoreceptor responses at this gestational age.[105]

### Fetal Responses that Increase Cerebral Oxygen Substrate Supply

An initial response to decreasing fetal oxygen delivery is an increase in fetal oxygen extraction, a mechanism capable of sustaining fetal oxygen delivery until the umbilical venous oxygen content falls to around 50% of normal. During fetal hypoxemia, flow to all organs is maintained relatively constant until the arterial oxygen content falls to around 50% of normal; before the development of metabolic acidosis, there are no significant changes in either fetal cardiac output or in umbilicoplacental perfusion. At circulating oxygen levels below about 50% of normal, oxygen extraction may persist but is unable to compensate fully for the decrease in oxygen delivery, and tissue oxygen consumption begins to fall.[102] At this point, several compensatory changes in the fetal circulation are initiated to optimize oxygen substrate delivery to the fetal brain, heart, and adrenals. Hypoxemia results in an increased shunting of umbilical venous blood into the ductus venosus,[106–108] and from here through the foramen ovale into the left heart and up to the brain.[88] At the same time, there is a marked increase in sympathetic tone, mediated in part by the chemoreceptor pathways and an increase in circulating catecholamines, which results in peripheral vasoconstriction and an increase in blood pressure, but decreased perfusion of the kidneys, liver, intestine, and musculoskeletal system.[88,109] This response is known as circulatory centralization, or the brain-sparing effect.[110] This centralization response is mediated by neural (mainly adrenergic), circulating (catecholamines, serotonin, and angiotensin-II), and local mechanisms (eg, nitric oxide [NO], prostaglandins).

### Intrinsic Cerebral Compensatory Responses to Fetal Hypoxia

In addition to the previously mentioned compensatory responses in the systemic circulation, cerebral vasodilation in response to acute hypoxia has been described in fetal models less than 0.7 weeks of gestation.[111,112] Within the brain, hypoxemia triggers a redistribution of cerebral perfusion, such that blood is redistributed preferentially to the most actively developing brain regions at the particular gestational age. Most data for fetal cerebral responses to hypoxia are derived from animal fetal models, and to a lesser extent from the premature infant (or ex utero fetus). In considering these data, several important points are worth noting. First, because these responses aim to restore adequate oxygen substrate delivery, lower baseline demands as occur in the more immature brain will require less striking compensatory responses during cerebral hypoxia. There are important species differences in the level of brain maturation at different gestational ages, and the cerebral hypoxic responses must be considered in this context. In the fetal sheep, the most commonly used species in these studies, both cerebral blood flow and oxygen consumption are reduced significantly at 0.6 weeks of gestation, being only a third of that in the near-term fetus.[113,114] Using data from prematurely born infants is suboptimal, because there are significant differences between the fetal and postnatal circulation. Adaptive responses in development are rapid, and consequently within a very short time, the premature extrauterine circulation is no longer representative of the gestational age equivalent fetal circulation.

During fetal hypoxemia, there is not only a global increase in cerebral blood flow but also a redistribution of blood flow within the brain, such that brainstem perfusion exceeds cerebellar perfusion, which in turn exceeds blood flow to the cerebrum[88,115] in the fetal brainstem. This robust vasodilatory response in the fetal brainstem makes it significantly more resistant to hypoxic injury than other brain regions.[116] These intrinsic cerebrovascular responses are part of a complex autoregulatory system aimed at maintaining metabolism in the most actively developing and physiologically critical brain structures. Although most if not all intrinsic vasoregulatory (autoregulatory) systems present in the mature brain begin to develop during the fetal period, their efficiency is related to the maturational level of the fetus.[117] Furthermore, unlike the mature brain, in which the endothelium is a major source of vasoregulatory substances, the endothelium plays a lesser role in the cerebrovascular response to hypoxia in the fetus.[118,119] A review of the multiple different vasoregulatory mechanisms in the fetal brain is beyond the scope of this article; instead, the discussion will be confined to the intrinsic cerebrovascular responses to hypoxemia. Hypoxic vasodilation is mediated by an interplay between different endogenous substances, including NO, adenosine, endogenous opioids, and adrenomedullin. Hypoxia also may have direct vasodilating effects at the muscularis of the cerebral resistance vessels. Furthermore, the regional differences in cerebral perfusion during hypoxemia likely result from a complex interplay between regional vasodilator synthesis and the generation of regional vasoconstrictor substances.[120] In the fetus, the complex interplay between cerebral vasoactive substances during hypoxemia is characterized incompletely.[121]

NO is an important mediator of hypoxic vasodilation in the mature brain. The hemodynamic importance of NO in the developing fetal circulation, however, remains incompletely understood. In the fetus, it appears that NO plays a tonic vasodilator role during normoxia,[122] but its role in hypoxic vasodilation remains unclear[113] and appears to differ across species.[123,124] In the developing fetal cerebral cortex, there is a threefold increase in neuronal nitric oxide synthatase (NOS) activity during late gestation.[122] As discussed previously, the ATP breakdown product adenosine mediates cerebral hypoxic vasodilation through an action on vascular adenosine (A2) receptors.[125,126] It additionally inhibits cerebral metabolism during hypoxia by stimulating presynaptic (A1) receptors.[127] Adenosine-mediated vasodilation is developed fully by 0.6 weeks of gestation in most species[111] and is thought to mediate about half the hyperemia during acute hypoxia.[127] Although hypoxia also increases prostaglandin levels,[128] the role for prostanoid vasodilation during hypoxia in the immature brain appears to be modest at best.[129]

## SUMMARY

Normal development of the fetal brain is heavily dependent on an oxygen substrate supply capable of supporting the energy demands of the complex structural and functional maturational processes. Consequently, oxygen substrate deprivation is a major cause of injury to the developing brain, with a broad spectrum of sequelae involving not only encephaloclastic lesions but also derailment of critical programmed developmental events. Although there are ongoing obstacles to the understanding of cerebral blood flow and metabolism in the human fetus, a growing number of innovative neurodiagnostic techniques are emerging (and are discussed elsewhere in this issue) that are likely to advance understanding and lead to meaningful brain-oriented fetal care in the future.

## ACKNOWLEDGMENTS

The author wishes to thank Ms. Shaye Moore for assistance in preparing this manuscript.

## REFERENCES

1. Opitz T, De Lima AD, Voigt T. Spontaneous development of synchronous oscillatory activity during maturation of cortical networks in vitro. J Neurophysiol 2002; 88(5):2196–206.

2. Allene C, Cattani A, Ackman JB, et al. Sequential generation of two distinct synapse-driven network patterns in developing neocorteax. J Neurosci 2008; 28(48):12851–63.

3. Heck N, Kilb W, Reiprich P, et al. GABA-A receptors regulate neocortical neuronal migration in vitro and in vivo. Cereb Cortex 2007;17(1):138–48.

4. Kostovic I, Judas M. Transient patterns of cortical lamination during prenatal life: do they have implications for treatment? Neurosci Biobehav Rev 2007;31(8): 1157–68.

5. Kostovic I, Judas M, Rados M, et al. Laminar organization of the human fetal cerebrum revealed by histochemical markers and magnetic resonance imaging. Cereb Cortex 2002;12(5):536–44.

6. Kostovic I, Jovanov-Milosevic N. The development of cerebral connections during the first 20–45 weeks' gestation. Semin Fetal Neonatal Med 2006;11(6): 415–22.

7. Kostovic I. Structural and histochemical reorganization of the human prefrontal cortex during perinatal and postnatal life. Prog Brain Res 1990;85:223–39.

8. Hansen K, Sung CJ, Huang C, et al. Reference values for second trimester fetal and neonatal organ weights and measurements. Pediatr Dev Pathol 2003;6(2): 160–7.

9. Huppi PS, Warfield S, Kikinis R, et al. Quantitative magnetic resonance imaging of brain development in premature and mature newborns. Ann Neurol 1998;43: 224–35.

10. Limperopoulos C, Soul JS, Gauvreau K, et al. Late gestation cerebellar growth is rapid and impeded by premature birth. Pediatrics 2005;115(3):688–95.

11. Hellström-Westas L, Rosen I, Svenningsen NW. Cerebral function monitoring during the first week of life in extremely small low birthweight (ESLBW) infants. Neuropediatrics 1991;22(1):27–32.

12. Klebermass K, Kuhle S, Olischar M, et al. Intra- and extrauterine maturation of amplitude-integrated electroencephalographic activity in preterm infants younger than 30 weeks of gestation. Biol Neonate 2006;89(2):120–5.

13. Dreyfus-Brisac C. The electroencephalogram of the premature infant. World Neurol 1962;3:5–15.

14. Lombroso CT. Neonatal polygraphy in full-term and premature infants: a review of normal and abnormal findings. J Clin Neurophysiol 1985;2(2):105–55.

15. Roche-Labarbe N, Wallois F, Ponchel E, et al. Coupled oxygenation oscillation measured by NIRS and intermittent cerebral activation on EEG in premature infants. Neuroimage 2007;36(3):718–27.

16. Milh M, Kaminska A, Huon C, et al. Rapid cortical oscillations and early motor activity in premature human neonates. Cereb Cortex 2007;17(7):1582–94.

17. Khazipov R, Sirota A, Leinekugel X, et al. Early motor activity drives spindle bursts in the developing somatosensory cortex. Nature 2004;432(7018): 758–61.

18. Blumberg MS, Lucas DE. Dual mechanisms of twitching during sleep in neonatal rats. Behav Neurosci 1994;108(6):1196–202.

19. Bocking AD, Harding R, Wickham PJ. Relationship between accelerations and decelerations in heart rate and skeletal muscle activity in fetal sheep. J Dev Physiol 1985;7(1):47–54.

20. Lowery CL, Eswaran H, Murphy P, et al. Fetal magnetoencephalography. Semin Fetal Neonatal Med 2006;11(6):430–6.

21. de Vries JI, Fong BF. Normal fetal motility: an overview. Ultrasound Obstet Gynecol 2006;27(6):701–11.

22. de Vries JI, Visser GH, Prechtl HF. The emergence of fetal behaviour. II. Quantitative aspects. Early Hum Dev 1985;12(2):99–120.
23. Nijhuis JG, Prechtl HF, Martin CB Jr, et al. Are there behavioural states in the human fetus? Early Hum Dev 1982;6(2):177–95.
24. Kostovic I, Judas M, Petanjek Z, et al. Ontogenesis of goal-directed behavior: anatomo-functional considerations. Int J Psychophysiol 1995;19(2):85–102.
25. Divon MY, Platt LD, Cantrell CJ, et al. Evoked fetal startle response: a possible intrauterine neurological examination. Am J Obstet Gynecol 1985;153(4):454–6.
26. Leader LR. Studies in fetal behaviour. Br J Obstet Gynaecol 1995;102(8):595–7.
27. Wolff T, Witkop CT, Miller T, et al. Folic acid supplementation for the prevention of neural tube defects: an update of the evidence for the US Preventive Services Task Force. Ann Intern Med 2009;150(9):632–9.
28. Wolf G. The function of cholesterol in embryogenesis. J Nutr Biochem 1999; 10(4):188–92.
29. Hahn JS, Hahn SM, Kammann H, et al. Endocrine disorders associated with holoprosencephaly. J Pediatr Endocrinol Metab 2005;18(10):935–41.
30. Dobyns WB, Elias ER, Newlin AC, et al. Causal heterogeneity in isolated lissencephaly. Neurology 1992;42(7):1375–88.
31. Inder TE, Huppi PS, Zientara GP, et al. The postmigrational development of polymicrogyria documented by magnetic resonance imaging from 31 weeks' postconceptional age. Ann Neurol 1999;45(6):798–801.
32. Lodygensky GA, Seghier ML, Warfield SK, et al. Intrauterine growth restriction affects the preterm infant's hippocampus. Pediatr Res 2008;63(4):438–43.
33. Tolsa CB, Zimine S, Warfield SK, et al. Early alteration of structural and functional brain development in premature infants born with intrauterine growth restriction. Pediatr Res 2004;56(1):132–8.
34. Geva R, Eshel R, Leitner Y, et al. Neuropsychological outcome of children with intrauterine growth restriction: a 9-year prospective study. Pediatrics 2006; 118(1):91–100.
35. Fattal-Valevski A, Leitner Y, Kutai M, et al. Neurodevelopmental outcome in children with intrauterine growth retardation: a 3-year follow-up. J Child Neurol 1999; 14(11):724–7.
36. Low JA, Handley-Derry MH, Burke SO, et al. Association of intrauterine fetal growth retardation and learning deficits at age 9 to 11 years. Am J Obstet Gynecol 1992;167(6):1499–505.
37. Licht DJ, Shera DM, Clancy RR, et al. Brain maturation is delayed in infants with complex congenital heart defects. J Thorac Cardiovasc Surg 2009;137(3): 529–36.
38. Akundi RS, Rivkees SA. Hypoxia alters cell cycle regulatory protein expression and induces premature maturation of oligodendrocyte precursor cells. PLoS ONE 2009;4(3):e4739.
39. Segovia KN, McClure M, Moravec M, et al. Arrested oligodendrocyte lineage maturation in chronic perinatal white matter injury. Ann Neurol 2008;63(4): 520–30.
40. Myatt L. Placental adaptive responses and fetal programming. J Physiol 2006; 572:25–30.
41. Nelson DM, Smith SD, Furesz TC, et al. Hypoxia reduces expression and function of system A amino acid transporters in cultured term human trophoblasts. Am J Physiol Cell Physiol 2003;284(2):C310–5.
42. Murphy VE, Smith R, Giles WB, et al. Endocrine regulation of human fetal growth: the role of the mother, placenta, and fetus. Endocr Rev 2006;27(2):141–69.

43. Wilkening RB, Anderson S, Martensson L, et al. Placental transfer as a function of uterine blood flow. Am J Physiol 1982;242(3):H429–36.
44. Stuart B, Drumm J, FitzGerald DE, et al. Fetal blood velocity waveforms in normal pregnancy. Br J Obstet Gynaecol 1980;87(9):780–5.
45. Trudinger BJ, Giles WB, Cook CM. Flow velocity waveforms in the maternal uteroplacental and fetal umbilical placental circulations. Am J Obstet Gynecol 1985;152(2):155–63.
46. Hemsen A. Biochemical and functional characterization of endothelin peptides with special reference to vascular effects. Acta Physiol Scand Suppl 1991;602:1–61.
47. Hemsen A, Gillis C, Larsson O, et al. Characterization, localization, and actions of endothelins in umbilical vessels and placenta of man. Acta Physiol Scand 1991;143(4):395–404.
48. van Huisseling H, Muijsers GJ, de Haan J, et al. Fetal hypertension induced by norepinephrine infusion and umbilical artery flow velocity waveforms in fetal sheep. Am J Obstet Gynecol 1991;165(2):450–5.
49. Paulick RP, Meyers RL, Rudolph AM. Vascular responses of umbilical–placental circulation to vasodilators in fetal lambs. Am J Physiol 1991;261:H9–14.
50. Paulick RP, Meyers RL, Rudolph CD, et al. Hemodynamic responses to alpha-adrenergic blockade during hypoxemia in the fetal lamb. J Dev Physiol 1991; 16(2):63–9.
51. Rosenfeld CR. Mechanisms regulating angiotensin II responsiveness by the uteroplacental circulation. Am J Physiol Regul Integr Comp Physiol 2001;281(4): R1025–40.
52. Gant NF, Daley GL, Chand S, et al. A study of angiotensin II pressor response throughout primigravid pregnancy. J Clin Invest 1973;52(11):2682–9.
53. Erkkola RU, Pirhonen JP. Uterine and umbilical flow velocity waveforms in normotensive and hypertensive subjects during the angiotensin II sensitivity test. Am J Obstet Gynecol 1992;166(3):910–6.
54. Iwamoto HS, Rudolph AM. Effects of angiotensin II on the blood flow and its distribution in fetal lambs. Circ Res 1981;48(2):183–9.
55. Hahn T, Barth S, Graf R, et al. Placental glucose transporter expression is regulated by glucocorticoids. J Clin Endocrinol Metab 1999;84(4):1445–52.
56. Krozowski Z, MaGuire JA, Stein-Oakley AN, et al. Immunohistochemical localization of the 11 beta-hydroxysteroid dehydrogenase type II enzyme in human kidney and placenta. J Clin Endocrinol Metab 1995;80(7):2203–9.
57. Murphy VE, Clifton VL. Alterations in human placental 11beta-hydroxysteroid dehydrogenase type 1 and 2 with gestational age and labour. Placenta 2003; 24(7):739–44.
58. Alfaidy N, Gupta S, DeMarco C, et al. Oxygen regulation of placental 11 beta-hydroxysteroid dehydrogenase 2: physiological and pathological implications. J Clin Endocrinol Metab 2002;87(10):4797–805.
59. Bonnin P, Fouron JC, Teyssier G, et al. Quantitative assessment of circulatory changes in the fetal aortic isthmus during progressive increase of resistance to umbilical blood flow. Circulation 1993;88(1):216–22.
60. Tchirikov M, Schroder HJ, Hecher K. Ductus venosus shunting in the fetal venous circulation: regulatory mechanisms, diagnostic methods, and medical importance. Ultrasound Obstet Gynecol 2006;27(4):452–61.
61. Kiserud T, Acharya G. The fetal circulation. Prenat Diagn 2004;24(13):1049–59.
62. Rosenberg AA, Koehler RC, Jones MD Jr. Distribution of cardiac output in fetal and neonatal lambs with acute respiratory acidosis. Pediatr Res 1984;18(8): 731–5.

63. Kenny JF, Plappert T, Doubilet P, et al. Changes in intracardiac blood flow veloc-ities and right and left ventricular stroke volumes with gestational age in the normal human fetus: a prospective Doppler echocardiographic study. Circula-tion 1986;74(6):1208–16.
64. Mahony L. Calcium homeostasis and control of contractility in the developing heart. Semin Perinatol 1996;20(6):510–9.
65. Mahony L. Calcium homeostasis and control of contractility in the developing heart. Semin Perinatol 1996;20(6):510–9.
66. Rudolph AM, Heymann MA. Cardiac output in the fetal lamb: the effects of spon-taneous and induced changes of heart rate on right and left ventricular output. Am J Obstet Gynecol 1976;124(2):183–92.
67. Saarikoski S. Functional development of adrenergic uptake mechanisms in the human fetal heart. Biol Neonate 1983;43:158–63.
68. Friedman WF. Neuropharmacologic studies of perinatal myocardium. Cardio-vasc Clin 1972;4(3):43–57.
69. Kuban KC, Gilles FH. Human telencephalic angiogenesis. Ann Neurol 1985; 17(6):539–48.
70. Kinnala A, Suhonen-Polvi H, Aarimaa T, et al. Cerebral metabolic rate for glucose during the first six months of life: an FDG positron emission tomography study. Arch Dis Child Fetal Neonatal Ed 1996;74(3):F153–7.
71. Powers WJ, Rosenbaum JL, Dence CS, et al. Cerebral glucose transport and metabolism in preterm human infants. J Cereb Blood Flow Metab 1998;18(6): 632–8.
72. Altman DI, Perlman JM, Volpe JJ, et al. Cerebral oxygen metabolism in newborns. Pediatrics 1993;92(1):99–104.
73. Altman DI, Powers WJ, Perlman JM, et al. Cerebral blood flow requirement for brain viability in newborn infants is lower than in adults. Ann Neurol 1988;24: 218–26.
74. Murthy MR, Rappoport DA. Biochemistry of the developing rat brain. II. Neonatal mitochondrial oxidations. Biochim Biophys Acta 1963;74:51–9.
75. Stanley CA, Anday EK, Baker L, et al. Metabolic fuel and hormone responses to fasting in newborn infants. Pediatrics 1979;64(5):613–9.
76. Vannucci SJ, Maher F, Simpson IA. Glucose transporter proteins in brain: delivery of glucose to neurons and glia. Glia 1997;21(1):2–21.
77. Maher F, Vannucci SJ, Simpson IA. Glucose transporter proteins in brain. FASEB J 1994;8(13):1003–11.
78. Vannucci SJ. Developmental expression of GLUT1 and GLUT3 glucose trans-porters in rat brain. J Neurochem 1994;62(1):240–6.
79. Cremer J, Cunningham V, Partridge W, et al. Kinetics of blood–brain barrier transport of pyruvate, lactate, and glucose in suckling, weanling, and adult rats. J Neurochem 1979;33:439–45.
80. Cremer JE. Substrate utilization and brain development. J Cereb Blood Flow Metab 1982;2(4):394–407.
81. Hellman J, Vannucci R, Nardis E. Blood–brain barrier permeability to lactic acid in the newborn dog: lactate as a cerebral metabolic fuel. Pediatr Res 1982;16: 40–4.
82. Duffy TE, Kohle SJ, Vannucci RC. Carbohydrate and energy metabolism in peri-natal rat brain: relation to survival in anoxia. J Neurochem 1975;24(2):271–6.
83. Swaab DF, Boer K. The presence of biologically labile compounds during ischemia and their relationship to the EEG in rat cerebral cortex and hypothal-amus. J Neurochem 1972;19(12):2843–53.

84. Yoxall CW, Weindling AM. Measurement of cerebral oxygen consumption in the human neonate using near infrared spectroscopy: cerebral oxygen consumption increases with advancing gestational age. Pediatr Res 1998;44(3):283–90.

85. Edelstone DI. Fetal compensatory responses to reduced oxygen delivery. Semin Perinatol 1984;8(3):184–91.

86. Carter AM. Factors affecting gas transfer across the placenta and the oxygen supply to the fetus. J Dev Physiol 1989;12(6):305–22.

87. Towell ME, Figueroa J, Markowitz S, et al. The effect of mild hypoxemia maintained for twenty-four hours on maternal and fetal glucose, lactate, cortisol, and arginine vasopressin in pregnant sheep at 122 to 139 days' gestation. Am J Obstet Gynecol 1987;157(6):1550–7.

88. Peeters LL, Sheldon RE, Jones MD Jr, et al. Blood flow to fetal organs as a function of arterial oxygen content. Am J Obstet Gynecol 1979;135(5):637–46.

89. Lutz PL. Mechanisms for anoxic survival in the vertebrate brain. Annu Rev Physiol 1992;54:601–18.

90. Bocking AD, White SE, Homan J, et al. Oxygen consumption is maintained in fetal sheep during prolonged hypoxaemia. J Dev Physiol 1992;17(4):169–74.

91. Richardson BS, Rurak D, Patrick JE, et al. Cerebral oxidative metabolism during sustained hypoxaemia in fetal sheep. J Dev Physiol 1989;11(1):37–43.

92. Rurak DW, Richardson BS, Patrick JE, et al. Blood flow and oxygen delivery to fetal organs and tissues during sustained hypoxemia. Am J Physiol 1990;258:R1116–22.

93. Rurak DW, Richardson BS, Patrick JE, et al. Oxygen consumption in the fetal lamb during sustained hypoxemia with progressive acidemia. Am J Physiol 1990;258:R1108–15.

94. Boddy K, Dawes GS, Fisher R, et al. Foetal respiratory movements, electrocortical and cardiovascular responses to hypoxaemia and hypercapnia in sheep. J Physiol 1974;243(3):599–618.

95. Natale R, Clewlow F, Dawes GS. Measurement of fetal forelimb movements in the lamb in utero. Am J Obstet Gynecol 1981;140(5):545–51.

96. Bocking AD, Harding R. Effects of reduced uterine blood flow on electrocortical activity, breathing, and skeletal muscle activity in fetal sheep. Am J Obstet Gynecol 1986;154(3):655–62.

97. Richardson BS. The effect of behavioral state on fetal metabolism and blood flow circulation. Semin Perinatol 1992;16(4):227–33.

98. Richardson BS, Carmichael L, Homan J, et al. Electrocortical activity, electroocular activity, and breathing movements in fetal sheep with prolonged and graded hypoxemia. Am J Obstet Gynecol 1992;167(2):553–8.

99. Blanco CE, Dawes GS, Hanson MA, et al. The response to hypoxia of arterial chemoreceptors in fetal sheep and newborn lambs. J Physiol 1984;351:25–37.

100. Bartelds B, van Bel F, Teitel DF, et al. Carotid, not aortic, chemoreceptors mediate the fetal cardiovascular response to acute hypoxemia in lambs. Pediatr Res 1993;34(1):51–5.

101. Boekkooi PF, Baan J Jr, Teitel D, et al. Chemoreceptor responsiveness in fetal sheep. Am J Physiol 1992;263:H162–7.

102. Itskovitz J, LaGamma EF, Rudolph AM. The effect of reducing umbilical blood flow on fetal oxygenation. Am J Obstet Gynecol 1983;145(7):813–8.

103. Itskovitz J, Goetzman BW, Rudolph AM. The mechanism of late deceleration of the heart rate and its relationship to oxygenation in normoxemic and chronically hypoxemic fetal lambs. Am J Obstet Gynecol 1982;142(1):66–73.

104. Gavilanes AW, Vles JS, von Siebenthal K, et al. Neonatal electrocortical brain activity and cerebral tissue oxygenation during nonacidotic, normocarbic, and normotensive graded hypoxemia. Clin Neurophysiol 2004;115(2):282–8.
105. Iwamoto HS, Kaufman T, Keil LC, et al. Responses to acute hypoxemia in fetal sheep at 0.6–0.7 gestation. Am J Physiol 1989;256:H613–20.
106. Jensen A, Roman C, Rudolph AM. Effects of reducing uterine blood flow on fetal blood flow distribution and oxygen delivery. J Dev Physiol 1991;15(6): 309–23.
107. Bristow J, Rudolph AM, Itskovitz J, et al. Hepatic oxygen and glucose metabolism in the fetal lamb. Response to hypoxia. J Clin Invest 1983;71(5):1047–61.
108. Itskovitz J, LaGamma EF, Rudolph AM. Effects of cord compression on fetal blood flow distribution and $O_2$ delivery. Am J Physiol 1987;252:H100–9.
109. Richardson B, Korkola S, Asano H, et al. Regional blood flow and the endocrine response to sustained hypoxemia in the preterm ovine fetus. Pediatr Res 1996; 40(2):337–43.
110. Wladimiroff JW, Tonge HM, Stewart PA. Doppler ultrasound assessment of cerebral blood flow in the human fetus. Br J Obstet Gynaecol 1986;93(5):471–5.
111. Kurth CD, Wagerle LC. Cerebrovascular reactivity to adenosine analogues in 0.6–0.7 gestation and near-term fetal sheep. Am J Physiol 1992;262:H1338–42.
112. Gleason CA, Hamm C, Jones MD Jr. Effect of acute hypoxia on brain blood flow and oxygen metabolism in immature fetal sheep. Am J Physiol 1990;258: H1064–9.
113. Harris AP, Helou S, Gleason CA, et al. Fetal cerebral and peripheral circulatory responses to hypoxia after nitric oxide synthase inhibition. Am J Physiol Regul Integr Comp Physiol 2001;281(2):R381–90.
114. Gleason CA, Hamm C, Jones MD Jr. Cerebral blood flow, oxygenation, and carbohydrate metabolism in immature fetal sheep in utero. Am J Physiol 1989; 256:R1264–8.
115. Cavazzuti M, Duffy T. Regulation of local cerebral blood flow in normal and hypoxic newborn dogs. Ann Neurol 1982;11:247–57.
116. Tolcos M, Harding R, Loeliger M, et al. The fetal brainstem is relatively spared from injury following intrauterine hypoxemia. Brain Res Dev Brain Res 2003; 143(1):73–81.
117. Bilger A, Nehlig A. Regional cerebral blood flow response to acute hypoxia changes with postnatal age in the rat. Brain Res Dev Brain Res 1993;76(2): 197–205.
118. Zurcher SD, Ong-Veloso GL, Akopov SE, et al. Maturational modification of hypoxic relaxation in ovine carotid and cerebral arteries: role of endothelium. Biol Neonate 1998;74(3):222–32.
119. Pearce WJ, Longo LD. Developmental aspects of endothelial function. Semin Perinatol 1991;15(1):40–8.
120. Bari F, Errico RA, Louis TM, et al. Differential effects of short-term hypoxia and hypercapnia on N-methyl-D-aspartate-induced cerebral vasodilatation in piglets. Stroke 1996;27(9):1634–9.
121. Pearce W. Hypoxic regulation of the fetal cerebral circulation. J Appl Physiol 2006;100(2):731–8.
122. Northington FJ, Tobin JR, Harris AP, et al. Developmental and regional differences in nitric oxide synthase activity and blood flow in the sheep brain. J Cereb Blood Flow Metab 1997;17(1):109–15.
123. Armstead WM. Opioids and nitric oxide contribute to hypoxia-induced pial arterial vasodialation in newborn pigs. Am J Physiol 1995;268:H226–32.

124. Wilderman MJ, Armstead WM. Role of neuronal NO synthase in relationship between NO and opioids in hypoxia-induced pial artery dilation. Am J Physiol 1997;273:H1807–15.

125. Blood AB, Hunter CJ, Power GG. The role of adenosine in regulation of cerebral blood flow during hypoxia in the near-term fetal sheep. J Physiol 2002;543: 1015–23.

126. Park TS, Van Wylen DG, Rubio R, et al. Increased brain interstitial fluid adenosine concentration during hypoxia in newborn piglet. J Cereb Blood Flow Metab 1987;7(2):178–83.

127. Blood AB, Hunter CJ, Power GG. Adenosine mediates decreased cerebral metabolic rate and increased cerebral blood flow during acute moderate hypoxia in the near-term fetal sheep. J Physiol 2003;553(3):935–45.

128. Ment LR, Stewart WB, Duncan CC, et al. Beagle puppy model of perinatal cerebral infarction. Regional cerebral prostaglandin changes during acute hypoxemia. J Neurosurg 1986;65(6):851–5.

129. Leffler CW, Parfenova H. Cerebral arteriolar dilation to hypoxia: role of prostanoids. Am J Physiol 1997;272:H418–24.

# Disorders of Placental Circulation and the Fetal Brain

Raymond W. Redline, MD[a,b,c,*]

**KEYWORDS**

- Cerebral palsy • Fetal vascular • Maternal vascular
- Placenta • Thromboinflammatory

Perinatally acquired neurologic abnormalities not related to congenital malformations or genetic syndromes primarily affect two groups: very low birth weight (<1.5 kg) and extremely low birth weight infants (<1 kg) who deliver prematurely because of a hostile intrauterine environment and are at risk for further injury because of immaturity of the central nervous system (CNS); and (2) term infants born with significant neurologic findings that persist into later life as cerebral palsy (CP) and other developmental disabilities. Both situations are characterized by poorly understood underlying genetic susceptibility factors and only slightly better understood acute stresses occurring at the time of parturition or in the early neonatal period.

The placenta is the sole provider of nutrients and oxygen to the developing fetus and also serves a significant protective function, buffering the effects of teratogenic exposures, such as infection, trauma, and various toxins during pregnancy. Like other organs, the placenta shows significant histopathologic changes when physiologic derangements lead to impaired function. The nature of these changes provides useful insight into the intermediary processes that act between underlying susceptibility and adverse exposures in the perinatal period, and in some cases placental abnormalities by themselves may explain adverse outcomes.

The placenta is essentially a vascular organ in which maternal blood from the uterine arteries is brought into contact with placental villi in the intervillous space.[1] Trophoblastic epithelium surrounding the villi mediates the transfer of oxygen and essential nutrients across a diffusion barrier that is normally quite thin, consisting only of the basement membranes of the trophoblast and the fetal villous capillary endothelium and the endothelial cells themselves (vasculosyncytial membrane). These fetal

a Department of Pathology, Case Western Reserve University School of Medicine, OH 44106, USA
b Department of Reproductive Biology, Case Western Reserve University School of Medicine, OH 44106, USA
c Pediatric and Perinatal Pathology, University Hospitals Case Medical Center, Cleveland, OH 44106, USA
* Corresponding author. Pathology, University Hospitals Case Medical Center, Cleveland, OH 44106, USA
E-mail address: raymondw.redline@UHhospitals.org

Clin Perinatol 36 (2009) 549–559
doi:10.1016/j.clp.2009.06.003
0095-5108/09/$ – see front matter

capillaries receive deoxygenated blood from the fetus by a branching system of arteries and arterioles originating from the paired umbilical arteries of the umbilical cord. Newly oxygenated fetal blood is then delivered to a network of gradually enlarging veins that drain into a single umbilical vein that runs through the umbilical cord. Proper functioning of the placenta depends on the patency and integrity of the maternal arteries, proper conductance of maternal blood through the intervillous space, exposure of maternal blood to the villous trophoblastic epithelium, maintenance of a normal diffusion distance between maternal and fetal blood at the interhemal membrane, patency and integrity of larger vessels in the villous tree, and unobstructed flow in the umbilical cord. An additional complicating factor is the potential for harmful blood-born mediators generated within abnormal placentas to be transmitted to the fetus by the umbilical vein. **Table 1** and **Fig. 1** summarize the types of placental lesions that have been associated with CNS damage, their time of onset relative to delivery, and their anatomic localization within the placenta. Details are discussed next.

## MATERNAL CIRCULATORY LESIONS
### Reduced Flow, Large Vessels

The arteries of the nongravid uterus are insufficient to supply the nutritional needs of the second- and third-trimester human fetus. In normal pregnancies, they are invaded and remodeled by extravillous trophoblast, leading to increased caliber, decreased contractility, and greatly increased flow volume. Failure of this process secondary to oxidative stress in early pregnancy underlies the clinical disorder preeclampsia and most cases of intrauterine growth restriction.[2] Generalized hypoperfusion or repeated episodes of ischemia and reperfusion can lead to decreased placental growth and a stereotypical set of placental histopathologic characteristics that include increased syncytial knots and intervillous fibrin, villous agglutination, and laminar necrosis of the placental membrane (findings consistent with maternal underperfusion).[3,4] Placentas with these findings have a decreased functional reserve to withstand periods of acute hypoxia which can cause fetal metabolic abnormalities affecting short- and long-term responses to stress. These placental findings have been directly associated with CP in extremely low birth weight infants.[5] Complete thrombotic occlusion of uterine arteries results in villous infarcts. Large villous infarcts have been associated with ischemic CNS lesions in stillborns.[6,7] Finally, episodes of acute maternal hypotension related to cardiac arrest, amniotic fluid embolus, or septic shock are among the so-called "sentinel events" that can directly cause fetal brain injury.

### Decreased Conductance, Intervillous Space

Transport of oxygen and nutrients by villous trophoblast depends on adequate conductance in the intervillous space. Excessive fibrin or fibrinoid deposition on the trophoblast surface and surrounding intervillous space interferes with conductance and can have profound effects on fetal growth and circulatory physiology. The most severe example of this process is known as "massive perivillous fibrinoid deposition" (maternal floor infarction). This idiopathic lesion has been associated with numerous adverse perinatal outcomes including miscarriage, stillbirth, intrauterine growth restriction, indicated preterm delivery, and long-term neurodisability.[8,9] Mothers with affected placentas have a very high recurrence rate approaching 60%. Autoimmunity and thrombophilic disorders have been implicated in some cases.[10] The underlying pathophysiology is unknown, but may involve an aberrant response to injury resulting in metaplasia of the villous trophoblast to a matrix-secreting

| Table 1 | |
| --- | --- |
| **Categorization of placental circulatory abnormalities related to brain injury** | |
| **Placental Lesions** | **Timing** |
| *Maternal circulation* | |
| Reduced flow, large vessels | |
|   Maternal hypotension | Acute |
|   Findings consistent with underperfusion | Chronic |
|   Villous infarcts | Chronic |
| Decreased conductance, intervillous space | |
|   Massive perivillous fibrinoid deposition | Chronic |
|   Villitis of unknown etiology with extensive perivillous fibrin | Chronic |
|   Placental malaria | Chronic |
|   Chronic histiocytic intervillositis | Chronic |
| Hemorrhages, retroplacental | |
|   Abruptio placenta | Acute |
|   Chronic abruption | Chronic |
| *Fetal circulation* | |
| Obstruction, umbilical cord | |
|   Complete total | Acute |
|   Partial/intermittent | |
|     Cord entanglements | Subacute |
|     Pathologic umbilical cord lesions | Subacute |
| Thromboinflammatory lesions, large vessels | |
|   Fetal thrombotic vasculopathy | Chronic |
|   Villitis of unknown etiology with obliterative fetal vasculopathy | Chronic |
|   Meconium-associated vascular necrosis | Subacute |
|   Chorioamnionitis with intense chorionic vasculitis | Subacute |
| Microcirculatory abnormalities | |
|   Diffuse villous edema | Subacute |
|   Diffuse villitis of unknown etiology | Chronic |
|   Distal villous immaturity | Chronic |
| Hemorrhages, fetal | |
|   Massive fetomaternal hemorrhage (capillary) | Subacute |
|   Fetal vessel rupture (large vessel) | Acute |

Estimated onset of lesion in most cases: acute, 0–6 h; subacute, 6 h–7 d; chronic, greater than 1 week.

extravillous trophoblast phenotype, which subsequently spreads to contiguous regions of the placenta. Other conditions associated with extensive perivillous fibrin include diffuse villitis of unknown etiology (VUE) (discussed later); maternal malarial infection; and a rare recurrent lesion known as "chronic histiocytic intervillositis."[11–13]

### Retroplacental Hemorrhage

The placenta is anchored to the maternal uterus by extracellular matrix secreted by extravillous trophoblast, which invade to the level of the superficial myometrium. Disruption of maternal arteries or veins can lead to a loss of uteroplacental integrity and the

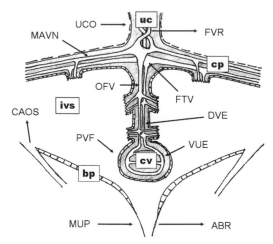

**Fig. 1.** Schematic view of the placenta with the anatomic site of injury for major placental circulatory lesions associated with CNS injury. Anatomic sites: bp, basal plate (maternal surface); cp, chorionic plate (fetal surface); cv, chorionic villi; ivs, intervillous space; uc, umbilical cord. Placental lesions: ABR, abruptio placenta; CAOS, chronic abruption oligohydramnios sequence; DVE, diffuse villous edema; FTV, fetal thrombotic vasculopathy; FVR, fetal vessel rupture; MAVN, meconium-associated vascular necrosis; MUP, maternal underperfusion; OFV, obliterative fetal vasculopathy associated with VUE; PVF, perivillous fibrin/fibrinoid deposition; UCO, umbilical cord obstruction; VUE, villitis of unknown etiology.

formation of retroplacental hematomas that separate the placenta from its maternal blood supply. Risk factors for arterial disruption include uterine rupture; trauma; preeclamptic arteriopathy; and vasospasm related to vasoactive drugs, such as cocaine or nicotine.[14,15] The clinical correlate of arterial disruption is abruptio placenta, which is another of the sentinel lesions that by themselves are sufficient to result in acute brain injury. Most of the venous drainage of the placenta is at the margin. Marginal retroplacental hemorrhages (marginal abruptions) are associated with sudden changes in amniotic fluid volume, low implantation, and acute chorioamnionitis.[16] Marginal abruption is an important cause of premature delivery, but has not been associated with adverse neurologic outcome. Marginal retroplacental hemorrhages that do not culminate in delivery can evolve into chronic peripheral separation with membrane hemosiderin deposition, a condition known clinically as the "chronic abruption-oligohydramnios sequence."[17–19] This syndrome, which is associated with chronic intermittent vaginal bleeding, has been associated with CP in term infants.[20,21]

## FETAL CIRCULATORY LESIONS
### Umbilical Cord Obstruction

The umbilical cord is the lifeline connecting placenta to fetus. Significant deformational forces including extrinsic compression, hypercoiling, or torsion of unprotected vessels at the insertion site may retard or prevent flow, particularly in the less well protected umbilical vein.[22–24] Decreased Wharton's jelly, seen with maternal underperfusion or other causes of fetal extracellular volume depletion, may also increase the risk of compression. Excessive cord length can lead to decreased flow by virtue of path length alone.[25,26] Prolonged partial or intermittent cord obstruction can occur secondary to either pathologic umbilical cord abnormalities or clinical cord entanglements, such as nuchal coils. The latter are quite common, being observed in approximately 30% of all term deliveries. Limited clinical evidence concentrating on sonographically confirmed persisting clinical cord entanglements has documented significant antenatal abnormalities in middle cerebral arterial flow by pulsed flow Doppler studies and postnatal neurodevelopmental problems in the infants when tested at 1 year of age.[27,28] Prolonged partial or intermittent cord obstruction may lead in some cases to the well-recognized neuropathologic pattern known as "partial prolonged asphyxia."[29] Pathologic findings suggestive of prolonged partial or intermittent cord obstruction in the context of a clinical or pathologic "cord at risk" include dilation of umbilical veins relative to arteries; fibrin deposition in the wall of large vessels (intimal fibrin cushions); and scattered small foci of terminal villi either lacking or having damaged capillaries.[30] Sustained complete total cord occlusion in liveborn infants is rare and seen primarily with cord prolapse or umbilical cord knots that tighten during fetal descent in the birth canal. Cord occlusion is another example of a sentinel event.

## Thromboinflammatory Lesions, Large Vessels

Large fetal vessels in the chorionic plate or stem villi are the site of injury for four distinct thromboinflammatory processes that are observed in 34% to 51% of all term infants with CP and related disorders compared with 5% to 10% of term infants whose placentas are submitted to pathology for other pregnancy complications.[21,30] These lesions are associated with neurologic impairment in infants with both normal and abnormal umbilical cord pH and 5-minute Apgar scores, suggesting that they may affect the CNS independently of acute hypoxia at the time of delivery. The most frequent of these lesions is fetal thrombotic vasculopathy, which is defined by the finding of extensive avascular villi secondary to upstream vascular occlusion.[31] The threshold for diagnosis is an average of greater than 15 villi per slide, and thrombi are observed in upstream vessels in one third or more of cases. Fetal thrombotic vasculopathy has also been associated with neonatal thrombocytopenia and thromboembolic disease.[32,33] Although fetal thrombophilic mutations and diabetes have been suggested as risk factors, only clinical or pathologic abnormalities of the umbilical cord have been specifically associated with this diagnosis.[32] Second most common of the large vessel thromboembolic lesions is VUE with obliterative fetal vasculopathy.[34] This lesion is characterized by chronic inflammation of distal villi that spreads to chorionic plate or stem villous vessels, leading to vasoocclusion, downstream avascular villi, and significant elevations in circulating neonatal chemokines.[35] VUE is caused by maternal lymphocytic infiltration of chorionic villi leading to manifestations of allograft rejection and graft-versus-host disease that may include maternal chimerism in fetal tissues.[36] The next most common lesion is meconium-associated vascular necrosis, characterized by apoptosis of vascular smooth muscle cells on the amnionic aspect of umbilical or chorionic plate vessels.[37,38] This lesion is associated with prolonged exposure to meconium, particularly in the context of oligohydramnios and intact membranes. Prolonged meconium exposure may also cause significant vasospasm of large fetal vessels, and in very rare cases can cause transmural necrosis of the umbilical vessel wall.[39,40] The least frequent of these lesions in term infants, chorioamnionitis with intense chorionic vasculitis, is actually the most frequent risk factor for CNS injury in very low birth weight infants.[41] Fetal inflammatory responses, such as intense chorionic vasculitis, have also been associated with increased levels of circulating cytokines and chemokines in the neonatal circulation.[42,43] Chorionic vasculitis may also lead to nonocclusive chorionic vessel thrombi, another significant risk factor for neurologic impairment in premature infants.

## Microcirculatory Abnormalities

Diffuse villous edema affecting immature intermediate villi is the strongest individual placental risk factor for later CP and abnormal neurocognitive performance at school age in premature infants.[5,41] Diffuse villous edema has also been associated with an increased incidence of respiratory distress syndrome and neonatal death.[44] Although more frequent in very immature placentas with chorioamnionitis, its effects of neurologic outcome are independent of these variables. Whether edema directly affects placental function by compressing arterioles and venules within immature intermediate villi, or is an indicator of systemic fetal microcirculatory failure, has not been established. Placental disorders that can increase the diffusion distance between trophoblast and fetal capillaries include distal villous immaturity with decreased vasculosyncytial membranes, a lesion commonly seen in diabetics, and high-grade (patchy or diffuse) VUE.[36,45] Finally, villous chorangiosis is a microcirculatory abnormality characterized by adaptive angiogenesis in terminal villi, sometimes in association with reduced oxygen delivery in such conditions as pregnancy at high altitude, smoking, or maternal anemia.[46-49] Villous chorangiosis is considered to be a marker for, rather than a cause of, placental dysfunction, and is not by itself a risk factor for neurologic impairment.

## Fetal Hemorrhage

Two distinct categories of fetal hemorrhage may be important for the development of neurologic abnormalities. The first, rupture of a large fetal vessel, is another of the sentinel lesions. These ruptures can be obvious, as in the case of a ruptured vasa previa, or more subtle, such as with rupture of an umbilical (Wharton's jelly hemorrhage) or chorionic plate (subamnionic hemorrhage vessels) before delivery of the fetus. These latter hemorrhages may also occur during the third stage of labor secondary to excessive traction on the umbilical cord following delivery of the fetus, so they should be considered as possibly significant only in infants with documented hypovolemia or anemia. The second category is massive fetomaternal hemorrhage secondary to disruption of smaller vessels in the distal villi, usually before labor.[50] Diagnosis is confirmed by enumeration of fetal blood cells in the maternal circulation by either Kleihauer-Betke staining or flow cytometry using antibodies directed against fetal hemoglobin. Fetomaternal hemorrhages have been associated with placental intervillous thrombi and often show a characteristic histopathologic pattern of constricted arterioles and dilated venules in mature intermediate villi.[51] Long-standing fetomaternal hemorrhages show increased circulating nucleated red blood cells and villous hydrops related to high-output congestive heart failure. These findings may also be seen with other types of severe fetal anemia. Increased circulating nucleated red blood cells, also serves as an indicator of protracted (6–12 hours or more) significant fetal hypoxia of any etiology and can be helpful in the evaluation of infants presenting with severe neurologic problems.[52]

## ADDITIONAL CONSIDERATIONS
### Localization

The anatomic site at which placental lesions occur is an important factor in their impact on risk of CNS injury. The subset of lesions affecting the large fetal vessels of the chorionic plate are particularly important.[53] These 8 to 10 major chorionic vessels carry approximately 40% of the fetal cardiac output. They lack anastomoses and are prone to develop irreversible vasoocclusion when subjected to pathologic injury or prolonged episodes of decreased flow. More common pathologic processes affecting other placental compartments, such as changes consistent with maternal underperfusion, chorioamnionitis, and VUE, have lesser effects on the risk of neurodisability in the absence of superimposed large fetal vessel disease.

## Severity

Several placental lesions show a dose-response relationship to risk of neurodisability. The total number of avascular villi is an important predictor of clinical complications in cases of fetal thrombotic vasculopathy.[31] Increasing magnitude of elevated circulating nucleated red blood cells correlates with a higher odds ratio for CNS complications.[21] Severity of the fetal inflammatory response is the critical determinant for the risk of neurologic injury with chorioamnionitis in both premature and term infants.[41] High-grade (diffuse or patchy) chronic villitis shows a stronger relationship to neurologic impairment than low-grade (focal or multifocal) chronic villitis, independent of the presence or absence of obliterative fetal vasculopathy.[21]

## Multiplicity

One of the strongest risk factors for CNS damage is the presence of multiple placental lesions. In the case of premature infants, the finding of multiple lesions was the only placental finding that predicted neurologic impairment independent of clinical risk factors after multivariate analysis.[54] In term infants, each additional placental lesion was synergistic, as demonstrated by significantly increased specificity relative to decreased sensitivity for predicting CNS injury.[21] In general, multiple placental lesions enhance risk only when they affect different physiologic compartments. For instance, a combination of lesions related to decreased flow in both the maternal and fetal circulations, such as increased syncytial knots and avascular villi, has a greater risk for adverse outcome than do separate lesions that affect only the maternal circulation, such as increased syncytial knots and multiple villous infarcts.

## Timing

Placental lesions may be separated into three temporal categories. Acute lesions reflect processes occurring within 6 hours of delivery, often sentinel events. Subacute lesions indicate processes of 6 hours to 7 days' duration, and chronic lesions indicate processes with an onset more than 1 week before delivery. Results in the analysis of neurologic impairment in term infants have shown that cases with a combination of chronic and subacute lesions are at increased risk compared with those having either multiple chronic or multiple subacute lesions.[21] One interpretation of this relationship is that adaptation to an earlier lesion decreases the ability of the placenta to cope with a subsequent lesion. A corollary is that underlying placental lesions impair the ability of the fetus or placenta to compensate for acute stress at the time of parturition, stresses that might not affect an otherwise normal infant. The underlying impairment could be as simple as the inability to provide additional substrate on demand (decreased placental reserve) or might be more complex involving biochemical preconditioning, as discussed next.

## Preconditioning

Preconditioning was initially described in the cardiovascular system, where prior non-damaging ischemia was found to reduce the extent of subsequent myocardial infarction on occlusion of the coronary arteries.[55] Similar phenomena have been described in the placenta, where there is some evidence that mild maternal underperfusion may decrease the risk of CNS injury in premature infants with preeclampsia or intrauterine growth restriction.[41] These cardiovascular and placental phenomena are both examples of negative preconditioning. Bacterial lipopolysaccharide shows both negative and positive CNS preconditioning.[56] Exposure to lipopolysaccharide 4 hours before carotid occlusion in newborn rats increases the extent of brain injury, whereas exposure 24 hours before insult is protective. Repetitive exposures to low doses of lipopolysaccharide over a 24-hour period are also deleterious.[57] Cytokines, such as interleukin-1β, can substitute for lipopolysaccharide, and excitotoxic agents, such as glutamate, can substitute for hypoxia in analogous murine models.[58,59] These experimental models have obvious relevance for human pregnancy, where bacterial products, cytokines, and activating ligands released from damaged placental tissues may be released into the fetal circulation during late pregnancy and modulate subsequent CNS responses to hypoxia, ischemia, oxidant stress, or other stressors in the peripartum period.

## SUMMARY

The authors recently completed a clinicopathologic analysis of placental lesions in a large cohort of term infants who subsequently developed CP.[30] A hierarchical approach was taken, starting with cases having a sentinel event, such as maternal hypotension, abruptio placenta, uterine rupture, umbilical cord prolapse, or early onset sepsis; these cases comprised 20% of the sample. Second in the hierarchy were the severe fetoplacental large-vessel lesions that both have profound effects on fetoplacental physiology and can be associated with the release of damaging thromboinflammatory mediators into the fetal circulation. These accounted for another 34% of the cohort. Third were chronic processes that can decrease placental reserve. Lesions in this category, including findings consistent with maternal underperfusion, high-grade chronic villitis without obliterative fetal vasculopathy, increased perivillous fibrinoid depositon, chronic abruption, and distal villous immaturity with decreased vasculosyncytial membranes, were present in another 23% of cases. The fourth category, placental indicators of protracted fetal hypoxia, such as increased circulating nucleated red blood cells and villous chorangiosis, accounted for another 15%, leaving only 8% lacking either a sentinel event or a significant placental pathologic lesion. These latter unexplained cases were more likely to have had an inadequate placental examination or peripartum complications, such as birth trauma and failed assisted vaginal delivery. Attesting to the importance of multiple placental lesions, 20% of the 54 cases with severe fetoplacental large-vessel lesions also had chronic processes affecting underlying placental reserve. Finally, 63% of all cases had clinical or pathologic evidence of umbilical cord compromise, a factor that was not included in the hierarchical classification.

In summary, placental lesions affecting the maternal and fetal perfusion of the placenta can act in both a direct and indirect manner to modulate the effects of underlying clinical diseases and peripartum stressors. Failure to consider fully these important intermediary processes may lead to an incomplete or misleading understanding of the etiology of CNS injury in any given case.

## REFERENCES

1. Kraus FT, Redline R, Gersell DJ, et al. Placental pathology. Washington, DC: American Registry of Pathology; 2004.
2. Pijnenborg R, Anthony J, Davey DA, et al. Placental bed spiral arteries in the hypertensive disorders of pregnancy. Br J Obstet Gynaecol 1991;98:648–55.

3. Redline RW, Boyd T, Campbell V, et al. Maternal vascular underperfusion: nosology and reproducibility of placental reaction patterns. Pediatr Dev Pathol 2004;7:237–49.

4. Stanek J, Al-Ahmadie HA. Laminar necrosis of placental membranes: a histologic sign of uteroplacental hypoxia. Pediatr Dev Pathol 2005;8(1):34–42.

5. Redline RW, Minich N, Taylor HG, et al. Placental lesions as predictors of cerebral palsy and abnormal neurocognitive function at school age in extremely low birth weight infants (<1 kg). Pediatr Dev Pathol 2007;10(4):282–92.

6. Burke CJ, Tannenberg AE. Prenatal brain damage and placental infarction: an autopsy study. Dev Med Child Neurol 1995;37:555–62.

7. Burke C, Gobe G. Pontosubicular apoptosis (necrosis) in human neonates with intrauterine growth retardation and placental infarction. Virchows Arch 2005; 446(6):640–5.

8. Andres RL, Kuyper W, Resnik R, et al. The association of maternal floor infarction of the placenta with adverse perinatal outcome. Am J Obstet Gynecol 1990;163: 935–8.

9. Adams-Chapman I, Vaucher YE, Bejar RF, et al. Maternal floor infarction of the placenta: association with central nervous system injury and adverse neurodevelopmental outcome. J Perinatol 2002;22(3):236–41.

10. Sebire NJ, Backos M, El Gaddal S, et al. Placental pathology, antiphospholipid antibodies, and pregnancy outcome in recurrent miscarriage patients. Obstet Gynecol 2003;101(2):258–63.

11. Redline RW, Abramowsky CR. Clinical and pathologic aspects of recurrent placental villitis. Hum Pathol 1985;16:727–31.

12. Ordi J, Ismail MR, Ventura PJ, et al. Massive chronic intervillositis of the placenta associated with malaria infection. Am J Surg Pathol 1998;22:1006–11.

13. Boyd TK, Redline RW. Chronic histiocytic intervillositis: a placental lesion associated with recurrent reproductive loss. Hum Pathol 2000;31:1389–92.

14. Williams MA, Lieberman E, Mittendorf R, et al. Risk factors for abruptio placentae. Am J Epidemiol 1991;134:965–72.

15. Ananth CV, Smulian JC, Vintzileos AM. Incidence of placental abruption in relation to cigarette smoking and hypertensive disorders during pregnancy: a meta-analysis of observational studies. Obstet Gynecol 1999;93(4):622–8.

16. Harris BA. Peripheral placental separation: a review. Obstet Gynecol Surv 1988; 43:577–81.

17. Redline RW, Wilson-Costello D. Chronic peripheral separation of placenta: the significance of diffuse chorioamnionic hemosiderosis. Am J Clin Pathol 1999; 111(6):804–10.

18. Naftolin F, Khudr G, Benirschke K, et al. The syndrome of chronic abruptio placentae, hydrorrhea, and circumallate placenta. Am J Obstet Gynecol 1973; 116:347–50.

19. Elliott JP, Gilpin B, Strong TH Jr, et al. Chronic abruption-oligohydramnios sequence. J Reprod Med 1998;43(5):418–22.

20. Nelson KB, Ellenberg JH. Antecedents of cerebral palsy: multivariate analysis of risk. N Engl J Med 1986;315:81–6.

21. Redline RW, O'Riordan MA. Placental lesions associated with cerebral palsy and neurologic impairment following term birth. Arch Pathol Lab Med 2000;124(12): 1785–91.

22. Spellacy WN, Graven H, Fisch RO. The umbilical cord complications of true knots, nuchal coils and cords around the body. Am J Obstet Gynecol 1966;94: 1136–42.

23. Kouyoumdijian A. Velamentous insertion of the umbilical cord. Obstet Gynecol 1980;56:737–42.
24. Machin GA, Ackerman J, Gilbert-Barness E. Abnormal umbilical cord coiling is associated with adverse perinatal outcomes. Pediatr Dev Pathol 2000;3(5): 462–71.
25. Labarrere C, Sebastiani M, Siminovich M, et al. Absence of Wharton's jelly around the umbilical cord; an unusual cause of perinatal mortality. Placenta 1985;6: 555–9.
26. Baergen RN, Malicki D, Behling C, et al. Morbidity, mortality, and placental pathology in excessively long umbilical cords: retrospective study. Pediatr Dev Pathol 2001;4(2):144–53.
27. Clapp JF III, Lopez B, Simonean S. Nuchal cord and neurodevelopmental performance at 1 year. J Soc Gynecol Investig 1999;6(5):268–72.
28. Clapp JF III, Stepanchak W, Hashimoto K, et al. The natural history of antenatal nuchal cords. Am J Obstet Gynecol 2003;189(2):488–93.
29. Myers RE. Four patterns of perinatal brain damage and their conditions of occurrence in primates. Adv Neurol 1975;10:223–34.
30. Redline RW. Cerebral palsy in term infants: a clinicopathologic analysis of 158 medicolegal case reviews. Pediatr Dev Pathol 2008;11(6):456–64.
31. Redline RW, Pappin A. Fetal thrombotic vasculopathy: the clinical significance of extensive avascular villi. Hum Pathol 1995;26:80–5.
32. Redline RW. Clinical and pathological umbilical cord abnormalities in fetal thrombotic vasculopathy. Hum Pathol 2004;35(12):1494–8.
33. Dahms BB, Boyd T, Redline RW. Severe perinatal liver disease associated with fetal thrombotic vasculopathy. Pediatr Dev Pathol 2002;5(1):80–5.
34. Redline RW, Ariel I, Baergen RN, et al. Fetal vascular obstructive lesions: nosology and reproducibility of placental reaction patterns. Pediatr Dev Pathol 2004;7:443–52.
35. Kim MJ, Romero R, Kim CJ, et al. Villitis of unknown etiology is associated with a distinct pattern of chemokine up-regulation in the feto-maternal and placental compartments: implications for conjoint maternal allograft rejection and maternal anti-fetal graft-versus-host disease. J Immunol 2009;182(6):3919–27.
36. Redline RW. Villitis of unknown etiology: noninfectious chronic villitis in the placenta. Hum Pathol 2007;38(10):1439–46.
37. Altshuler G. Some placental considerations related to neurodevelopmental and other disorders. J Child Neurol 1993;8(1):78–94.
38. King EL, Redline RW, Smith SD, et al. Myocytes of chorionic vessels from placentas with meconium associated vascular necrosis exhibit apoptotic markers. Hum Pathol 2004;35:412–7.
39. Altshuler G, Hyde S. Meconium-induced vasocontraction: a potential cause of cerebral and other fetal hypoperfusion and of poor pregnancy outcome. J Child Neurol 1989;4:137–42.
40. Burgess AM, Hutchins GM. Inflammation of the lungs, umbilical cord and placenta associated with meconium passage in utero: review of 123 autopsied cases. Pathol Res Pract 1996;192(11):1121–8.
41. Redline RW, Wilson-Costello D, Borawski E, et al. Placental lesions associated with neurologic impairment and cerebral palsy in very low birth weight infants. Arch Pathol Lab Med 1998;122:1091–8.
42. Rogers BB, Alexander JM, Head J, et al. Umbilical vein interleukin-6 levels correlate with the severity of placental inflammation and gestational age. Hum Pathol 2002;33(3):335–40.

43. Yoon BH, Romero R, Yang SH, et al. Interleukin-6 concentrations in umbilical cord plasma are elevated in neonates with white matter lesions associated with periventricular leukomalacia. Am J Obstet Gynecol 1996;174:1433–40.
44. Naeye RL, Maisels J, Lorenz RP, et al. The clinical significance of placental villous edema. Pediatrics 1983;71:588–94.
45. Stallmach T, Hebisch G, Meier K, et al. Rescue by birth: defective placental maturation and late fetal mortality. Obstet Gynecol 2001;97(4):505–9.
46. Altshuler G. Chorangiosis: an important placental sign of neonatal morbidity and mortality. Arch Pathol Lab Med 1984;108(1):71–4.
47. Soma H, Watanabe Y, Hata T. Chorangiosis and chorangioma in three cohorts of placentas from Nepal, Tibet and Japan. Reprod Fertil Dev 1996;7:1533–8.
48. Kadyrov M, Kosanke G, Kingdom J, et al. Increased fetoplacental angiogenesis during first trimester in anaemic women. Lancet 1998;352(9142):1747–9.
49. Pfarrer C, Macara L, Leiser R, et al. Adaptive angiogenesis in placentas of heavy smokers. Lancet 1999;354(9187):1390.
50. de Almeida V, Bowman JM. Massive fetomaternal hemorrhage: Manitoba experience. Obstet Gynecol 1994;83(3):323–8.
51. Kaplan C, Blanc WA, Elias J. Identification of erythrocytes in intervillous thrombi: a study using immunoperoxidase identification of hemoglobins. Hum Pathol 1982;13:554–7.
52. Redline RW. Elevated circulating fetal nucleated red blood cells and placental pathology in term infants who develop cerebral palsy. Hum Pathol 2008;39(9): 1378–84.
53. Redline RW. Severe fetal placental vascular lesions in term infants with neurologic impairment. Am J Obstet Gynecol 2005;192:452–7.
54. Redline R, Wilson-Costello D, Borawski E, et al. The relationship between placental and other perinatal risk factors for neurologic impairment in very low birth weight children. Pediatr Res 2000;47:721–6.
55. Murry CE, Jennings RB, Reimer KA. Preconditioning with ischemia: a delay of lethal cell injury in ischemic myocardium. Circulation 1986;74(5):1124–36.
56. Hagberg H, Dammann O, Mallard C, et al. Preconditioning and the developing brain. Semin Perinatol 2004;28(6):389–95.
57. Duncan JR, Cock ML, Scheerlinck JP, et al. White matter injury after repeated endotoxin exposure in the preterm ovine fetus. Pediatr Res 2002;52(6):941–9.
58. Dommergues MA, Patkai J, Renauld JC, et al. Proinflammatory cytokines and interleukin-9 exacerbate excitotoxic lesions of the newborn murine neopallium. Ann Neurol 2000;47(1):54–63.
59. Rousset CI, Kassem J, Olivier P, et al. Antenatal bacterial endotoxin sensitizes the immature rat brain to postnatal excitotoxic injury. J Neuropathol Exp Neurol 2008; 67(10):994–1000.

# Disorders of the Fetal Circulation and the Fetal Brain

Catherine Limperopoulos, PhD[a,b,c,d,*]

KEYWORDS

- Fetal • Brain • Circulation • Congenital heart disease
- Magnetic resonance imaging

Normal brain growth and development in the fetus is a function of adequate supply of oxygen-substrate delivery, which depends in turn on the volume and content of blood that is delivered to the brain. This oxygen-substrate supply system relies on several critical factors throughout gestation, including an intact maternal and placental circulation as well as a normal fetal brain circulation. Moreover, fetal blood flow is influenced by intrinsic and extrinsic factors, including the structure of the heart, the impedance of the distal vascular beds, changes in placental vascular resistance, cardiac contractibility, vessel compliance, and blood viscosity.[1] Normal fetal brain growth is fostered by preferential streaming of oxygen and glucose from the umbilical venous return to the brain. However, the ability to fulfill this role may depend on normal fetal circulatory pathways and compensatory responses. With abnormal development of the cardiovascular system, the pathways favoring the streaming of oxygen-substrate–rich perfusion to the brain may be disrupted. Intrinsic autoregulatory mechanisms in the fetus have been shown to alter cerebrovascular resistance in order to counteract changes in oxygen delivery and preserve energy requirements. However, in addition to disturbances in placental exchange, disturbances in cerebral blood flow can result from impaired placental circulation or fetal cardiovascular circulation, and

This work was supported in part by Sickkids Foundation and the Canadian Institutes of Health Research. C.L. is supported by the Canada Research Chairs Program, Canada Research Chair in Brain and Development.

a Department of Neurology and Neurosurgery, McGill University, 2300 Tupper Street, Montreal, QC H3H 1P3, Canada

b Department of Pediatrics, McGill University, 2300 Tupper Street, Montreal, Quebec QC H3H 1P3, Canada

c Fetal-Neonatal Neurology Research Group, Department of Neurology, Children's Hospital Boston and Harvard Medical School, 300 Longwood Avenue, Boston, MA 02115, USA

d Montreal Children's Hospital, Pediatric Neurology, 2300 Tupper Street A-334, Montreal, Quebec, H3H 1P3, Canada

* Corresponding author. Montreal Children's Hospital, Pediatric Neurology, 2300 Tupper Street A-334, Montreal, Quebec, H3H 1P3.

E-mail address: catherine.limperopoulos@mcgill.ca

Clin Perinatol 36 (2009) 561–577

doi:10.1016/j.clp.2009.07.005

perinatology.theclinics.com

0095-5108/09/$ – see front matter © 2009 Elsevier Inc. All rights reserved.

play an important role in the genesis of prenatal cerebrovascular injury and impaired fetal brain growth.

Consequently, in the fetus with congenital heart disease (CHD), decreased cerebral oxygen or substrate supply may place the developing fetus at risk for aberrant brain growth and development in utero. Recent advances in fetal imaging techniques of the heart and brain are providing novel quantitative biomarkers for advancing the understanding of the multifaceted nature and timing of brain injury in the developing fetus with CHD. This article reviews evidence for early life brain injury in this population, and explores the underlying mechanisms of fetal blood flow dynamics and the role of developmental brain disturbances in utero.

## CONGENITAL HEART DISEASE AND BRAIN INJURY

Recent advances and ongoing refinements in diagnostic and surgical techniques have greatly enhanced the survival of young infants with complex CHD, even those lesions previously considered lethal or extremely debilitating. Open heart surgery in the newborn is now routine in many large centers, and is increasingly performed in younger and less mature neonates. Thus, infants at greatest risk for brain injury now survive. Consequently, a new profile of neurologic dysfunction has emerged among survivors, reflecting the effects of early life hemodynamic disturbances rather than the consequences of chronic hypoxia.

Concurrent with these recent trends, there is a burgeoning literature demonstrating that early neurologic sequelae in these new survivors of CHD are associated with a spectrum of long-term developmental disabilities, estimated between 25% and 50% and including motor, cognitive, learning, social, and behavioral difficulties.[2-8] Until recently, studies have focused largely on intraoperative cerebral hypoxic-ischemic insult as the principal mechanism for neurologic dysfunction in young infants with CHD.[9-14] However, patient-specific risk factors such as type of CHD, genetic syndromes, and polymorphisims of the gene for apolipoprotein E have also been linked with adverse long-term outcome.[15,16] A growing body of evidence is showing that preoperative brain injury is implicated in the pathogenesis of neurologic sequelae in newborns with CHD. These data are summarized here.

## EVIDENCE OF ABNORMAL NEUROLOGY AT BIRTH
### Functional Evidence

#### Neurologic examination
In recent years, there has been accumulating evidence for an alarmingly high prevalence of neurologic compromise already evident before neonatal surgical correction.[17-23] In fact, more than half of newborns with CHD show evidence of neurologic abnormality before open heart surgery, including muscle tone abnormalities, jitteriness, motor asymmetries, poor behavioral state regulation, feeding difficulties, and absent suck. Furthermore, up to 36% of neonates with CHD are reported to be microcephalic preoperatively, despite birth weights appropriate for gestational age,[6,24 26] suggesting impaired brain growth of fetal onset.

#### Electrophysiology
Available electrophysiological[17,19] data have also emphasized the potential for antenatal onset neurologic dysfunction in the fetus with CHD. Preoperative electroencephalographic abnormalities have been documented in up to 44% of newborns, characterized more frequently by moderate and diffuse disturbances in background

activity rather than epileptiform activity.[18] Somatosensory evoked potential abnormalities have been reported in up to 41% of newborns.[24]

## Structural Evidence

There is growing recognition that infants with CHD are at risk for abnormal neurologic structure before the hazards of open heart surgery. These data are summarized in **Table 1**. Cranial ultrasound studies performed before surgery have demonstrated a 40% to 60% incidence of brain abnormalities in full-term infants with CHD.[27,28] The most common abnormalities include cerebral atrophy (41%), widened ventricular or subarachnoid spaces (26%), linear echodensities of the deep gray matter (20%), intraventricular hemorrhage (16%), and parenchymal echodensities (16%).[27] In one report, newborns with aortic coarctation or hypoplastic left heart syndrome (HLHS) were at greatest risk for cerebral abnormalities (63%).[27] In another report, cerebral atrophy and deep gray linear echodensities were reported in over two-thirds (71%) of newborns with coarctation of the aorta and ventricular septal defects.[28] The investigators speculate that these abnormalities were the result of intrauterine impairment of cerebral perfusion due to the limited perfusion of the preductal aorta with this lesion.

Recent magnetic resonance imaging (MRI) studies have provided evidence for a high prevalence of brain injury before cardiac surgery, particularly in infants with critical CHD lesions (eg, HLHS, transposition of the great arteries [TGA]), those with low preoperative oxygenation and a longer time to surgery, and those undergoing invasive diagnostic procedures (eg, balloon-atrial septostomy).[29–31] A range of abnormalities has been described including intracranial hemorrhage, cerebral venous thromboses, thromboembolisms, infarctions, ventriculomegaly and dilation of the subarachnoid spaces consistent with cerebral atrophy, white matter injury in the form of periventricular leukomalacia, and gray matter injury.[29,32–36]

In addition to structural evidence, decreased preoperative cerebral blood flow has been shown in newborns with CHD and has been linked with periventricular leukomalacia, using pulsed arterial spin-label perfusion MRI.[26] The presence of anaerobic metabolism as measured by elevated lactate levels via magnetic resonance spectroscopy (MRS) has also been reported in up to 50% of newborns with CHD, particularly in those with TGA and single ventricle physiology.[34,35,37–39] A recent report described delayed anatomic brain development with structural immaturity in term neonates with HLHS and TGA,[40] which corroborates previous findings of decreased pyramidal tract maturation using diffusion tensor tractography[41] and biochemical immaturity of the white matter using MRS.[37]

The high incidence of periventricular leukomalacia in the newborn with CHD suggests an increased vulnerability of the white matter, possibly of the oligodendrocyte progenitors.[37,40,42] It has been suggested that in the infants with CHD oligodendrocyte immaturity (and thus vulnerability) may persist much later into gestation, even into the postnatal period after term delivery,[40] placing the newborn with CHD at increased risk of injury.

Taken together, these converging lines of investigation support the notion that neurologic dysfunction associated with CHD may originate in the fetal period. To date, the predictive value of these acute preoperative MRI abnormalities has not been determined.

## Predictive Value of Preoperative Neurologic Status

In recent years, several reports have suggested that neurologic abnormalities evident in the preoperative neonatal period are important determinants of adverse long-term outcome in this population. In one study, 55% of the variance in long-term outcome could be explained by preoperative factors.[22] Preoperative neurologic abnormalities,

**Table 1**
**Summary of preoperative neuroimaging abnormalities in newborns with CHD**

| Study | Year | Sample Size | Type of CHD | Preoperative Findings |
|---|---|---|---|---|
| **Cranial Ultrasound (US)** | | | | |
| van Houten et al[28] | 1996 | 49 CHD 42 controls | Mixed | 59% US abnormalities 27% cerebral atrophy; 20% linear echodensities (basal ganglia and thalamus); 16% IVH; 8% periventricular echodensities; 8% intraparenchymal echodensities; 4% subarachnoid hemorrhage; 2% subarachnoid space enlargement |
| Te Pas et al[27] | 2005 | 50 | Mixed | 42% US abnormalities 26% widened ventricular and/or subarachnoid spaces; 8% acute ischemic changes; 6% lenticulostriate vasculopathy; 2% basal nuclei calcifications |
| **Magnetic resonance imaging (MRI)** | | | | |
| Ashwal et al[38] | 1996 | 9 | Mixed | 44% 33% cerebral edema; 11% hemorrhage |
| McConnell et al[33] | 1990 | 15 | MIXED | 33% MRI abnormalities 33% ventriculomegaly and dilatation of the subarachnoid spaces |
| Mahle et al[34] | 2002 | 24 | Mixed | 42% MRI abnormalities 17% open operculum; 17% PVL; 8% infarction; 4% hemorrhage 53% presence of lactate on magnetic resonance spectroscopy |
| Ashwal et al[39] | 2003 | 11 | Mixed | 36% MRI abnormalities 36% cerebral atrophy/ encephalomalacia |
| Tavani et al[32] | 2003 | 24 | Mixed | 52% subdural bleeding of the infratentorium 33% small hemorrhages in the choroid plexus; 29% supratentorial subdural bleeding; 5% parenchymal hemorrhage; 5% occipital horn hemorrhage |
| Miller et al[35] | 2004 | 10 CHD 5 controls | TGA | 40% MRI abnormalities 20% stroke, 10% germinal matrix hemorrhage, 10% hemorrhage and stroke Higher lactate/choline and lower NAA/choline in CHD versus controls |

(continued on next page)

| Table 1 (continued) | | | | |
|---|---|---|---|---|
| Study | Year | Sample Size | Type of CHD | Preoperative Findings |
| **Cranial Ultrasound (US)** | | | | |
| Licht et al[26] | 2004 | 25 | Mixed | 53% developmental and/or acquired brain lesions 29% PVL; 16%incomplete closure of the operculum 20% low cerebral blood flow (pulsed arterial spin-label perfusion imaging) |
| McQuillen et al[29] | 2006 | 29 | TGA | 41% MRI abnormalities 17% focal infarcts; 7% focal white matter injury; 3% IVH: 14% combined lesions |
| Partridge et al[41] | 2006 | 25 | Mixed | Fractional anisotropy maturation rate was found to be the lowest in newborns with preoperative injury |
| McQuillen et al[36] | 2007 | 62 | Mixed | 39% MRI abnormalities 21% stroke; 18% white matter injury; 8% IVH |
| Miller et al[37] | 2007 | 41 CHD 16 controls | TGA, single ventricle | 41% MRI abnormalities with TGA 31% stroke; 10% white matter injury; 7% intraventricular hemorrhage. 50% MRI abnormalities with single ventricle 8% stroke; 8% white matter injury Lower NAA/choline in CHD versus controls Decreased average diffusivity in CHD versus controls Decreased mean fractional anisotropy in CHD versus controls |
| Petit et al[31] | 2009 | 26 | TGA | 38% MRI abnormalities 38% PVL |
| Licht et al[40] | 2009 | 42 | HLHS, TGA | 31% MRI abnormalities 86% incomplete closure of the opercular space; 21% PVL; 10% stroke |

*Abbreviations:* CHD, congenital heart disease; HLHS, hypoplastic left heart syndrome; IVH, intraventricular hemorrhage; NAA, *N*-acetyl aspartate PVL, periventricular leukomalacia; TGA, transposition of the great arteries.

including abnormal neurologic examination and microcephaly, have been shown to be a significant predictor for later persistent neurodevelopmental morbidity, including neuromotor and cognitive impairments, functional limitations in day-to-day activities, and quality of life in the years following cardiac surgery.[2,4,5,19,23,43]

## ADVANCES IN IMAGING OF THE FETUS: MOVING BEYOND THE FETAL HEART
### Advances in Fetal Echocardiography

Advances in fetal cardiac imaging technologies have facilitated the earlier and more accurate detection of cardiac abnormalities in the developing fetus. Fetal echocardiography is now widely used for the prenatal diagnosis of CHD, and has had a far-reaching impact on the care of high-risk fetuses.[44–47] Ultrasound screening for CHD has increased the percentage of cases that are detected prenatally and allowed for improved counseling of families regarding the remaining fetal course, the postnatal prognosis, and interventions that may be required. As a consequence, fetal echocardiography has contributed to the significant increase in survival rates and decrease in termination rates as well as the number of neonatal deaths, and has directly affected the location, timing, or route of delivery.

### Advances in Fetal Brain MRI

An exciting new area in fetal research has been the application of MRI in the living fetus, providing previously unavailable insights into the development of the fetal brain. Specifically, advanced in vivo 3-dimensional volumetric MRI techniques allow quantitative measurements of the rate and progression of in utero brain development.[48–51] In healthy control fetuses, the relationship between increasing total brain volume and gestational age has been described, with a concurrent decrease in cerebrospinal fluid (Limperopoulos, unpublished data, 2008) (**Fig. 1**).[51] The ability now to quantify volumetric brain growth in the healthy fetus has enabled the study of timing and progression of impaired brain growth in the compromised fetus.

Proton magnetic resonance spectroscopy ($^1$H-MRS) is another powerful noninvasive tool for monitoring cerebral metabolism in the fetus in vivo. MRS allows measurement of specific brain metabolites including N-acetyl aspartate (NAA), reflecting development of dendrites and synapses as well as mitochondrial metabolism; creatine (Cr), indicating cellular energy metabolism; choline (Cho), a marker of myelination (**Fig. 2**); and lactate, representing anaerobic metabolism. Normative fetal MRS studies have reported the in vivo metabolic maturation of the fetal brain from 22 to 39 weeks of gestation.[52–56] Creatine is evident as early as 22 weeks of gestation, along with a small NAA peak, and the ratio of NAA:Cho increases fourfold over the third trimester in healthy control fetuses (**Fig. 3**).[51] This increase in NAA:Cho ratio likely reflects the accelerated development of dendrites during the third trimester.[55] Unlike the preterm infant ex utero, lactate has not been reported in the healthy fetus in utero[55,56] The availability of normative $^1$H-MRS data for fetal brain metabolites provides a valuable reference for measurement of cerebral metabolites in the high-risk fetal brain.

Another exciting development is that microstructural development of the fetal brain can now be measured in vivo using diffusion-weighted imaging (DWI) and diffusion tensor imaging (DTI). DWI and DTI studies are based on the preferential diffusion of water molecules in a magnetic field. DWI has enabled the detection of acute ischemic

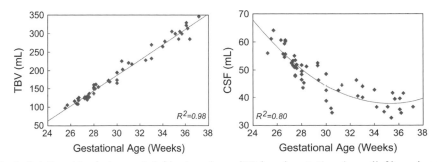

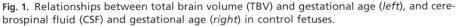

**Fig. 1.** Relationships between total brain volume (TBV) and gestational age (*left*), and cerebrospinal fluid (CSF) and gestational age (*right*) in control fetuses.

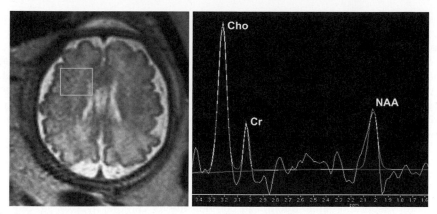

**Fig. 2.** Proton magnetic resonance spectroscopy (TE 144 ms) acquired in a 35-week gestational age fetus with voxel positioned in the right cerebral hemisphere. Identifiable peaks on MR spectra include *N*-acetyl aspartate (NAA), creatine (Cr), and choline (Cho).

changes in the brain, whereas DTI is used to quantify the impact of early injury on subsequent microstructural organization of the developing brain. Apparent diffusion coefficient (ADC) and fractional anisotropy (FA) maps can now be readily acquired in the fetus.[57–61] Normative values of fetal brain ADC and FA have been established, which allows detection of pathologic changes in the compromised fetal brain.[57–61]

These advances in fetal MRI techniques collectively provide the tools necessary to study for the first time the development of the fetal brain in conditions of abnormal fetal circulation.

## EVIDENCE OF IMPAIRED FETAL CIRCULATION AND BRAIN DEVELOPMENT IN CONGENITAL HEART DISEASE
### *Fetal Circulation and Congenital Heart Disease*

The inception of Doppler ultrasound in the mid 1970s led to numerous studies on fetal blood flow and uteroplacental hemodynamics, and led to its establishment as the principal diagnostic and prognostic tool in pregnancies complicated by uteroplacental insufficiency.[62] Fetal brain growth and development is dependent on adequate substrate and oxygen delivery. Under normal conditions, fetal perfusion provides optimal oxygen and substrate delivery to the transverse aorta and the cerebral circulation. In the presence of fetal hypoxia, autoregulatory mechanisms result in

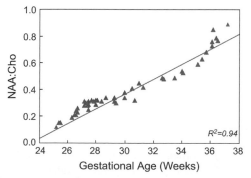

**Fig. 3.** Relationship between NAA:Cho ratio and gestational age in control fetuses.

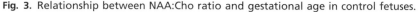

a redistribution of fetal circulation to maintain optimal cerebral oxygen-substrate supply, known as the "brain-sparing effect."[63] These mechanisms are discussed in detail elsewhere in this issue.

Pulsatility index in the middle cerebral artery (MCA PI) has been used as a surrogate measure of impedance to cerebral blood flow. The ability to reliably measure fetal blood flow has permitted the evaluation of regional alterations in arterial resistance in the fetus with CHD, and has enabled researchers to begin to address the following critical question: Do fetuses with CHD experience alterations in cerebrovascular blood flow dynamics in utero?

Alterations in cerebral vascular resistance may occur in fetuses with CHD for 2 principal reasons. First, a lower oxygen content of blood is delivered to the brain, given that CHD may be associated with intermixing of oxygenated and deoxygenated blood. As a result, the oxygen content of blood delivered to the brain may be low, causing cerebral vasodilation in an attempt to compensate for cerebral hypoxemia. Studies have shown that fetuses with CHD are significantly more likely to experience reduced cerebrovascular impedance, and that this reduced impedance.[64,65] For example, the work by Jouannic and colleagues[65] reported significantly lower MCA PI in fetuses with TGA, and the investigators hypothesized that decreased MCA PI was an indication of hypoxemia or hypercapnea in regions perfused by the preisthmus aorta.

Second, changes in cerebral impedance may be associated with decreased cerebral perfusion. In fetuses with a normal 2-ventricle heart anatomy, intracardiac streaming causes the preferential delivery of highly oxygenated ductus venosus blood across the foramen ovale to the left atrium and ventricle, ascending aorta, and cerebral circulation.[66] This occurrence has been shown to be reduced or altogether absent in the fetus with obstructive lesions such as HLHS. Kaltman and colleagues[67] reported significantly lower cerebral vascular resistance in fetuses with HLHS, a cardiac lesion where cerebral perfusion is supplied retrograde through the ductus arteriosus. In contrast, left-sided obstructive CHD with preserved antegrade perfusion did not show cerebral flow redistribution, presumably because of normal or near normal aortic oxygen content and relatively normal cerebral oxygen delivery. In contrast, in a recent report by Guorong and colleagues,[68] no significant differences in MCA PI values were found between CHD diagnostic groups (eg, left-sided obstructive lesions, right-sided obstructive lesions, and mixed type of CHD). The investigators postulated that this finding was due to the severity of obstructive lesions, which was inversely related to the amount of cerebral blood delivery. This study also reported that fetuses with CHD complicated by congestive heart failure have a significantly lower MCA PI than controls, which negatively impacted cerebrovascular blood flow dynamics. The investigators speculate that the lower MCA PI evident in fetuses with congestive heart failure represents a marker of cerebral vasodilation that is attributable to cerebral hypoxemia and limited perfusion.[68]

Significant differences have also been reported in umbilical artery pulsatility indices between fetuses with CHD and controls, possibly due to changes in pulsatility of the descending aorta blood flow.[69,70] However, considerable controversy persists regarding the prognostic value of umbilical arterial blood flow velocity waveforms in the fetus with isolated CHD[67,69,71,72]; further research is clearly needed on this topic.

### Fetal Brain Development Using Ultrasound

A paucity of studies has examined the impact of in utero alterations in cerebral-systemic hemodynamics on brain growth in fetuses with CHD; the data are conflicting and are presented here.

A prospective study[72] of 36 fetuses with CHD compared with normal controls demonstrated that a decreased umbilical artery to middle cerebral artery pulsatility index was associated with a reduced head circumference in a significant number of fetuses with CHD. A recent retrospective study described normal and proportional head size in fetuses with HLHS at mid-gestation; however, 50% showed a significant decrease in head growth (50% reduction in head circumference percentile) and 22% were found to be growth restricted during the latter part of gestation.[73] Of note, umbilical artery resistance index was reported to be normal for gestational age in all cases, suggesting that growth restriction was not due to placental insufficiency and that there was no relationship between head size or head growth and aortic atresia or absence of antegrade blood flow. These emerging data underscore the considerable controversy that exists regarding the relative contribution of cardiovascular hemodynamics on brain development in the fetus with CHD.

In summary, studies to date that have examined cerebrovascular impedance in fetuses with CHD have been mostly retrospective, with measurements taken at single time points during gestation; in addition, studies have examined heterogeneous groups of infants. Consequently, meaningful comparisons and overall generalizability of the findings are limited. Serial, prospective observational studies, with clearly defined cohorts that examine the evolving systemic-cerebral hemodynamic profile of fetuses with CHD throughout gestation, are sorely lacking.

### Fetal MRI in the Fetus with Congenital Heart Disease

To date, only one MRI study has examined volumetric brain growth and metabolism in a consecutive series of second- and third-trimester fetuses with CHD and healthy control fetuses in vivo.[51] In this study, brain volume and metabolism were compared prospectively between 55 fetuses with different types of CHD and 50 normal fetuses ranging from 25 to 37 weeks' gestational age using 3-D volumetric MRI and $^1$H-MRS. The results of this study have shown for the first time in vivo evidence of abnormal brain growth and metabolism in third-trimester fetuses with CHD. The data are summarized here.

Although no differences in brain volumes were detected between controls and CHD fetuses during the second trimester, a significant progressive impairment of parenchymal brain volumetric growth, particularly in fetuses with reduced systemic ventricular outflow or other major central arterial abnormalities, was documented during the third trimester. A lower cerebroplacental resistance ratio was also associated with lower brain volume in CHD fetuses. These data suggest that the fetal compensatory ("brain sparing") mechanisms described earlier are at best temporizing, and fail during severe or sustained hypoxemia.

In vivo $^1$H-MRS studies in the same cohort demonstrated that the NAA:Cho ratio increased progressively over the second and third trimester in control fetuses and fetuses with CHD. However, this increase was significantly and progressively slower with increasing gestational age in fetuses with CHD compared with controls. Absence of antegrade flow in the aortic arch was found to be an independent predictor of a lower NAA:Cho ratio (**Fig. 4**). Moreover, lactate was identified in 20% of fetuses (5 with HLHS and 2 with TGA), whereas none of the control fetuses had detectable cerebral lactate. Based on the expected distribution and mixing of umbilical venous blood passing through the anomalous cardiac pathways and reaching the brain, fetuses were categorized into those with estimated cerebral oxygen-substrate delivery that was either normal or decreased. Among fetuses with CHD, when controlling for gestational age and total brain volume, the NAA:Cho ratio was independently and significantly lower in those fetuses with lower estimated cerebral

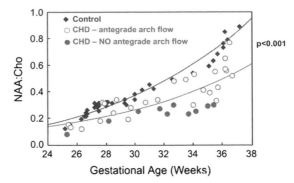

**Fig. 4.** Relationship between NAA:Cho ratio and gestational age. Control fetuses are indicated with diamonds. Fetuses with CHD are indicated with circles (those with absence of antegrade blood flow in the transverse aortic arch are solid and others are open).

oxygen-substrate delivery, as well as those with lactate (**Fig. 5**). These data suggest impaired neuroaxonal development and cerebral metabolism in fetuses with CHD, and severely perturbed central cerebrovascular hemodynamics. Fetuses with decreased antegrade systemic ventricular outflow showed the greatest impairment in brain volumetric growth, abnormal NAA:Cho ratio, and the presence of lactate, supporting the notion that in this subgroup of fetuses, cerebral oxygen-glucose substrate delivery failed to meet the increasing substrate requirements during a critical period of normal brain development.

Finally, preliminary diffusion tensor analyses in a subset of fetuses with CHD show significantly higher ADC values and concomitant lower FA values in the frontal and posterior white matter regions compared with controls (**Fig. 6**) (Limperopoulos, unpublished data, 2008). An analysis of the relationship between disturbed white matter architecture in fetuses with CHD and systemic hemodynamics is currently underway.

Together, these data support the theory that impaired substrate delivery to the brain of fetuses with abnormally developing cardiovascular systems may mediate abnormal brain growth, microstructural development, and metabolism in fetuses with CHD.

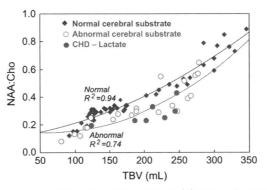

**Fig. 5.** Relationship between NAA:Cho ratio, TBV, and lactate. Congenital heart disease (CHD) fetuses with normal cerebral substrate are indicated with diamonds, and those with abnormal cerebral substrate are indicated with open circles. Fetuses with CHD that showed presence of lactate are indicated with solid circles.

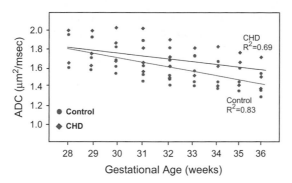

**Fig. 6.** Relationship between apparent diffusion coefficients (ADC) and gestational age in the posterior white matter region. Control fetuses are indicated with circles. Fetuses with CHD are indicated with diamonds.

Assessment of the long-term predictive value of impaired fetal brain growth and metabolism in these subjects is currently underway.

## POTENTIAL MECHANISMS FOR FETAL BRAIN MALDEVELOPMENT

Potential mechanisms for the antenatal onset of neurologic dysfunction in infants with CHD are likely multifactorial, and may include primary genetic and dysgenetic conditions (described later), secondary disruptions of fetal brain development, and acquired encephaloplastic lesions due to, for example, acute or chronic oxygen-glucose deprivation. In most cases the fetal diagnosis of CHD is made by fetal echocardiogram between 16 and 24 weeks of gestation. Although many of the major events in brain development have occurred by 24 weeks of gestation, several critical events have yet to commence or be completed. Most importantly, these later gestational events place an escalating demand on the developing cardiovascular system for delivery of oxygen and energy substrates. Given the high energy demands during brain development, the potential for disturbed oxygen-substrate supply due to CHD presents a major threat to the developing fetus.

Although the peak period for prosencephalic development is between 8 and 12 weeks, corpus callosum development is only completed around 20 weeks of gestation. The sylvian fissure appears around 14 weeks and develops over the subsequent 10 to 12 weeks, such that by week 19 the insula begins to form over the rest of gestation, and the insula surface is gradually covered by caudal to rostral opercularization. It is thus of particular interest that disorders of callosal development[74,75] and incomplete insular closure[76,77] are particularly prevalent among infants with CHD. In fact, incomplete closure of the operculum has recently been reported in approximately 90% of newborns with TGA and HLHS.[40] It is noteworthy that the opercular region includes the buccal, glottic, and esophageal structures, and receptive and expressive language areas,[40] and that opercular abnormalities have been associated with feeding and language impairments.[78]

Between 20 and 24 weeks of gestation, a burst of developmental activity results in a dramatic increase in fetal brain weight.[79,80] Although neuronal proliferation is in large part complete by 20 weeks of gestation, and neuronal migration has been active for some time before that, neuronal migration continues until at least 25 weeks of gestation and perhaps longer. Between 25 and 40 weeks of gestation, several critical developmental events occur, including neuronal arborization, synaptogenesis, programmed cell death, and reorganization of synaptic connections. Many of the primary cerebral gyri and sulci become defined between 26 and 28 weeks of gestation, with secondary and tertiary gyration occurring later, that is, between 40 and 44 weeks of gestation. In addition, at around 30 weeks of gestation myelination in the cerebral hemispheres begins to accelerate, and continues for the rest of gestation and well beyond.[81,82] This critical period is associated with rapid brain growth, with an almost threefold increase from 120 g at 28 weeks of gestation to 350 g at term.[79] This accelerated third trimester growth has also been corroborated by quantitative MRI studies in preterm infants ex utero.[83,84]

### Primary Genetic and Dysgenetic Disorders of Brain Development

This article focuses primarily on disturbances in oxygen and energy substrate supply in CHD as a cause for impaired brain development. Of course, the role for primary genetic and dysgenetic mechanisms of brain maldevelopment cannot be underestimated in this population, but a detailed discussion of this topic is beyond the scope of this article. However, in summary, the prevalence of brain dysgenesis in children with CHD approaches 30% in autopsy studies.[74,75,85,86] Furthermore, the risk of cerebral dysgenesis seems to be related to the underlying cardiac lesion. Newborns with HLHS seem to be at greater risk for associated developmental brain lesions, ranging in severity from microdysgenesis to gross cerebral malformations, such as agenesis of the corpus callosum and holoprosencephaly.[74] Extracardiac anomalies are more frequent in children with CHD than in the general population, even in the absence of a demonstrable chromosomal, single gene, or contiguous gene defects.[74,75,86] In fact, certain genetic syndromes predictably involve combined malformations of the heart and brain, such as the chromosome 22 deletion spectrum, which includes the velocardiofacial and DiGeorge syndromes. With ongoing advances in fetal MRI, the relationship between cardiac and brain dysgenesis will become more clearly defined.

### SUMMARY

A growing body of evidence points to a high prevalence of neurologic abnormalities in the newborn with CHD before surgical intervention. These data suggest an antenatal onset for impaired brain development. Furthermore, these preoperative neonatal abnormalities are associated with wide-ranging, long-term developmental disabilities. In vivo data in the fetus with CHD support a fetal onset for these neurologic disturbances. The causes of abnormal brain development in the fetus with CHD are undoubtedly multifactorial, and likely include genetic and environmental factors that mediate the timing, severity, and progression of the insult.

Recent technological advances in cardiac and brain imaging techniques are revolutionizing the ability to study the living fetus. Advances in quantitative MRI that have provided valuable insights into brain development in premature infants ex utero have now been successfully applied to the fetus in vivo. These techniques are providing unprecedented access to features of brain growth and development in this population. Should these approaches fulfill their promise, it is likely that in future early detection of compromised brain development will help guide rational management decisions for these fetuses.

### REFERENCES

1. Degani S. Fetal cerebrovascular circulation: a review of prenatal ultrasound assessment. Gynecol Obstet Invest 2008;66(3):184–96.

2. Limperopoulos C, Majnemer A, Shevell MI, et al. Predictors of developmental disabilities after open heart surgery in young children with congenital heart defects. J Pediatr 2002;141(1):51–8.
3. Wernovsky G, Shillingford AJ, Gaynor JW. Central nervous system outcomes in children with complex congenital heart disease. Curr Opin Cardiol 2005;20(2): 94–9.
4. Majnemer A, Limperopoulos C, Shevell M, et al. Long-term neuromotor outcome at school entry of infants with congenital heart defects requiring open-heart surgery. J Pediatr 2006;148(1):72–7.
5. Majnemer A, Limperopoulos C, Shevell M, et al. Health and well-being of children with congenital cardiac malformations, and their families, following open-heart surgery. Cardiol Young 2006;16(2):157–64.
6. Shillingford AJ, Ittenbach RF, Marino BS, et al. Aortic morphometry and microcephaly in hypoplastic left heart syndrome. Cardiol Young 2007;17(2):189–95.
7. Shillingford AJ, Glanzman MM, Ittenbach RF, et al. Inattention, hyperactivity, and school performance in a population of school-age children with complex congenital heart disease. Pediatrics 2008;121(4):e759–67.
8. Bellinger DC. Are children with congenital cardiac malformations at increased risk of deficits in social cognition? Cardiol Young 2008;18(1):3–9.
9. Bellinger DC, Wypij D, du Plessis AJ, et al. Developmental and neurologic effects of alpha-stat versus pH-stat strategies for deep hypothermic cardiopulmonary bypass in infants. J Thorac Cardiovasc Surg 2001;121(2):374–83.
10. Bellinger DC, Wypij D, duDuplessis AJ, et al. Neurodevelopmental status at eight years in children with dextro-transposition of the great arteries: the Boston Circulatory Arrest Trial. J Thorac Cardiovasc Surg 2003;126(5):1385–96.
11. Newburger JW, Jonas RA, Soul J, et al. Randomized trial of hematocrit 25% versus 35% during hypothermic cardiopulmonary bypass in infant heart surgery. J Thorac Cardiovasc Surg 2008;135(2):347–54, 54, e1–4.
12. Wypij D, Newburger JW, Rappaport LA, et al. The effect of duration of deep hypothermic circulatory arrest in infant heart surgery on late neurodevelopment: the Boston Circulatory Arrest Trial. J Thorac Cardiovasc Surg 2003;126(5):1397–403.
13. Wypij D, Jonas RA, Bellinger DC, et al. The effect of hematocrit during hypothermic cardiopulmonary bypass in infant heart surgery: results from the combined Boston hematocrit trials. J Thorac Cardiovasc Surg 2008;135(2): 355–60.
14. Jonas RA, Wypij D, Roth SJ, et al. The influence of hemodilution on outcome after hypothermic cardiopulmonary bypass: results of a randomized trial in infants. J Thorac Cardiovasc Surg 2003;126(6):1765–74.
15. Gaynor JW, Wernovsky G, Jarvik GP, et al. Patient characteristics are important determinants of neurodevelopmental outcome at one year of age after neonatal and infant cardiac surgery. J Thorac Cardiovasc Surg 2007;133(5):1344–53, 53, e1–3.
16. Zeltser I, Jarvik GP, Bernbaum J, et al. Genetic factors are important determinants of neurodevelopmental outcome after repair of tetralogy of Fallot. J Thorac Cardiovasc Surg 2008;135(1):91–7.
17. Limperopoulos C, Majnemer A, Shevell MI, et al. Neurologic status of newborns with congenital heart defects before open heart surgery. Pediatrics 1999;103(2): 402–8.
18. Limperopoulos C, Majnemer A, Shevell MI, et al. Neurodevelopmental status of newborns and infants with congenital heart defects before and after open heart surgery. J Pediatr 2000;137(5):638–45.

19. Limperopoulos C, Majnemer A, Shevell MI, et al. Functional limitations in young children with congenital heart defects after cardiac surgery. Pediatrics 2001; 108(6):1325–31.

20. Newburger JW, Jonas RA, Wernovsky G, et al. A comparison of the perioperative neurologic effects of hypothermic circulatory arrest versus low-flow cardiopulmonary bypass in infant heart surgery. N Engl J Med 1993;329:1057–64.

21. Clancy RR, McGaurn SA, Goin JE, et al. Allopurinol neurocardiac protection trial in infants undergoing heart surgery using deep hypothermic circulatory arrest. Pediatrics 2001;108(1):61–70.

22. Robertson CM, Joffe AR, Sauve RS, et al. Outcomes from an interprovincial program of newborn open heart surgery. J Pediatr 2004;144(1):86–92.

23. Fuller S, Nord AS, Gerdes M, et al. Predictors of impaired neurodevelopmental outcomes at one year of age after infant cardiac surgery. Eur J Cardiothorac Surg 2009;36(1):40–7.

24. Limperopoulos C, Majnemer A, Rosenblatt B, et al. Multimodality evoked potential findings in infants with congenital heart defects. J Child Neurol 1999;14(11): 702–7.

25. Manzar S, Nair AK, Pai MG, et al. Head size at birth in neonates with transposition of great arteries and hypoplastic left heart syndrome. Saudi Med J 2005;26(3): 453–6.

26. Licht DJ, Wang J, Silvestre DW, et al. Preoperative cerebral blood flow is diminished in neonates with severe congenital heart defects. J Thorac Cardiovasc Surg 2004;128(6):841–9.

27. Te Pas AB, van Wezel-Meijler G, Bokenkamp-Gramann R, et al. Preoperative cranial ultrasound findings in infants with major congenital heart disease. Acta Paediatr 2005;94(11):1597–603.

28. van Houten J, Rothman A, Bejar R. High incidence of cranial ultrasound abnormalities in full-term infants with congenital heart disease. Am J Perinatol 1996; 13(1):47–53.

29. McQuillen PS, Hamrick SE, Perez MJ, et al. Balloon atrial septostomy is associated with preoperative stroke in neonates with transposition of the great arteries. Circulation 2006;113(2):280–5.

30. Cheng TO. That balloon atrial septostomy is associated with preoperative stroke in neonates with transposition of the great arteries is another powerful argument in favor of therapeutic closure of every patent foramen ovale. Am J Cardiol 2006; 98(2):277–8.

31. Petit CJ, Rome JJ, Wernovsky G, et al. Preoperative brain injury in transposition of the great arteries is associated with oxygenation and time to surgery, not balloon atrial septostomy. Circulation 2009;119(5):709–16.

32. Tavani F, Zimmerman RA, Clancy RR, et al. Incidental intracranial hemorrhage after uncomplicated birth: MRI before and after neonatal heart surgery. Neuroradiology 2003;45(4):253–8.

33. McConnell JR, Fleming WH, Chu WK, et al. Magnetic resonance imaging of the brain in infants and children before and after cardiac surgery. A prospective study. Am J Dis Child 1990;144(3):374–8.

34. Mahle WT, Tavani F, Zimmerman RA, et al. An MRI study of neurological injury before and after congenital heart surgery. Circulation 2002;106(12 Suppl 1): I109–14.

35. Miller SP, McQuillen PS, Vigneron DB, et al. Preoperative brain injury in newborns with transposition of the great arteries. Ann Thorac Surg 2004; 77(5):1698–706.

36. McQuillen PS, Barkovich AJ, Hamrick SE, et al. Temporal and anatomic risk profile of brain injury with neonatal repair of congenital heart defects. Stroke 2007;38(2 Suppl):736–41.
37. Miller SP, McQuillen PS, Hamrick S, et al. Abnormal brain development in newborns with congenital heart disease. N Engl J Med 2007;357(19):1928–38.
38. Ashwal S, Holshouser B, Schell R, et al. Proton magnetic resonance spectroscopy in the evaluation of children with congenital heart disease and acute central nervous system injury. J Thorac Cardiovasc Surg 1996;112:403–14.
39. Ashwal S, Holshouser BA, del Rio MJ, et al. Serial proton magnetic resonance spectroscopy of the brain in children undergoing cardiac surgery. Pediatr Neurol 2003;29(2):99–110.
40. Licht DJ, Shera DM, Clancy RR, et al. Brain maturation is delayed in infants with complex congenital heart defects. J Thorac Cardiovasc Surg 2009;137(3): 529–36 [discussion 36–7].
41. Partridge SC, Vigneron DB, Charlton NN, et al. Pyramidal tract maturation after brain injury in newborns with heart disease. Ann Neurol 2006;59(4):640–51.
42. du Plessis AJ. Neurologic complications of cardiac disease in the newborn. Clin Perinatol 1997;24(4):807–26.
43. Gaynor JW, Gerdes M, Zackai EH, et al. Apolipoprotein E genotype and neurodevelopmental sequelae of infant cardiac surgery. J Thorac Cardiovasc Surg 2003; 126(6):1736–45.
44. Kovalchin JP, Silverman NH. The impact of fetal echocardiography. Pediatr Cardiol 2004;25(3):299–306.
45. Yeu BK, Chalmers R, Shekleton P, et al. Fetal cardiac diagnosis and its influence on the pregnancy and newborn—a tertiary centre experience. Fetal Diagn Ther 2008;24(3):241–5.
46. Mellander M. Perinatal management, counselling and outcome of fetuses with congenital heart disease. Semin Fetal Neonatal Med 2005;10(6):586–93.
47. Russo MG, Paladini D, Pacileo G, et al. Changing spectrum and outcome of 705 fetal congenital heart disease cases: 12 years, experience in a third-level center. J Cardiovasc Med (Hagerstown) 2008;9(9):910–5.
48. Grossman R, Hoffman C, Mardor Y, et al. Quantitative MRI measurements of human fetal brain development in utero. Neuroimage 2006;33(2):463–70.
49. Kazan-Tannus JF, Dialani V, Kataoka ML, et al. MR volumetry of brain and CSF in fetuses referred for ventriculomegaly. AJR Am J Roentgenol 2007;189(1):145–51.
50. Guizard N, Lepag C, Fonov V, et al. Development of a fetal brain atlas from multiaxial MR acquisitions. Paper presented at: Proceedings, 16th Scientific Meeting, International Society for Magnetic Resonance in Medicine, 2008. Toronto, Ontario, May 3–9, 2008.
51. Limperopoulos C, Tworetzky W, McElhinney DB, et al. Brain volume and metabolism in fetuses with congenital heart disease: evaluation with quantitative magnetic resonance imaging and spectroscopy. Circulation, in press.
52. Kok RD, van den Bergh AJ, Heerschap A, et al. Metabolic information from the human fetal brain obtained with proton magnetic resonance spectroscopy. Am J Obstet Gynecol 2001;185(5):1011–5.
53. Kok RD, van den Berg PP, van den Bergh AJ, et al. Maturation of the human fetal brain as observed by [1]H MR spectroscopy. Magn Reson Med 2002;48(4): 611–6.
54. Fenton BW, Lin CS, Macedonia C, et al. The fetus at term: in utero volume-selected proton MR spectroscopy with a breath-hold technique—a feasibility study. Radiology 2001;219(2):563–6.

55. Girard N, Gouny SC, Viola A, et al. Assessment of normal fetal brain maturation in utero by proton magnetic resonance spectroscopy. Magn Reson Med 2006; 56(4):768–75.
56. Girard N, Fogliarini C, Viola A, et al. MRS of normal and impaired fetal brain development. Eur J Radiol 2006;57(2):217–25.
57. Bui T, Daire JL, Chalard F, et al. Microstructural development of human brain assessed in utero by diffusion tensor imaging. Pediatr Radiol 2006;36(11):1133–40.
58. Schneider JF, Confort-Gouny S, Le Fur Y, et al. Diffusion-weighted imaging in normal fetal brain maturation. Eur Radiol 2007;17(9):2422–9.
59. Righini A, Bianchini E, Parazzini C, et al. Apparent diffusion coefficient determination in normal fetal brain: a prenatal MR imaging study. AJNR Am J Neuroradiol 2003;24(5):799–804.
60. Baldoli C, Righini A, Parazzini C, et al. Demonstration of acute ischemic lesions in the fetal brain by diffusion magnetic resonance imaging. Ann Neurol 2002;52(2): 243–6.
61. Erdem G, Celik O, Hascalik S, et al. Diffusion-weighted imaging evaluation of subtle cerebral microstructural changes in intrauterine fetal hydrocephalus. Magn Reson Imaging 2007;25(10):1417–22.
62. Rizzo G, Arduini D, Romanini C, et al. Doppler echocardiographic assessment of atrioventricular velocity waveforms in normal and small-for-gestational-age fetuses. Br J Obstet Gynaecol 1988;95(1):65–9.
63. Vyas S, Nicolaides KH, Bower S, et al. Middle cerebral artery flow velocity waveforms in fetal hypoxaemia. Br J Obstet Gynaecol 1990;97(9):797–803.
64. Modena A, Horan C, Visintine J, et al. Fetuses with congenital heart disease demonstrate signs of decreased cerebral impedance. Am J Obstet Gynecol 2006;195(3):706–10.
65. Jouannic JM, Benachi A, Bonnet D, et al. Middle cerebral artery Doppler in fetuses with transposition of the great arteries. Ultrasound Obstet Gynecol 2002;20(2):122–4.
66. Edelstone DI, Rudolph AM. Preferential streaming of ductus venosus blood to the brain and heart in fetal lambs. Am J Phys 1979;237(6):H724–9.
67. Kaltman JR, Di H, Tian Z, et al. Impact of congenital heart disease on cerebrovascular blood flow dynamics in the fetus. Ultrasound Obstet Gynecol 2005;25(1): 32–6.
68. Guorong L, Shaohui L, Peng J, et al. Cerebrovascular blood flow dynamic changes in fetuses with congenital heart disease. Fetal Diagn Ther 2009;25(1): 167–72.
69. Meise C, Germer U, Gembruch U. Arterial Doppler ultrasound in 115 second- and third-trimester fetuses with congenital heart disease. Ultrasound Obstet Gynecol 2001;17(5):398–402.
70. Berg C, Kremer C, Geipel A, et al. Ductus venosus blood flow alterations in fetuses with obstructive lesions of the right heart. Ultrasound Obstet Gynecol 2006;28(2):137–42.
71. Al-Gazali W, Chapman MG, Chita SK, et al. Doppler assessment of umbilical artery blood flow for the prediction of outcome in fetal cardiac abnormality. Br J Obstet Gynaecol 1987;94(8):742–5.
72. Donofrio MT, Bremer YA, Schieken RM, et al. Autoregulation of cerebral blood flow in fetuses with congenital heart disease: the brain sparing effect. Pediatr Cardiol 2003;24(5):436–43.
73. Hinton RB, Andelfinger G, Sekar P, et al. Prenatal head growth and white matter injury in hypoplastic left heart syndrome. Pediatr Res 2008;64:364–9.

74. Glauser T, Rorke L, Weinberg P, et al. Congenital brain anomalies associated with the hypoplastic left heart syndrome. Pediatrics 1990;85(6):984–90.
75. Glauser T, Rorke L, Weinberg P, et al. Acquired neuropathologic lesions associated with the hypoplastic left heart syndrome. Pediatrics 1990;85(6):991–1000.
76. Bingham PM, Zimmerman RA, McDonald-McGinn D, et al. Enlarged sylvian fissures in infants with interstitial deletion of chromosome 22q11. Am J Med Genet 1997;75(4):538–43.
77. Bingham PM, Lynch D, McDonald-McGinn D, et al. Polymicrogyria in chromosome 22 deletion syndrome. Neurology 1998;51(5):1500–2.
78. Chen CY, Zimmerman RA, Faro S, et al. MR of the cerebral operculum: abnormal opercular formation in infants and children. AJNR Am J Neuroradiol 1996;17(7): 1303–11.
79. Hansen K, Sung CJ, Huang C, et al. Reference values for second trimester fetal and neonatal organ weights and measurements. Pediatr Dev Pathol 2003;6(2): 160–7.
80. Awoust J, Levi S. Neurological maturation of the human fetus. Ultrasound Med Biol 1983;(suppl 2):583–7.
81. Volpe JJ. Neurology of the newborn. 5th edition. Philadelphia: Saunders Elsevier; 2008.
82. Haynes RL, Folkerth RD, Keefe RJ, et al. Nitrosative and oxidative injury to premyelinating oligodendrocytes in periventricular leukomalacia. J Neuropathol Exp Neurol 2003;62(5):441–50.
83. Huppi PS, Warfield S, Kikinis R, et al. Quantitative magnetic resonance imaging of brain development in premature and mature newborns. Ann Neurol 1998;43: 224–35.
84. Limperopoulos C, Soul JS, Gauvreau K, et al. Late gestation cerebellar growth is rapid and impeded by premature birth. Pediatrics 2005;115(3):688–95.
85. Jones M. Anomalies of the brain and congenital heart disease: a study of 52 necropsy cases. Pediatr Pathol 1991;11:721–36.
86. Miller G, Vogel H. Structural evidence of injury or malformation in the brains of children with congenital heart disease. Semin Pediatr Neurol 1999;6(1):20–6.

# Fetal Hypoxia Insults and Patterns of Brain Injury: Insights from Animal Models

Alistair Jan Gunn, MBChB, PhD[a,b,c,*], Laura Bennet, PhD[a]

KEYWORDS

- Perinatal asphyxia • Hypoxic-ischemic encephalopathy
- Fetal sheep • Premature delivery • Neuronal loss
- Repeated hypoxia

Acute neonatal encephalopathy remains a significant cause of death and long-term disability.[1] Despite the highly adverse outcomes of moderate to severe encephalopathy around birth[2] the predictive value for cerebral palsy of abnormal fetal heart rate patterns is consistently weak.[3] Indeed, even measures of total oxygen debt such as base deficit (BD) or lactate show only a broad relationship with later encephalopathy. For example, profound acidosis (BD>18 mmol/L at 30 minutes of life) was associated with moderate to severe encephalopathy in nearly 80% of patients,[4] and no cases occur with mild BDs below approximately 10–12 mmol/L.[4,5] However, it is striking that Low and colleagues found that less than half of babies born with cord blood BDs over 16 mmol/L (and pH <7.0) developed significant encephalopathy, and that encephalopathy still occurred, although at low frequency (10% of cases), in cases with moderate metabolic acidosis of between 12 and 16 mmol/L.[5] These data contrast with the presence of (very) non-reassuring fetal heart rate tracings and severe metabolic acidosis in those infants who do go on to develop neonatal encephalopathy.[2,6]

Early onset neonatal encephalopathy is important, because it is the key link between exposure to asphyxia and subsequent neurodevelopmental impairment.[7] Newborns with mild encephalopathy are completely normal to follow-up, while all of those with severe (stage III) encephalopathy die or have severe handicap. In contrast, only half of those with moderate (stage II) hypoxic–ischemic encephalopathy develop

---

[a] Department of Physiology, Faculty of Medical and Health Sciences, University of Auckland, Private Bag 92019, 85 Park Road, Grafton, Auckland 1023, New Zealand
[b] Department of Paediatrics, Faculty of Medical and Health Sciences, University of Auckland, Private Bag 92019, 85 Park Road, Grafton, Auckland 1023, New Zealand
[c] Paediatric Endocrinology Service, Starship Children's Hospital, 2 Park Road, Grafton, Auckland 1023, New Zealand
* Corresponding author. Department of Physiology, Faculty of Medical and Health Sciences, University of Auckland, Private Bag 92019, Auckland, New Zealand.
E-mail address: aj.gunn@auckland.ac.nz (A.J. Gunn).

Clin Perinatol 36 (2009) 579–593
doi:10.1016/j.clp.2009.06.007

handicap. However, even those who do not develop cerebral palsy have increased risk of learning and more subtle neurologic problems in later childhood.[8] This strongly infers that much of the variation in outcome is related to the immediate insult period.

This article focuses on recent developments that help shed light on the factors that determine whether the brain is or is not damaged after apparently similar asphyxial insults. In part, this variation is simply because the fetus is spectacularly good at defending itself against such insults. Thus, it appears that injury occurs only in a very narrow window between intact survival and death. The fetus's ability to defend itself though is modified by multiple factors including the depth, duration, and repetition of the insult, the gestational age, sex and condition of the fetus, and its environment, and particularly pyrexia and exposure to sensitizing factors such as infection/inflammation.

Most of the studies discussed here were undertaken in chronically instrumented fetal sheep. The sheep is a highly precocial species, whose neural development around 0.8–0.85 of gestation approximates that of the term human.[9,10] Earlier gestations have also been studied; the 0.7 gestation fetus is broadly equivalent to the late preterm infant at 30 to 34 weeks, before the onset of cortical myelination, while at 0.6 gestation the sheep fetus is similar to the 26 to 28 week gestation human.

## WHAT INITIATES NEURONAL INJURY?

It is useful to consider what is required to trigger injury of brain cells, independent of the fetus's cardiovascular defenses.[11] At the most fundamental level, injury requires a period of insufficient delivery of oxygen and substrates such as glucose (and in the fetus other aerobic substrates such as lactate) such that neurons (and glia) cannot maintain homeostasis. If oxygen is reduced but substrate delivery is effectively maintained (ie, pure or nearly pure hypoxia), the cells adapt in two ways. First, they can to some extent reduce non-obligatory energy consumption, initially switching to lower energy requiring states and then, as an insult becomes more severe, completely suppressing neuronal activity, at a threshold above that which causes neuronal depolarization.[12] This reduced activity is actively mediated by inhibitory neuromodulators such as adenosine.[13] Second, they can use anaerobic metabolism to support their production of high-energy metabolites for a time. The use of anaerobic metabolism is of course very inefficient since anaerobic glycolysis produces lactate and only 2 ATP, whereas aerobic glycolysis produces 38 ATP. Thus glucose reserves are rapidly consumed, and a metabolic acidosis develops due to accumulation of lactic acid, with local and systemic consequences such as impaired vascular tone and cardiac contractility.[11]

In contrast, under conditions of combined reduction of oxygen and substrate the neuron's options are much more limited, as not only is less oxygen available, but there is also much less glucose for anaerobic metabolism. This may occur during either pure ischemia (reduced tissue blood flow) and even more critically during conditions of hypoxia–ischemia, ie, both reduced oxygen content, and reduced total blood flow. Under these conditions depletion of high energy metabolites will occur much more rapidly and profoundly than during hypoxia alone, while at the same time there may actually be less metabolic acidosis both because there is much less glucose being delivered for metabolism to lactate, and because the insult is evolving more quickly. This is important, since the fetus is commonly exposed to hypoxia–ischemia due to hypoxic cardiac compromise.

These concepts help to explain the consistent observation discussed below that across multiple paradigms in the fetus most cerebral injury after acute insults occurs in association with hypotension and consequent tissue hypoperfusion or ischemia.

Technically, asphyxia is defined as the combination of impaired respiratory gas exchange (ie, hypoxia and hypercapnia) accompanied by the development of metabolic acidosis. To understand much of the apparent variation in outcome it is critical to keep in mind that this definition tells us much about things that can be measured relatively easily (blood gases and systemic acidosis) and essentially nothing about blood pressure or perfusion of the brain.

## CEREBRAL INJURY: AN 'EVOLVING' PROCESS

The seminal concept to emerge from both experimental and clinical studies is that brain cell death does not necessarily occur during hypoxia-ischemia (the 'primary' phase of injury), but rather that the injurious event may precipitate a cascade of biochemical processes leading to delayed cell death hours or even days afterwards (the 'secondary' phase). Experimental studies have demonstrated the existence of both a primary phase of energy failure during hypoxia–ischemia, a 'latent' phase during which oxidative metabolism normalizes, followed by secondary failure of oxidative metabolism in piglets,[14] immature rats,[15] and the fetal sheep.[16] Consistent with these studies, although some newborn infants exposed to profound asphyxia show no initial recovery of oxidative metabolism after birth and typically have very severe brain injury and high mortality,[17] in many other cases infants show initial, transient recovery of cerebral oxidative metabolism followed by a secondary deterioration, with cerebral energy failure from 6 to 15 hours after birth.[17,18] The severity of secondary energy failure correlates closely with the severity of neurodevelopmental outcome at 1 and 4 years of age.[18] Critically, for understanding labor insults, experimental studies show that a single 'sub-threshold' insult that causes either minor or no neural injury can lead to a phase of increased vulnerability to further insults in a similar window of around 6 or more hours.[19–21]

## MILD TO MODERATE HYPOXIA IS NOT INJURIOUS

The fetus can fully adapt to mild to moderate reductions in oxygen tension without injury, from normal values of greater than 20 mm Hg down to 10 to 12 mm Hg.[22,23] The late gestation fetal sheep fetus shows an initial transient, moderate bradycardia followed by tachycardia and an increase in blood pressure, typically accompanied by a minor initial increase in circulating lactate.[22,23] There is a rapid peripheral vasoconstriction reducing blood flow to peripheral organs such as the gut, lungs, skin and muscle, in favor of the brain, heart and adrenal gland.[23] Thanks to this increased blood flow to the brain that helps to restore oxygen delivery, greater oxygen extraction, and a switch to lower frequency EEG states with approximately a 20% reduction in oxygen consumption,[24] brain oxygen consumption is maintained at normal values. If the hypoxia is sustained, the fetus can fully adapt essentially indefinitely as shown by normalization of heart rate and blood pressure and the return of normal sleep state cycling. However, redistribution of blood flow is maintained,[25,26] resulting in reduced somatic growth.

## ASPHYXIA, HYPOTENSION AND HYPOXIC-ISCHEMIC BRAIN INJURY

Asphyxia by definition involves both hypoxia and hypercapnia with metabolic acidosis. It is important to appreciate that experimental studies of asphyxia have typically involved a greater depth of hypoxia than is possible using maternal inhalational hypoxia. Brief, total clamping of the uterine artery or umbilical cord leads to a rapid reduction of fetal oxygenation within a few minutes.[27–29] In contrast, gradual partial occlusion induces a slow fetal metabolic deterioration without the initial fetal cardiovascular responses of bradycardia and hypertension; this is a function of the speed and relative depth of hypoxia that was attained.[30] During profound asphyxia, corresponding with a severe reduction of uterine blood flow to 25% or less and a fetal arterial oxygen content of less than 1 mmol/L, the fetus responds very differently than during mild to moderate hypoxia. Typically, we can distinguish two phases: an initial, rapid chemoreflex-mediated period of compensation,[31–34] followed by progressive hypoxic-decompensation, ultimately terminated by profound systemic hypotension with cerebral hypoperfusion (**Fig. 1**).[28,29,35]

Term and preterm fetuses alike respond to asphyxia in a qualitatively similar manner, albeit the preterm fetuses can survive for much longer without injury.[35–37] A wide range of studies suggest that it is the period of hypotension during severe asphyxia that is associated with cerebral injury across paradigms, likely because of the close relationship between maintenance of fetal blood pressure during severe asphyxia and changes in brain perfusion (carotid blood flow [CaBF]) as shown in **Fig. 1**. In these fetuses, MAP initially rose with intense peripheral vasoconstriction; at this time CaBF was maintained at around baseline values, but with profound suppression of EEG activity.[13,35] Microsphere studies have shown that although total brain flow did not change, within the brain blood flow is diverted away from the cerebrum and increased in the brain stem.[38] As umbilical cord occlusion was continued MAP eventually fell. The key mediators of hypotension include impaired cardiac function secondary to hypoxia, acidosis, depletion of myocardial glycogen and cardiomyocyte injury[39] and loss of the initial peripheral vasoconstriction.[35,40] Once MAP fell below baseline, carotid blood flow fell in parallel, consistent with the known relatively narrow low range of autoregulation of cerebrovasculature in the fetus,[27] and there is loss of redistribution of flow within the brain.[38]

In the near-term fetus neural injury has been commonly reported in areas such as the parasagittal cortex, the dorsal horn of the hippocampus, and the cerebellar neocortex after a range of insults including pure ischemia,[41] prolonged single complete umbilical cord occlusion,[28] prolonged partial asphyxia[30,42,43] and repeated brief umbilical cord occlusion (eg, as illustrated in the bottom panel of **Fig. 2**).[44] These areas are 'watershed' zones within the borders between major cerebral arteries, where perfusion pressure is least, and in both adults and children lesions in these areas are typically seen after systemic hypotension.[45]

There are some data suggesting that limited, or localized white or gray matter injury may occur even when significant hypotension is not seen,[30,43] particularly when hypoxia is very prolonged.[46] Clearly it remains possible that regional hypoperfusion may have occurred or that perfusion was insufficient for particular, highly metabolically active regions. Nevertheless, the magnitude of damage reported after insults without hypotension is modest[46] and there is a strong correlation between either the depth or duration of hypotension and the amount of neuronal loss within individual studies of acute asphyxia (**Fig. 3**).[42–44,47] This is also seen between similar asphyxial paradigms causing severe fetal acidosis, which have been manipulated to either cause fetal hypotension[42] or not.[30] In fetal lambs exposed to prolonged severe partial asphyxia induced by partial occlusion of the uterine artery, neuronal loss occurred only in fetuses in whom one or more episodes of acute hypotension occurred.[42] In contrast, in a similar study where an equally 'severe' insult was induced gradually and titrated to maintain normal or elevated blood pressure throughout the insult no neuronal loss was seen except in the cerebellum.[30]

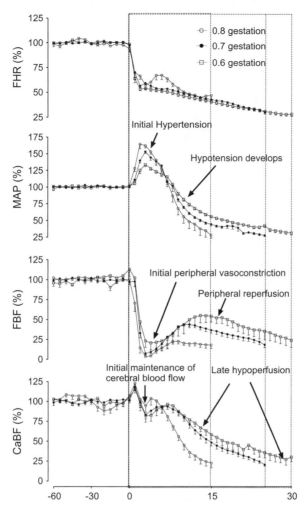

**Fig. 1.** Changes in fetal heart rate (FHR, bpm, top panel), mean arterial pressure (MAP, mm Hg, second panel), femoral blood flow (FBF, ml/min, third panel) and carotid blood flow (CaBF, ml/min, bottom panel) in 0.6 (□), 0.7 (●) and 0.85 gestation (○) fetuses during complete umbilical cord occlusion. FHR, MAP, FBF and CaBF data represent one minute averages and are expressed as percentage of baseline. The period of umbilical cord occlusion for each group is indicated by the rectangles. Data are mean ± SE (*Data from* Wassink G, Bennet L, Booth LC, et al. The ontogeny of hemodynamic responses to prolonged umbilical cord occlusion in fetal sheep. J Appl Physiol 2007;103(4):1311–7).

## BASAL GANGLIA INJURY: CARDIOVASCULAR COLLAPSE AND REPEATED INSULTS?

Although the watershed-type injuries described above are a commonly recognized clinical MRI pattern, basal ganglia and thalamic damage is widely recognized. It is typically associated with more severe or "sentinel" events at birth,[48] and with more severe neurodevelopmental disability.[49] Although the basal ganglia seem to be relatively mildly affected in the experimental settings mentioned above, the clinical association with more severe acute events at birth[49,50] raises the possibility that it may be

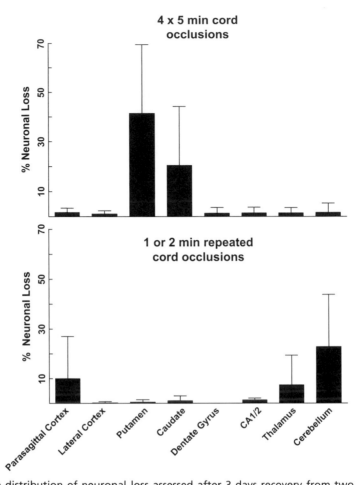

**Fig. 2.** The distribution of neuronal loss assessed after 3 days recovery from two different paradigms of repeated prenatal asphyxia in near-term fetal sheep. The top panel shows the effect of five minute episodes of umbilical cord occlusion, repeated four times, at intervals of 30 minutes. There is marked neuronal loss in the putamen and caudate nucleus, which are nuclei of the striatum. The bottom panel shows the effects of brief umbilical cord occlusions repeated at frequencies consistent with established labor, either 1 minute every 2.5 minutes or 2 minutes every 5 minutes. Occlusions were terminated after a variable time, when the fetal blood pressure fell below 20 mm Hg for two successive occlusions. This insult led to damage in the watershed regions of the parasagittal cortex and cerebellum with sparing of the striatum. CA 1/2 and the dentate gyrus are regions of the hippocampus. Data are mean ± SD and derived from de Haan et al.[44,47]

a function of more severe cardiovascular collapse. Blood to the brain during the initial adaptation to asphyxia is not distributed evenly, but rather reduced to the cortex and increased in the basal ganglia/thalamus and brainstem.[38] This suggests that in part the apparent sparing of the basal ganglia and other critical deep nuclei during many insults reflects this greater residual perfusion, and that it must fail during profound hypotension, which would expose the deep nuclei to overt ischemia.[51]

Another contributing factor is suggested by the experimental association between relatively widely spaced, but prolonged episodes of asphyxia and selective neuronal

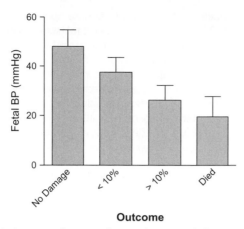

**Outcome**

**Fig. 3.** The relationship between hypotension and neuronal damage. The severity of fetal systemic hypotension during asphyxia induced by partial common uterine artery occlusion is closely related to the degree of neuronal loss and risk of death in the near-term fetal sheep. BP (blood pressure). (*Data from* Gunn AJ, Parer JT, Mallard EC, et al. Cerebral histologic and electrocorticographic changes after asphyxia in fetal sheep. Pediatr Res 1992;31(5):486–91).

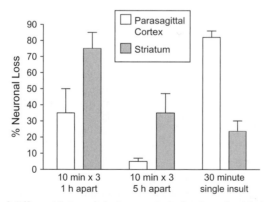

**Fig. 4.** The effects of different intervals between periods of cerebral ischemia insults on the distribution of cerebral damage the near-term fetal sheep. Cerebral ischemia induced by bilateral occlusion of the carotid arteries was applied either for 10 minutes, repeated three times at intervals of either 1 or 5 hours, or for a single continuous episode of 30 minutes. The divided insults were associated with a preponderance of damage in the striatum, whereas a single episode of 30 minutes of carotid occlusion was associated with severe cortical neuronal loss. When the interval was increased to 5 hours, cortical damage was nearly completely abolished, but there was still substantial neuronal loss in the striatum (*Data from* Mallard EC, Williams CE, Gunn AJ, et al. Frequent episodes of brief ischemia sensitize the fetal sheep brain to neuronal loss and induce striatal injury. Pediatr Res 1993;33(1):61–5).

damage to the striatal nuclei (putamen and caudate nucleus, see **Fig. 2**, top).[21,44,52] Further, whereas a single 30 minute period of cerebral ischemia leads to predominantly parasagittal cortical neuronal loss, with only moderate injury to the dorsolateral striatum, when the insult was divided into three episodes of 10 minutes of ischemia, a greater proportion of striatal injury was seen relative to cortical neuronal loss (**Fig. 4**).[19] Intriguingly, significant striatal involvement was also seen after prolonged partial asphyxia in which distinct episodes of bradycardia and hypotension occurred.[42]

The striatum is not in a watershed zone but rather within the territory of the middle cerebral artery. Thus it is likely that the pathogenesis of striatal involvement in the near-term fetus is related to the precise timing of the relatively prolonged episodes of asphyxia and not to more severe local hypoperfusion. The mechanism is unclear, however, the relatively greater striatal damage with greater spacing between insults[19] suggests that it is in part a consequence of the evolving neural dysfunction and sensitivity triggered by noninjurious single insults, and thus speculatively, with slower recovery of this period of sensitivity to further insults in the basal ganglia than the cortex. Further, we should note that the inhibitory striatal neurons were primarily damaged by repeated ischemia,[21] raising the possibility that this enhanced injury is related in part to abnormal excitatory inputs to these neurons.

## PRE-EXISTING METABOLIC STATUS, AND CHRONIC HYPOXIA

While the original studies of factors influencing the degree and distribution of brain injury, primarily by Myers,[53] focused on metabolic status, the issue remains controversial. There is evidence, for example, that hyperglycemia during hypoxia-ischemia reduces damage in the infant rat whereas it was associated with greater damage in adult rats,[54,55] but had no effect in the piglet.[56] These differences may reflect species specific maturational differences in the activity of cerebral glucose transporters.[55] The most common metabolic disturbance to the fetus is intrauterine growth retardation (IUGR) associated with placental dysfunction. Although clinically IUGR is usually associated with a greater risk of brain injury, recent studies have suggested that the risk of encephalopathy has fallen markedly over time.[6] One interpretation of this finding is that the apparently increased sensitivity to injury is mostly due to reduced aerobic reserves, leading to early onset of systemic compromise during labor.

Consistent with this hypothesis, chronically hypoxic fetuses from multiple pregnancies developed much more severe, progressive metabolic acidosis than previously normoxic fetuses during brief (1 minute) umbilical cord occlusions repeated every 5 minutes (pH $7.07 \pm 0.14$ vs $7.34 \pm 0.07$) and hypotension (a nadir of $24 \pm 2$ mm Hg vs $45.5 \pm 3$ mm Hg after 4 hours of repeated occlusion).[57] The fetuses with pre-existing hypoxia were smaller on average, and had lower blood glucose values and higher $PaCO_2$ values. Similarly, in normally grown fetuses, 5 days of induced chronic hypoxemia was associated with increased striatal damage after acute exposure to repeated umbilical cord occlusion for 5 minutes every 30 minutes for a total of four occlusions.[52] Together, these data support the clinical concept that fetuses with chronic placental insufficiency are vulnerable even to relatively infrequent periods of additional hypoxia in early labor.

Less obvious adverse intrauterine events may also modify fetal responses to hypoxia. There is considerable interest on the effects of stimuli such as maternal undernutrition and steroid exposure, particularly at critical times in pregnancy, not only on the fetal responses to challenges to its environment such as hypoxia, but also on risks for adverse health outcomes in adult life.[58] Intriguingly, mild maternal undernutrition that does not alter fetal growth may still affect development of the fetal hypothalamic-pituitary-adrenal function, with reduced pituitary and adrenal responsiveness to moderate hypoxia.[59] There is some evidence that exposure to glucocorticoids may also detrimentally alter the responses to hypoxia.[60]

## BRAIN MATURITY

The effect of maturation on sensitivity to injury is of great importance, for two reasons. First, in recent years improvements in obstetric and pediatric management have resulted in significantly increased survival of preterm infants from 24 weeks of gestation, with continuing very high rates of physical disabilities and long-term learning, cognitive and behavioral problems.[61] Second, many infants may sustain neural injuries well before birth, including a significant number of infants with cerebral palsy.[62] The characteristic patterns of cerebral injury in the preterm fetus differ from those seen at term or after birth, with preferential injury of subcortical structures and white matter.

Their high rate of disability intuitively suggests that premature infants are more vulnerable to hypoxic damage than at term. Recent experimental studies now show that in fact the premature fetus is *less* vulnerable to a given duration of asphyxia than at term, and further that tolerance to hypoxia-ischemia falls with postnatal age.[36] For example, the premature sheep fetus at 90 days gestation (term is 147 days), before the onset of cortical myelination, can tolerate extended periods of up to 20 minutes of umbilical cord occlusion without neuronal loss.[37,63] The very prolonged cardiac survival during profound asphyxia (up to 30 minutes, see **Fig. 1**)[35] corresponds with the peak in cardiac glycogen levels that occurs near mid-gestation in the sheep and other species including man.[64]

Interestingly, while the preterm fetal response to mild to moderate hypoxia appears to be different to that seen at term,[65] the overall pattern of cardiovascular and cerebrovascular response during severe asphyxia is very similar to that seen in more mature fetuses, with sustained bradycardia, accompanied by circulatory centralization, initial hypertension, then a progressive fall in pressure.[35,66–68] As also reported in the term fetus, there was no increase in blood flow to the brain during this initial phase, and again this was due to a significant increase in vascular resistance rather than to hypotension. Compared with the term fetus, 0.6 and 0.7 gestation fetuses showed significantly slower suppression of EEG activity at the start of umbilical cord occlusion.[35,68] Speculatively, this delay is indicative of the relative anerobic tolerance of the preterm brain. As shown in **Fig. 1**, as in the term fetus, once blood pressure begins to fall blood flow to the brain falls in parallel.[35] The fall in pressure is partly a function of continuing fall in fetal heart and thus of combined ventricular output[35] and partly the loss of redistribution of blood flow with a rise in femoral blood flow (FBF). Similar responses are also seen in the kidney and gut.[66,67]

In the latter half of the maximum survivable interval of asphyxia in the preterm fetus there is progressive failure of combined ventricular output, with a fall in both central and peripheral perfusion, both associated with falling blood pressure. This phase is much less likely to be seen for any significant duration in the term fetus as cardiac glycogen stores are depleted more quickly at term.[64] Thus, at 0.6 gestation the majority of fetuses survive up to 30 minutes of complete umbilical cord occlusion.[68] In contrast, term fetuses are unable to survive such prolonged periods of sustained hypotension, and typically will recover spontaneously from up to a maximum of 10–12 minutes of cord occlusion, whereas after a 15 minute period of complete occlusion the majority of fetuses either die or require active resuscitation with adrenaline after release of occlusion.[28,29,35] Thus, as a consequence of this extended survival during severe asphyxia, the premature fetus is exposed to extremely prolonged and profound hypotension and hypoperfusion. At 0.6 gestation, for example, no injury occurs after 20 minutes of complete umbilical cord occlusion even though hypotension is already present as shown in **Fig. 1**,[63] but severe subcortical injury occurs if the occlusion is continued for 30 minutes.[37] It may be speculated that during this final 10 minutes of asphyxia there is a catastrophic failure of redistribution of blood flow within the fetal brain, which places previously protected areas of the brain such as the brainstem at risk of injury,[53] consistent with clinical observations.[50]

## TEMPERATURE AND HYPOXIA-ISCHEMIA

Brain temperature during and after hypoxia-ischemia potently modulates outcome. Whereas hypothermia during experimental cerebral ischemia is consistently associated with potent, dose-related, long-lasting neuroprotection,[69] hyperthermia of even 1 to 2°C extends and markedly worsens damage, and promotes pan-necrosis.[70,71] The impact of cerebral cooling or warming the brain by only a few degrees is disproportionate to the known changes in brain metabolism (approximately a 5% change in oxidative metabolism per °C),[72] suggesting that changes in temperature modulate the secondary factors that mediate or increase ischemic injury. Mechanisms that are likely to be involved in the worsening of ischemic injury by hyperthermia include greater release of oxygen free radicals and excitatory neurotransmitters such as glutamate, enhanced toxicity of glutamate on neurons, increased dysfunction of the blood brain barrier, and accelerated cytoskeletal proteolysis.[69]

These data logically lead to the concept that although mild pyrexia during labor might not necessarily be harmful in most cases, in those fetuses also exposed to an acute hypoxic-ischemic event it would be expected to accelerate and worsen the development of encephalopathy. Case control and case series studies strongly suggest that maternal pyrexia is indeed associated with an approximately four fold increase in risk for unexplained cerebral palsy, or newborn encephalopathy.[73]

Clearly, this association could potentially be mediated by maternal infection or by the fetal inflammatory reaction. However, maternal pyrexia was a major component of the operational definition of chorio-amnionitis in all of these studies, and in several studies pyrexia was either considered sufficient for diagnosis even in isolation, or was the only criterion.[73] Consistent with the hypothesis that pyrexia can have a direct adverse effect, in a case control study of 38 term infants with early onset neonatal seizures, in whom sepsis or meningitis were excluded, and 152 controls, intrapartum fever was associated with a comparable 3.4-fold increase in the risk of unexplained neonatal seizures in a multifactorial analysis.[74]

In newborn rodents recent studies suggest intriguingly that exposure to mild infection or inflammation can sensitize the brain, so that short or milder periods of hypoxia-ischemia, which do not normally injure the developing brain, can trigger severe damage.[75–77] The effect is complex and time dependent. A low dose of LPS given either shortly (four or six hours) or well before (72 hours or more) hypoxia in rat pups was associated with *increased* injury ('sensitization').[76,78] In contrast, when given at an intermediate time (24 hours) before hypoxia-ischemia, LPS actually *reduced* injury ('tolerance').[78] In mice, fetal exposure to endotoxin affected the responses to hypoxia-ischemia even in adulthood, with both reduced and increased injury, in different regions.[75] Thus, given that profound asphyxia or septic shock causing acute injury around the time of birth are only seen in a minority of preterm infants, these data raise the intriguing possibility that sensitization by infection/inflammation may compromise the fetus such that even normally non injurious periods of hypoxia can be transformed into a damaging event.

## SUMMARY

The experimental studies reviewed above, and clinical experience,[5] strongly suggest that there is, and can be, no close, intrinsic pathophysiological relationship between the severity of metabolic acidosis, and fetal compromise. Peripheral acidosis is primarily a consequence of peripheral vasoconstriction, and reflects peripheral oxygen debt, which occurs during redistribution of combined ventricular output. Thus severe acidosis may accompany both successful protection of the brain, and catastrophic failure.[44] Conversely, brief but intense insults such as complete cord occlusion may cause brain injury in association with comparatively modest acidosis.[13] In contrast, we now know that there are very strong relationships both within and between paradigms between the development and severity of fetal blood pressure and impairment of cerebral perfusion, and the development of subsequent cerebral injury. The impact of hypotension is directly related to both its depth and cumulative duration in relationship to the brains' metabolic requirements given its developmental stage.

How this hypoxia-ischemia triggers different patterns of injury is not fully understood, but key factors include profound hypotension and the pattern of the insult. The link between profound hypotension/hypoperfusion during asphyxia and subcortical damage in the preterm fetus likely reflects compromise of the initial intracerebral redistribution of blood flow from the forebrain to the subcortical areas. Of particular interest to clinicians, it is striking that repeated, relatively prolonged episodes of asphyxia or ischemia (5 to 10 minutes) are associated with selective basal ganglia damage, and that the proportion of basal ganglia damage relative to cortical injury increases as the interval between insults is increased. This relationship emphasizes the importance of interaction between even relatively benign, non-injurious individual periods of hypoxia-ischemia in labor that can lead to regionally specific, compounding damage.

## ACKNOWLEDGMENTS

The authors' work reported in this review has been supported by the Health Research Council of New Zealand, Lottery Health Board of New Zealand, the Auckland Medical Research Foundation, and the March of Dimes Birth Defects Trust.

## REFERENCES

1. Gunn AJ, Gunn TR. Changes in risk factors for hypoxic-ischaemic seizures in term infants. Aust N Z J Obstet Gynaecol 1997;37(1):36–9.
2. Wyatt JS, Gluckman PD, Liu PY, et al. Determinants of outcomes after head cooling for neonatal encephalopathy. Pediatrics 2007;119(5):912–21.
3. Nelson KB, Dambrosia JM, Ting TY, et al. Uncertain value of electronic fetal monitoring in predicting cerebral palsy. N Engl J Med 1996;334(10):613–8.
4. Wayenberg JL. Threshold of metabolic acidosis associated with neonatal encephalopathy in the term newborn. J Matern Fetal Neonatal Med 2005;18(6): 381–5.
5. Low JA, Lindsay BG, Derrick EJ. Threshold of metabolic acidosis associated with newborn complications. Am J Obstet Gynecol 1997;177(6):1391–4.
6. Westgate JA, Gunn AJ, Gunn TR. Antecedents of neonatal encephalopathy with fetal acidaemia at term. BJOG 1999;106(8):774–82.
7. MacLennan A, for the International Cerebral Palsy Task Force, Gunn AJ, et al. A template for defining a causal relation between acute intrapartum events and cerebral palsy: international consensus statement. BMJ 1999;319(7216):1054–9.

8. Robertson CM, Finer NN. Long-term follow-up of term neonates with perinatal asphyxia. Clin Perinatol 1993;20(2):483–500.

9. Barlow RM. The foetal sheep: morphogenesis of the nervous system and histochemical aspects of myelination. J Comp Neurol 1969;135(3):249–62.

10. McIntosh GH, Baghurst KI, Potter BJ, et al. Foetal brain development in the sheep. Neuropathol Appl Neurobiol 1979;5(2):103–14.

11. Bennet L, Westgate J, Gluckman PD, et al. Fetal responses to asphyxia. In: Stevenson DK, Sunshine P, editors. Fetal and neonatal brain injury: mechanisms, management, and the risks of practice. 2nd edition. Cambridge: Cambridge University Press; 2003. p. 83–110.

12. Hossmann KA. Pathophysiology and therapy of experimental stroke. Cell Mol Neurobiol 2006;26(7–8):1057–83.

13. Hunter CJ, Bennet L, Power GG, et al. Key neuroprotective role for endogenous adenosine A1 receptor activation during asphyxia in the fetal sheep. Stroke 2003; 34(9):2240–5.

14. Lorek A, Takei Y, Cady EB, et al. Delayed ("secondary") cerebral energy failure after acute hypoxia-ischemia in the newborn piglet: continuous 48-hour studies by phosphorus magnetic resonance spectroscopy. Pediatr Res 1994;36(6): 699–706.

15. Blumberg RM, Cady EB, Wigglesworth JS, et al. Relation between delayed impairment of cerebral energy metabolism and infarction following transient focal hypoxia-ischaemia in the developing brain. Exp Brain Res 1997;113(1): 130–7.

16. Williams CE, Gunn A, Gluckman PD. Time course of intracellular edema and epileptiform activity following prenatal cerebral ischemia in sheep. Stroke 1991; 22(4):516–21.

17. Azzopardi D, Wyatt JS, Cady EB, et al. Prognosis of newborn infants with hypoxic-ischemic brain injury assessed by phosphorus magnetic resonance spectroscopy. Pediatr Res 1989;25(5):445–51.

18. Roth SC, Baudin J, Cady E, et al. Relation of deranged neonatal cerebral oxidative metabolism with neurodevelopmental outcome and head circumference at 4 years. Dev Med Child Neurol 1997;39(11):718–25.

19. Mallard EC, Williams CE, Gunn AJ, et al. Frequent episodes of brief ischemia sensitize the fetal sheep brain to neuronal loss and induce striatal injury. Pediatr Res 1993;33(1):61–5.

20. Mallard EC, Williams CE, Johnston BM, et al. Increased vulnerability to neuronal damage after umbilical cord occlusion in fetal sheep with advancing gestation. Am J Obstet Gynecol 1994;170(1 Pt 1):206–14.

21. Mallard EC, Williams CE, Johnston BM, et al. Repeated episodes of umbilical cord occlusion in fetal sheep lead to preferential damage to the striatum and sensitize the heart to further insults. Pediatr Res 1995;37(6):707–13.

22. Giussani DA, Spencer JAD, Hanson MA. Fetal and cardiovascular reflex responses to hypoxaemia. Fetal Matern Med Rev 1994;6:17–37.

23. Jensen A, Garnier Y, Berger R. Dynamics of fetal circulatory responses to hypoxia and asphyxia. Eur J Obstet Gynecol Reprod Biol 1999;84(2):155–72.

24. Lee SJ, Hatran DP, Tomimatsu T, et al. Fetal cerebral blood flow, electrocorticographic activity, and oxygenation: responses to acute hypoxia. J Physiol 2009; 587(Pt 9):2033–47.

25. Richardson BS, Bocking AD. Metabolic and circulatory adaptations to chronic hypoxia in the fetus. Comp Biochem Physiol A Mol Integr Physiol 1998;119(3): 717–23.

26. Danielson L, McMillen IC, Dyer JL, et al. Restriction of placental growth results in greater hypotensive response to alpha-adrenergic blockade in fetal sheep during late gestation. J Physiol 2005;563(Pt 2):611–20.

27. Parer JT. Effects of fetal asphyxia on brain cell structure and function: limits of tolerance. Comp Biochem Physiol A Mol Integr Physiol 1998;119(3):711–6.

28. Mallard EC, Gunn AJ, Williams CE, et al. Transient umbilical cord occlusion causes hippocampal damage in the fetal sheep. Am J Obstet Gynecol 1992; 167(5):1423–30.

29. Bennet L, Peebles DM, Edwards AD, et al. The cerebral hemodynamic response to asphyxia and hypoxia in the near- term fetal sheep as measured by near infrared spectroscopy. Pediatr Res 1998;44(6):951–7.

30. de Haan HH, van Reempts JL, Vles JS, et al. Effects of asphyxia on the fetal lamb brain. Am J Obstet Gynecol 1993;169(6):1493–501.

31. Barcroft J. Researches in prenatal life. London, Oxford: Blackwell Scientific Publications Ltd; 1946.

32. Giussani DA, Spencer JA, Moore PJ, et al. Afferent and efferent components of the cardiovascular reflex responses to acute hypoxia in term fetal sheep. J Physiol 1993;461:431–49.

33. Itskovitz J, Rudolph AM. Denervation of arterial chemoreceptors and baroreceptors in fetal lambs in utero. Am J Physiol 1982;242(5):H916–20.

34. Bartelds B, van Bel F, Teitel DF, et al. Carotid, not aortic, chemoreceptors mediate the fetal cardiovascular response to acute hypoxemia in lambs. Pediatr Res 1993;34(1):51–5.

35. Wassink G, Bennet L, Booth LC, et al. The ontogeny of hemodynamic responses to prolonged umbilical cord occlusion in fetal sheep. J Appl Physiol 2007;103(4):1311–7.

36. Gunn AJ, Quaedackers JS, Guan J, et al. The premature fetus: not as defenseless as we thought, but still paradoxically vulnerable? Dev Neurosci 2001; 23(3):175–9.

37. George S, Gunn AJ, Westgate JA, et al. Fetal heart rate variability and brainstem injury after asphyxia in preterm fetal sheep. Am J Physiol Regul Integr Comp Physiol 2004;287(4):R925–33.

38. Jensen A, Hohmann M, Kunzel W. Dynamic changes in organ blood flow and oxygen consumption during acute asphyxia in fetal sheep. J Dev Physiol 1987; 9(6):543–59.

39. Gunn AJ, Maxwell L, de Haan HH, et al. Delayed hypotension and subendocardial injury after repeated umbilical cord occlusion in near-term fetal lambs. Am J Obstet Gynecol 2000;183(6):1564–72.

40. Bennet L, Booth LC, Ahmed-Nasef N, et al. Male disadvantage? Fetal sex and cardiovascular responses to asphyxia in preterm fetal sheep. Am J Physiol Regul Integr Comp Physiol 2007;293(3):R1280–6.

41. Gunn AJ, Gunn TR, de Haan HH, et al. Dramatic neuronal rescue with prolonged selective head cooling after ischemia in fetal lambs. J Clin Invest 1997;99(2): 248–56.

42. Gunn AJ, Parer JT, Mallard EC, et al. Cerebral histologic and electrocorticographic changes after asphyxia in fetal sheep. Pediatr Res 1992;31(5):486–91.

43. Ikeda T, Murata Y, Quilligan EJ, et al. Physiologic and histologic changes in near-term fetal lambs exposed to asphyxia by partial umbilical cord occlusion. Am J Obstet Gynecol 1998;178(1 Pt 1):24–32.

44. de Haan HH, Gunn AJ, Williams CE, et al. Brief repeated umbilical cord occlusions cause sustained cytotoxic cerebral edema and focal infarcts in near-term fetal lambs. Pediatr Res 1997;41(1):96–104.

45. Torvik A. The pathogenesis of watershed infarcts in the brain. Stroke 1984;15(2): 221–3.
46. Rees S, Mallard C, Breen S, et al. Fetal brain injury following prolonged hypoxemia and placental insufficiency: a review. Comp Biochem Physiol A Mol Integr Physiol 1998;119(3):653–60.
47. de Haan HH, Gunn AJ, Williams CE, et al. Magnesium sulfate therapy during asphyxia in near-term fetal lambs does not compromise the fetus but does not reduce cerebral injury. Am J Obstet Gynecol 1997;176(1 Pt 1):18–27.
48. Okereafor A, Allsop J, Counsell SJ, et al. Patterns of brain injury in neonates exposed to perinatal sentinel events. Pediatrics 2008;121(5):906–14.
49. Miller SP, Ramaswamy V, Michelson D, et al. Patterns of brain injury in term neonatal encephalopathy. J Pediatr 2005;146(4):453–60.
50. Barkovich AJ, Sargent SK. Profound asphyxia in the premature infant: imaging findings. Am J Neuroradiol 1995;16(9):1837–46.
51. Jensen A, Lang U, Kunzel W. Microvascular dynamics during acute asphyxia in chronically prepared fetal sheep near term. Adv Exp Med Biol 1987;220:127–31.
52. Pulgar VM, Zhang J, Massmann GA, et al. Mild chronic hypoxia modifies the fetal sheep neural and cardiovascular responses to repeated umbilical cord occlusion. Brain Res 2007;1176:18–26.
53. Myers RE. Experimental models of perinatal brain damage: relevance to human pathology. In: Gluck L, editor. Intrauterine asphyxia and the developing fetal brain. Chicago: Year Book Medical; 1977. p. 37–97.
54. Simpson IA, Carruthers A, Vannucci SJ. Supply and demand in cerebral energy metabolism: the role of nutrient transporters. J Cereb Blood Flow Metab 2007; 27(11):1766–91.
55. Vannucci SJ, Maher F, Simpson IA. Glucose transporter proteins in brain: delivery of glucose to neurons and glia. Glia 1997;21(1):2–21.
56. LeBlanc MH, Huang M, Vig V, et al. Glucose affects the severity of hypoxic-ischemic brain injury in newborn pigs. Stroke 1993;24(7):1055–62.
57. Westgate J, Wassink G, Bennet L, et al. Spontaneous hypoxia in multiple pregnancy is associated with early fetal decompensation and greater T wave elevation during brief repeated cord occlusion in near-term fetal sheep. Am J Obstet Gynecol 2005;193(4):1526–33.
58. McMillen IC, Robinson JS. Developmental origins of the metabolic syndrome: prediction, plasticity, and programming. Physiol Rev 2005;85(2):571–633.
59. Hawkins P, Steyn C, McGarrigle HH, et al. Effect of maternal nutrient restriction in early gestation on responses of the hypothalamic-pituitary-adrenal axis to acute isocapnic hypoxaemia in late gestation fetal sheep. Exp Physiol 2000;85(1):85–96.
60. Jellyman JK, Gardner DS, Edwards CM, et al. Fetal cardiovascular, metabolic and endocrine responses to acute hypoxaemia during and following maternal treatment with dexamethasone in sheep. J Physiol 2005;567(Pt 2):673–88.
61. Committee on Understanding Premature Birth and Assuring Healthy Outcomes. In: Behrman RE, Butler AS, editors. Preterm birth: causes, consequences, and prevention. Washington, DC: Institute of Medicine of the National Academies; 2007.
62. Badawi N, Felix JF, Kurinczuk JJ, et al. Cerebral palsy following term newborn encephalopathy: a population-based study. Dev Med Child Neurol 2005;47(5): 293–8.
63. Keunen H, Blanco CE, van Reempts JL, et al. Absence of neuronal damage after umbilical cord occlusion of 10, 15, and 20 minutes in midgestation fetal sheep. Am J Obstet Gynecol 1997;176(3):515–20.

64. Shelley HJ. Glycogen reserves and their changes at birth and in anoxia. Br Med Bull 1961;17:137–43.
65. Iwamoto HS, Kaufman T, Keil LC, et al. Responses to acute hypoxemia in fetal sheep at 0.6–0.7 gestation. Am J Physiol 1989;256(3 Pt 2):H613–20.
66. Quaedackers JS, Roelfsema V, Hunter CJ, et al. Polyuria and impaired renal blood flow after asphyxia in preterm fetal sheep. Am J Physiol Regul Integr Comp Physiol 2004;286(3):R576–83.
67. Bennet L, Quaedackers JS, Gunn AJ, et al. The effect of asphyxia on superior mesenteric artery blood flow in the premature sheep fetus. J Pediatr Surg 2000;35(1):34–40.
68. Bennet L, Rossenrode S, Gunning MI, et al. The cardiovascular and cerebrovascular responses of the immature fetal sheep to acute umbilical cord occlusion. J Physiol 1999;517(Pt 1):247–57.
69. Gunn AJ, Thoresen M. Hypothermic neuroprotection. NeuroRx 2006;3(2):154–69.
70. Busto R, Dietrich WD, Globus MY, et al. Small differences in intraischemic brain temperature critically determine the extent of ischemic neuronal injury. J Cereb Blood Flow Metab 1987;7(6):729–38.
71. Minamisawa H, Smith ML, Siesjo BK. The effect of mild hyperthermia and hypothermia on brain damage following 5, 10, and 15 minutes of forebrain ischemia. Ann Neurol 1990;28(1):26–33.
72. Laptook AR, Corbett RJ, Sterett R, et al. Quantitative relationship between brain temperature and energy utilization rate measured in vivo using 31P and 1H magnetic resonance spectroscopy. Pediatr Res 1995;38(6):919–25.
73. Gunn AJ, Bennet L. Is temperature important in delivery room resuscitation? Semin Neonatol 2001;6(3):241–9.
74. Lieberman E, Eichenwald E, Mathur G, et al. Intrapartum fever and unexplained seizures in term infants. Pediatrics 2000;106(5):983–8.
75. Wang X, Hagberg H, Nie C, et al. Dual role of intrauterine immune challenge on neonatal and adult brain vulnerability to hypoxia-ischemia. J Neuropathol Exp Neurol 2007;66(6):552–61.
76. Eklind S, Mallard C, Leverin AL, et al. Bacterial endotoxin sensitizes the immature brain to hypoxic–ischaemic injury. Eur J Neurosci 2001;13(6):1101–6.
77. Larouche A, Roy M, Kadhim H, et al. Neuronal injuries induced by perinatal hypoxic-ischemic insults are potentiated by prenatal exposure to lipopolysaccharide: animal model for perinatally acquired encephalopathy. Dev Neurosci 2005; 27(2–4):134–42.
78. Eklind S, Mallard C, Arvidsson P, et al. Lipopolysaccharide induces both a primary and a secondary phase of sensitization in the developing rat brain. Pediatr Res 2005;58(1):112–6.

# Fetal Effects of Psychoactive Drugs

Amy L. Salisbury, PhD[a,c,d,]*, Kathryn L. Ponder, BS[b,c],
James F. Padbury, MD[b,c], Barry M. Lester, PhD[a,c,d]

**KEYWORDS**

- Cocaine • Methamphetamine • SSRI
- Maternal depression • Fetal behavior

There has been a long-standing concern with the fetal effects of psychoactive drug use by pregnant women. This article describes the effects of three drugs with similar molecular targets that involve monoaminergic transmitter systems. These stimulants include the illegal drugs cocaine and methamphetamine (MA) and the class of selective serotonin reuptake inhibitors (SSRIs) used to treat maternal depression during pregnancy. Discussed are the mechanisms of action of each drug, including a possible common epigenetic mechanism for their effects on the developing child. Also discussed are fetal neurobehavioral techniques that may be useful in the early detection of the effects of in utero drug exposure.

In the past three decades, the concept of behavioral teratology[1] expanded the field of teratology to examine behavioral effects in the neonate caused by acute exposure to substances in utero, including environmental, nutritional, and drug exposures.[2,3] The developmental consequences of prenatal exposure to a toxic substance may include central nervous system (CNS) insult related to the period during gestation of the exposure. Damaging effects of drugs on the developing brain are quite different from those in the adult brain; often resulting in prevention of normal formation of various brain areas.[4] The effects of exposure during the first half of gestation impact processes related to cytogenesis and histogenesis, whereas effects during the second half of gestation relate to brain growth and differentiation. During this

This work was supported by National Institutes of Health grants MH6547 (Salisbury) and P20RR018728 (Padbury).

[a] Department of Pediatrics, Brown Center for the Study of Children at Risk, Women and Infants Hospital of Rhode Island, 101 Dudley Street, Providence, RI 02905, USA

[b] Warren Alpert Medical School of Brown University, Box G-A, Providence, RI 02912, USA

[c] Department of Pediatrics, Warren Alpert Medical School of Brown University, Box G-A, Providence, RI 02912, USA

[d] Department of Psychiatry, Warren Alpert Medical School of Brown University, Box G-A, Providence, RI 02912, USA

* Corresponding author. Department of Pediatrics, Brown Center for the Study of Children at Risk, Women and Infants Hospital of Rhode Island, 101 Dudley Street, Providence, RI 02905.
*E-mail address:* amy_salisbury@brown.edu (A.L. Salisbury).

Clin Perinatol 36 (2009) 595–619
doi:10.1016/j.clp.2009.06.002
0095-5108/09/$ – see front matter © 2009 Elsevier Inc. All rights reserved.

perinatology.theclinics.com

organizational phase in the second half of gestation, progressive events (neuroblast proliferation and migration, axonal projection, and synaptogenesis) and regressive events (programmed cell death and selective elimination of processes) affect the maturation of brain circuitry. Toxic influences during this period may dramatically alter brain development but may also alter the regressive events that underlie the capacity of the developing brain to compensate for injury.[4]

Recent years have seen further expansion of the principles of behavioral teratology to examine exposure effects on the human fetus at the time of the exposure. Epigenetic and organismic models of developmental theory suggest that true understanding of a developing system can occur with the study of its organization of form and structure as it moves toward a teleologic state.[5,6] This includes examination of the mutual influences of genes, physiology, and behavior as well as the physical, cultural, and social environments of the organism.[6] The use of such models are applicable to the study of outcomes from prenatal psychoactive drug exposure.

Increasing evidence from preclinical, prospective clinical, and epidemiologic studies suggests that many biologic factors acting during prenatal life are associated with adult disease and long-term neurobehavioral abnormalities[7-17] and behavioral disorders.[18-21] The notion that the development of common adult cardiovascular and metabolic disorders is linked to factors during prenatal development was originally known as the "Barker" or "fetal origins hypothesis."[7,9,10] Although these early studies related low birth weight to adult disease, it is generally accepted that low birth weight per se is not at the heart of these disorders, but that there are common factors that influence intrauterine growth and adult physiologic systems.[22] The fetal origins observations are caused, in part, by environmental factors acting early in life that affect developing systems, altering structure and function. It has been suggested that the biologic purpose of this programming is to alter the set-points or hard-wire physiologic systems to prepare the fetus for optimal adaptation to the postnatal environment.[23]

Because the postnatal environment is not always as anticipated, the degree to which these systems can adapt and adjust to a range of environments and conditions may predict later outcomes. Therefore, longitudinal study of the organism and contexts beginning before or at the time of exposure, and of long-term outcomes, is essential to understanding developmental trajectories related to substance exposures.

## COCAINE

In the 1980s, cocaine became one of the most frequently abused illicit drugs during pregnancy and also one of the most studied with regard to its potential teratologic and neurodevelopmental effects on the developing fetus and child. Although early catastrophic predictions about the long-term outcome of prenatally cocaine-exposed children were exaggerated, concern remains about more subtle effects[24] that may affect development, particularly in childhood and adolescence.

The neurochemical and vasoconstrictive effects of cocaine have been well documented. Cocaine acts primarily at the presynaptic level to block reuptake of the monoaminergic neurotransmitters dopamine, norepinephrine, and serotonin[25,26] by specific, presynaptic plasma membrane transporters.[27] These transporters are expressed in discrete pathways of the CNS, on postganglionic sympathetic neurons, and in the adrenal medulla. These pharmacologic actions lead to elevated circulating catecholamine levels and exaggerated sympathetic responses including hypertension, tachycardia, vasoconstriction, agitation, euphoria, and excitation. These effects are particularly profound in the fetus in which elevated sympathetic tone has been demonstrated.[28–31] Cocaine affects neuronal formation, proliferation, and early connectivity,[32–34] and disrupts neuronal migration and resulting cortical architecture.[35–38] Cocaine also affects the expression of transcription factors (immediate early genes) along dopaminergic[39,40] and serotonergic pathways.[41] Because monoamine neurotransmitter receptors (NA, 5-HT, and dopamine) are present early in corticogenesis, areas highly expressing these neurotransmitter systems may be especially susceptible to elevated synaptic monoamine neurotransmitter levels secondary to cocaine's main effect of blocking catecholamine reuptake at the presynaptic level.[42–44] Also, because monoamine neurotransmitters play a key trophic role in brain development,[45] prenatal cocaine may alter normal mechanisms that modulate neuronal growth.[42]

The effects of cocaine on fetal development have also been attributed to vasoconstrictive mechanisms. Uptake inhibitors, such as cocaine (and amphetamines and SSRIs), which block catecholamine transport[28,46] and decrease placental blood flow, reduce the supply of oxygen and nutrients to the fetus. Fetal hypoxemia and possibly ischemic injury can compromise brain development. Blood flow to the developing brain can also be reduced by cocaine-related noradrenergic effects on the developing fetal vasculature.[47,48] Norepinephrine and particularly the monoamine serotonin (5-HT) exert vasoconstrictive effects on the umbilical vein, thereby reducing blood flow from the placenta to the fetus.[49,50] Furthermore, the vascular response to 5-HT is potentiated by uptake inhibition.[51,52] Vasoconstriction at the uteroplacental complex coupled with anorexic effects of cocaine could explain the increase in intrauterine growth retardation that has been reported in cocaine-exposed infants.[53]

In addition to neurochemical and vasoconstrictive effects, cocaine may also act as an intrauterine stressor that alters fetal programming through epigenetic mechanisms that might alter the offspring's developmental trajectory.[54] In this model, cocaine alters the expression of key candidate genes and gene networks important to placental function in late gestation, specifically norepinephrine transporter (NET)[55] and a steroid metabolic enzyme, 11β-hydroxysteroid dehydrogenase-2 (11β-HSD-2). Placental NET and 11β-HSD-2 protect the fetus from excess catecholamines and glucocorticoids, which have harmful effects on the fetus.[56] 11β-HSD-2 in particular converts maternal cortisol to inert cortisone, protecting the developing fetus from exposure to maternal cortisol.[57] Placental expression of 11β-HSD-2 is downregulated by norepinephrine, which is in turn regulated by NET.[58] Prenatal cocaine exposure is associated with downregulation of NET,[59,60] which leads to increased circulating catecholamines, downregulation of 11β-HSD-2, and chronic fetal hypercortisolism. These changes in placental gene expression may be caused by epigenetic mechanisms including DNA methylation, as suggested by the findings in **Figs. 1** and **2**.[54] **Fig. 1** shows decreased 11β-HSD-2 expression in mothers who used cocaine (N = 4) or cigarettes (N = 4) or were depressed (N = 3), compared with 17 controls. The altered expression of these two key candidate genes is likely associated with changes in networks of genes involved in critical placental functions that maintain physiologic homeostasis in utero and otherwise promote intrauterine growth, development, and preparation for postnatal life. **Fig. 2** suggests that these changes in placental gene expression are associated with methylation of placental genomic DNA, particularly in promoter regions. These findings in **Fig. 2** are based on the same group of subjects with pregnancies complicated by cocaine, nicotine, and depression, and controls, shown in **Fig. 1**. The relative incorporation of cytosine used to measure methylation was comparable in promoter and genomic DNA in the cocaine- and nicotine-exposed subjects, suggesting hypermethylation of the promoter regions of DNA that contain CpG islands. This hypermethylation of DNA suggests gene silencing related to in utero cocaine exposure.

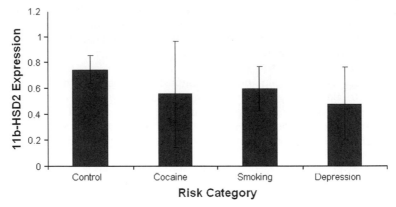

**Fig. 1.** Mean 11β-HSD-2 expression in risk groups. (*Adapted from* Lester B, Padbury J. The third pathophysiology of prenatal cocaine exposure. Dev Neurosci 2009;31:23–35; with permission.)

A substantial literature exists on the relationships between varying circadian cortisol levels and stress responses and child development[61] including infants with prenatal cocaine exposure.[62–64] Preclinical studies suggest effects of prenatal cocaine exposure on the developing monoaminergic system, resulting in both structural and functional changes to circuitry subserving functions, such as arousal, regulation, and reactivity.[43,65] Human infant studies show effects of prenatal cocaine exposure on arousal, hypertonicity and excitability, acoustic cry characteristics,[66] and auditory brain response.[67] At school age these children show more behavior problems[68] and they are more likely referred for special education services.[69] On functional neuroimaging (fMRI) they show differences in the right inferior frontal cortex and caudate during response inhibition, suggesting cocaine effects on brain systems involved in the regulation of attention and response inhibition.[70] This set of cognitive abilities is referred to as "executive function" and is particularly important as children reach school age. A recent review of 42 follow-up studies of cocaine-exposed children suggested

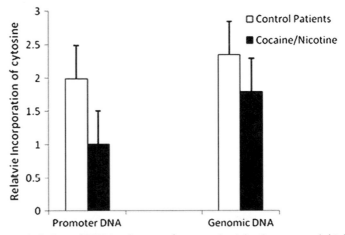

**Fig. 2.** Hypermethylation of DNA in placentas from cocaine/nicotine exposed. (*Adapted from* Lester B, Padbury J. The third pathophysiology of prenatal cocaine exposure. Dev Neurosci 2009;31:23–35; with permission.)

that executive function and behavior problems were major domains affected by prenatal cocaine exposure.[71] Fetal programming effects that alter the intrauterine neuroendocrine environment may be a marker for long-term behavioral consequences of prenatal cocaine exposure.

## METHAMPHETAMINE

MA is the dominant drug problem in the Western and Midwestern portions of the United States, second only to alcohol and marijuana,[72] and is the most widely abused drug worldwide.[73,74] The number of adults age 12 and over who have tried MA once in their lifetime has increased to 5.3% in 2007 from 4.3% in 1999 and 2.5% in 1997.[75] This increase has led to the concern that MA is the growing drug of choice for adults in the United States, including pregnant women.[76–78]

Although there is controversy about the nature and extent of the MA problem in the United States, including exaggerations reminiscent of the cocaine "epidemic," there is little argument that MA is a dangerous drug that substantially challenges policy-makers, health care professionals, social service providers, and the law enforcement community,[79] and there is little information about MA use by pregnant women.

MA is a CNS stimulant of the sympathetic nervous system with neurotoxic potential for developing monoaminergic systems. As the first cousin of amphetamine with the addition of a methyl radical, MA exerts its action by releasing dopamine and serotonin, blocking monoamine reuptake mechanisms, and inhibiting monoamine oxidase.[80] The mechanism of action most likely occurs by increasing synaptic concentrations of the neurotransmitters dopamine and norepinephrine[80] either by direct release from storage vesicles or by inhibition of reuptake.[81,82] MA may enhance synaptic catechol-amine levels by inhibiting monoamine oxidase, the enzyme responsible for the oxidation of norepinephrine and serotonin.[83] MA acts on the dopamine transporter that mediates the inward transmission of dopamine in the neuron. The action of MA on dopamine transporter releases dopamine and inhibits reuptake of dopamine from the presynaptic terminals, increasing dopamine activity.[84] MA also decreases sero-tonin (5-HT) uptake and densities of binding sites.[85] MA has been shown to be neuro-toxic to mature dopaminergic and serotonergic axons and axon terminal arbors,[86] and potentially neurotoxic to mature glutaminergic axons.[87] The cellular and molecular mechanisms implicated in the neurotoxicity induced by MA on mature neurons include the production of reactive oxygen species and nitric oxide, p53 activation resulting in apoptosis, and mitochondrial dysfunction.[88] Less is known about the mechanisms involved in MA-induced toxicity in the developing CNS; however, the early and wide-spread influence of serotonergic, dopaminergic, and glutaminergic systems on neuronal growth and connectivity suggests that prenatal exposure to MA may result in alterations in developing neural circuitry.[87]

Amphetamines are considered noncatecholamine sympathomimetics because they lack catecholamine structure yet have sympathomimetic actions.[89] These structural characteristics are important because they account for the wide distribution and long duration of action of amphetamine. MA also has vasoconstrictive effects[90] result-ing in decreased uteroplacental blood flow and fetal hypoxia.[91] In addition, MA has anorexic effects on the mother. These maternal-placental effects could affect fetal development to the previously mentioned monoaminergic effects. Weight control may also help explain the popularity of MA with women, including pregnant women.

Unfortunately, the scant human literature that is available on the effects of prenatal MA exposure is beset by methodologic problems.[92] Recent, more reliable findings showed that MA-exposed infants, although born at term, are more likely to be small for gestational age.[93] Newborn neurobehavioral effects were reminiscent of cocaine-exposed infants showing effects on arousal and physiologic stress.[94] In addition, these findings showed a dose-response relationship between amphetamine metabolites in meconium and newborn neurobehavior.

In preclinical work, administration of MA to laboratory animals results in profound and long-lasting toxicity to the developing CNS. Brain studies in the ovine model have found MA increases fetal blood pressure and decreases fetal oxyhemoglobin saturation and arterial pH.[91,95] In rodents, MA is toxic to dopaminergic and serotonergic neurons.[96,97] Damage to dopamine terminals[98,99] is thought to reflect irreversible terminal degeneration.[100] Positron emission tomography studies in abstinent MA users demonstrated decreased dopamine transporters, suggesting long-lasting neurotoxicity caused by MA abuse.[101]

Neurotoxic effects of prenatal MA exposure on serotonergic neurons produce neurochemical alternations in the CNS[102,103] thought to be associated with learning impairment, behavioral deficits,[103] increased motor activity,[104] enhanced conditioned avoidance responses,[105] and postural motor movements[106] seen in MA-exposed animals. Rhesus monkeys showed reduced brain monoamines 4 years after the last drug exposure.[107]

Administration of MA to laboratory animals also results in motor[108] and learning and memory impairment.[109] Studies with rats have shown a range of physical, motor, neurotransmitter, and behavioral effects in MA-exposed offspring. These include increased maternal and offspring mortality, retinal eye defects,[104,110,111] cleft palate and rib malformations,[111] and decreased rate of physical growth and delayed motor development.[105,110] MA exposure to pregnant dams showed effects on spatial learning in their adult offspring.[106] Spatial learning and attenuated corticosterone response was found in rats with prenatal MA exposure.[112] In pregnant mice, MA caused dopaminergic nerve terminal degeneration and long-term motor deficits in offspring.[113]

Consistent with the fetal programming model described previously, the human placenta may also be a direct target for MA. MA causes inhibition of the norepinephrine and serotonin transporters, suggesting cellular mechanisms by which MA could affect the developing fetus.[114] Blockage of these transporters increases the concentrations of norepinephrine and serotonin, resulting in constriction of blood vessels and decreased blood flow to the placenta. Also, placental NET downregulation resulting from MA could lead to increases in circulating catecholamines, downregulation of 11β-HSD-2, and chronic fetal hypercortisolism,[28,59] which could affect behavior through alteration of the hypothalamic-pituitary-adrenal axis, especially arousal regulation and attention.[43]

## SELECTIVE SEROTONIN REUPTAKE INHIBITORS

Each year at least 600,000 infants born in the United States are exposed to maternal major depressive disorder during gestation, which is associated with newborn medical and neurobehavioral deficits and long-term emotional, behavioral, and social problems in the child. Pharmacologic treatment of major depressive disorder during pregnancy remains the most common form of treatment. The current first-line choice of clinicians for somatic therapies during pregnancy is SSRIs and dual-action serotonin and norepinephrine reuptake inhibitors (referred to collectively here as SRIs) because of their lower side-effect profiles and relatively low risk to the fetus.[115,116] Over the past two decades, the use of newer antidepressants has dramatically increased over the use of tricyclic antidepressants and monoamine oxidase inhibitors. A survey of national patterns of antidepressant medication prescribed by physicians from 1987 to 2001 reported that SRIs were prescribed in 69% of office visits for depression in 2001.[117] Similarly, another study reported that in 2000, 65% of all antidepressants prescribed by primary care providers were SSRIs (fluoxetine, sertraline, paroxetine, fluvoxamine, and citalopram); newer antidepressants, including serotonin and norepinephrine reuptake inhibitors, such as venlafaxine, comprised an additional 17% of antidepressants prescribed.[118] A recent study examining antidepressant treatment rates during pregnancy found that at least 37% of depressed pregnant women choose to take antidepressant medications during pregnancy.[119] Another large study conducted retrospectively from 1996 to 2005 showed the use of SRIs during pregnancy to have a steady increase from 1.5% in 1996 to 6.2% of all pregnant women in 2005.[120]

SRIs block the presynaptic reuptake of serotonin (5-HT) by binding to the serotonin transporter (SERT). Some of the SRIs also bind to NET. SERT and NET are responsible for the reuptake and transport of 5-HT and norepinephrine out of the synapse. Inhibition of SERT and NET activity by SRIs prolongs neurotransmitter signaling. Fluoxetine has also recently been found to antagonize $5-HT_{2c}$ receptors. The antidepressant mechanisms of SRIs and many other psychoactive drugs remain unclear, but are presumed to be a result of the enhanced serotonergic neurotransmission at postsynaptic receptors, the effect on intracellular signal transduction cascades, and the modulation of other neurotransmitters.[121]

SRIs and their metabolites have been detected in both umbilical cord blood and amniotic fluid. The potency of serotonin placental passage, expressed as a ratio of medication concentration in cord blood to maternal serum, ranged from 0.29 (sertraline and paroxetine) to 0.89 (citalopram and fluoxetine).[122] A study of cord:maternal serum levels found roughly equivalent values for fluoxetine, sertraline, and paroxetine and their metabolites (0.52–0.67), whereas the concentration for the SRI venlafaxine was 1.1.[123] SRIs have also been found in amniotic fluid, representing another source of exposure because the fetus swallows an increasing amount of amniotic fluid throughout pregnancy.[124] Administration of fluoxetine to pregnant ewes was associated with a transient decrease in uterine artery blood flow, perhaps caused by serotonin activity following administration.[125] Immediately following fluoxetine administration, there was an increase in plasma serotonin concentrations. With prolonged exposure, however, plasma serotonin levels declined. Serotonin acts as a vasoconstrictor, therefore a transient elevation in serotonin might explain a temporary decrease in uterine artery blood flow. Changes in serotonin levels throughout development in exposed offspring may be one mechanism by which SRI medication influences adverse effects.

The serotonergic system develops early in gestation and is likely to be influenced by serotonin levels in all trimesters of pregnancy.[126] Serotonin is widely distributed throughout the central and peripheral nervous systems and is involved in the development of multiple brain areas.[126–129] Alterations in the 5-HT system during development are associated with changes in somatosensory processing, motor output, and emotional responses.[130,131] Recent evidence suggests that components of the serotonin system are critical to the development of neurobehavioral systems involved in mood, anxiety, aggression, and substance abuse.[131,132]

The serotonin system includes at least 14 receptors, multiple enzymes, and transporter proteins that exert influence on 5-HT metabolism, release, and reuptake. The serotonin transporter gene 5-HTT (SLC6A4) encodes for the transporter protein. The promoter region of the gene contains two common polymorphic alleles, a short or "S" allele with 14 repeated elements, and a long or "L" allele with 16 repeated elements. The variant region has been labeled the "serotonin transporter linked poly-morphic region."[133] Functionally, the deletion polymorphism ("s", or short allele) seems to cause a reduction in basal and stimulated transcription activity, 5-HTT mRNA, and 5-HT binding and uptake.[134] Individuals with the S allele (S/S or S/L) have been more susceptible to stress, depression, anxiety, suicidal ideation, and irritable temperament. Longitudinal research suggests a gene-environment interaction, in that those with the S allele are more susceptible to depression given stressful conditions.[135] Allelic differences have also been linked to responsiveness to antidepressant medication.[136]

A recent meta-analysis of the effects of SRIs on pregnancy and fetal physical development included published reports from 1995 through August of 2005.[137] The findings of the meta-analysis are in agreement with most of the previous reviews that did not find an increased risk of major, cardiovascular, or minor malformations, but did find an increased risk of spontaneous abortion.[138,139] The findings are in disagreement with reports of a higher rate of major cardiac malformations and persistent pulmonary hypertension of the newborn for infants exposed to SRIs compared with other antidepressant medications and controls.[140,141]

Lower birth weight, younger gestational age at birth, and lower Apgar scores have been reported with SRI exposure.[142] Similar results were seen with third-trimester exposure of fluoxetine but not with first- or second-trimester exposure.[138] Lower birth weight has been associated with higher doses of fluoxetine compared with lower doses or other SRIs,[143] whereas other studies failed to find birth weight differences between early and late SRI exposed infants[144] or between SRI exposed and nonexposed infants.[145,146]

Recent evidence supports acute effects of SRI exposure on neonatal neurobehavior. Several reviews were published in 2005 looking at recent case reports, database analyses, and cohort studies on the effects of SRI exposure on neonatal outcomes.[147–150] In general, a cluster of symptoms was observed in newborns that were prenatally exposed to SRIs. These symptoms include irritability, tremors, jitteriness, trouble feeding, agitation, respiratory distress, and poor sleep. Other symptoms reported include convulsions, abnormal posturing, and shivering.[151,152] These symptoms have been reported most often in infants exposed to paroxetine, but all SRIs have been indicated,[138,149,150] and the symptoms were originally described as a syndrome called "poor neonatal adaptation," which included respiratory difficulties, jitteriness, poor motor tone, hypothermia, hypoglycemia, weak or absent cry, and trouble feeding.[138] Since that time, frequent reports of "poor neonatal adaptation" have been seen in the literature. Data from a 2006 review suggest that 30% of SRI-exposed neonates have symptoms consistent with "neonatal abstinence syndrome," a condition often described in newborns withdrawing from other (mostly opioid) prenatal drug exposures.[153–156] The long-term outcomes associated with these apparently transient symptoms following delivery have only just begun to be studied. The few empirical studies have shown SRIs related to increased active sleep[157] and decreased facial and behavioral responses to acute pain in the first week postnatally and at 2 months of age, suggesting a blunting of pain reactivity.[158,159] SRI-exposed infants were found to have decreased basal cortisol levels in the early evening compared with nonexposed infants at 3 months of age, although this effect was not related to prenatal exposure level or current SRI level measured in infant plasma.[160] A related paper suggested that third-trimester maternal mood, rather than SRI exposure, is related to increased infant hypothalamic-pituitary-adrenal reactivity and that this effect is mediated by increased methylation of NR3C1 (human glucocorticoid receptor gene).[161] In a recent review of studies on the long-term development of children with prenatal SSRI exposure, 11 studies (306 children) suggested no impairment with exposure, and two studies (81 children) suggested mild adverse effects.[148]

It is also possible that SRIs affect fetal neurobehavior. Studies of SRI effects on sleep state development in the fetus are limited to the work of Morrison and colleagues,[162] who examined fetal sheep after fluoxetine exposure and found a significant decrease in fetal rapid eye movement sleep. By contrast, a study of sleep state in the first 2 to 3 days postnatally reported more active sleep, more arousals, and more activity during sleep in SSRI-exposed newborns.[157] It is possible that the increase in rapid eye movement sleep reported after birth by Zeskind and Stephens[157] was compensatory following rapid eye movement sleep deprivation based on the fetal sheep data.[163] This finding could be caused by the fact that serotonergic neurons in the dorsal raphe nucleus seem to be involved in the "turning-off" of active sleep and are a central monoamine involved in the regulation of ultradian rhythms.[164] The initial action of antidepressant medications is to enhance postsynaptic transmission of serotonin. It is reasonable to expect that SRI exposure initially decreases the amount of active sleep. Another possibility is that the newborn effects are related to the discontinuation of the SRIs following delivery.

The effects of SRIs on fetal neurobehavior can be studied by incorporating fetal actocardiography with ultrasound observations of fetal behavior.[165–168] The fetal neurobehavior coding system is a method of fetal neurobehavioral observation and scoring that includes measurement of fetal heart rate, motor activity, behavioral state, and responsiveness to external or extrauterine stimuli.[169] A fetal actocardiograph provides measurement of fetal heart rate, fetal heart patterns, and motor activity. The use of ultrasound technology enables visualization of the fetus to observe specific fetal action patterns, quality and amplitude of movements, and eye movements. Ultrasound technology coupled with fetal actocardiography allows for a comprehensive assessment of fetal neurobehavior. **Table 1** presents the behavioral variables coded in the fetal neurobehavior coding system.

Effects of SRIs on fetal neurobehavior coding system neurobehavioral measures are shown in **Figs. 3** and **4**. Fetal behavioral and physiologic data were collected simultaneously by a research nurse certified in obstetric ultrasound and fetal heart rate monitoring. The data were obtained using an ultrasound machine with a 3.75-MHz transducer and an actocardiograph. The time of the recordings was standardized to between 12 noon and 5:00 PM to account for possible variability in fetal activity levels at different times of the day.[170] The participants were asked to fast for at least 1.5 hours before their scheduled appointment to increase their appetite. On arrival to the appointment, the participants were given a small meal, standardized for calories and content, to standardize the immediate nutritional influence on fetal activity. Participants were asked about their smoking and nutritional and caffeine intake on the day of the observation to account for the potential acute effects of caffeine and nicotine on fetal behavior. Baseline behaviors and heart rate were collected for the first 40 minutes. A single, 3-second vibroacoustic stimulus was applied to the maternal abdomen during the first quiescent period following the 40-minute baseline period. Recording continued for 20 minutes post–vibroacoustic stimulus presentation. Additionally, a vibroacoustic stimulus control trial was conducted in the baseline period to control for maternal reaction to the vibroacoustic stimulus. Research assistants trained on the fetal neurobehavior coding system and blinded to maternal condition conducted the coding of fetal behaviors. Coders use the specialized software to score digital recording files for fetal movements and behaviors in 10-second epochs. The presence or absence of isolated limb and head movements, gross body movements,

**Table 1**
Fetal behaviors coded from ultrasound recordings in the fetal neurobehavior coding system

| Summary Variable | Variable | Description |
|---|---|---|
| Fetal eye movement | Present | Clear movement of the pupil or eyelid |
| | Absent | A clear view of the eye is obtained and there is no movement |
| Fetal breathing movements | Regular | Displacement of the diaphragm with outward movement of the abdomen |
| | Vigorous | Fetal breathing movements that are large enough to move the entire fetus' body |
| | Hiccup | Consists of a jerky, repetitive contraction of the diaphragm |
| General body movements | Smooth | Pattern of movement involving smooth, simultaneous movement of a limb, trunk, and head that results in change in plane |
| | Jerky | General body movement that involves jerky movements of limbs or entire body |
| | Incomplete | General body movement that is not fluid or coordinated and does not result in change in plane |
| | Flexion | Flexion of the trunk |
| Patterned body movements | Stretch | A single event including a back extension or upward movement of the shoulder with simultaneous retroflexion or rotation of the head typically includes a pause at the peak of the movement with subsequent relaxation |
| | Backarche | Extension of the trunk and maintenance in this position for greater than 1 second |
| | Startle | A quick, generalized movement, involving abduction or extension of the limbs with or without movement of the trunk and head, followed by a return to a resting position |
| | Fidget | Nearly continuous limb movements that are not part of general body movement or other patterned movement |

| | | |
|---|---|---|
| Head movements | Rotation | Movement of the head in the lateral plane for at least a 30-degree angle from starting position |
| | Extension | A small movement of the head that extends upward in the vertical plane |
| | General | Small movement of the head that is not an extension or rotation |
| Mouthing movements | Rhythmic | Rhythmic bursts of jaw opening and closing at least four times in 5 seconds (sucking) |
| | Nonrhythmic | Mouth opening and closing that is isolated or limited to less than four at one time, often with tongue protrusion or lapping (drinking) |
| | Yawning | The timing of a yawn is similar to a stretch that includes prolonged wide opening of the jaws followed by relaxation; often accompanied by a stretch or subsequent general body movement |
| Limb movements | Smooth | Limbs move from origin to destination without backtracking |
| | Jerky | A movement of an extremity in which the movement is generally forceful and/or abrupt in nature. |
| | Indeterminate | Unable to determine quality of movement |
| | Lower limb | Lower limb is partially out of view; movement is obvious but unable to determine quality. |
| | Multiple | Repetitive limb movement in the same plane in a single epoch |
| | Hand to face | The hand slowly touches the face or mouth |
| | Tremor | Small rhythmic, jerky movement of an extremity |

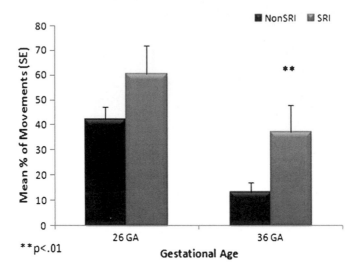

**Fig. 3.** Fetal jerky movements.

and behavior patterns were scored within each 10-second epoch. All movements were categorized as smooth, jerky, or indeterminate, with high interrater reliability. The actocardiograph data were scored for mean fetal heart rate, fetal heart rate accelerations, and fetal movement measures.[167,171]

In **Figs. 3** and **4**, the data are shown for fetuses (N = 60) exposed and unexposed to SRIs, with maternal depression scores used as a covariate. Fetuses in both groups demonstrated the expected developmental decrease in jerky movements from 26 to 36 weeks' gestational age; however, fetuses exposed to SRIs had more jerky movements at both gestational ages (see **Fig. 3**). The SRI-exposed fetuses did not show the anticipated developmental increase in fetal breathing movements at 36 weeks'

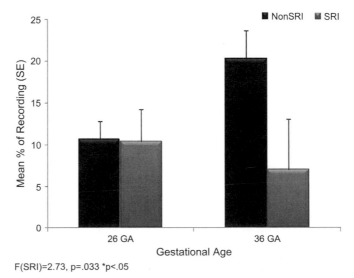

F(SRI)=2.73, p=.033 *p<.05

**Fig. 4.** Fetal breathing movements.

gestational age, and they had significantly fewer fetal breathing movements than non-SRI fetuses (see **Fig. 4**).

## BIOGENIC AMINE TRANSPORTERS

Some of the adverse effects on the fetus of the three uptake inhibitors reviewed here (cocaine, MA, and SRIs) may be caused by their action on blocking catecholamine transport, especially serotonin (5-HT). Catecholamines also exert vasoconstrictive effects on the umbilical vein, thereby reducing blood flow from the placenta to the fetus.[49,50] Furthermore, the vascular response to 5-HT is potentiated by uptake inhibition.[51,52] Because the umbilical cord is not innervated, transporter-dependent uptake by the placenta is also protecting the umbilical-placental circulation from deleterious effects of these neurotransmitters.[172,173]

Nonetheless, regulation of the placental capacity for catecholamine uptake should not be viewed solely in the context of protecting the fetus from exaggerated elevations in catecholamines or serotonin. Endogenous catecholamines are critical to fetal and neonatal growth, development, and survival. This conclusion is supported by studies in mice in which the gene for tyrosine hydroxylase[174,175] or dopamine β-hydroxylase[176,177] has been disrupted. Most fetuses homozygous for the disruption of either gene die during embryonic development. Small proportions (5%–10%) of fetuses survive, suggested to be rescue of the lethal phenotype by passage of maternal catecholamines across the placenta. 5-HT is also important at critical stages of development. 5-HT is present in early embryos and has been suggested to be maternal in origin.[178] Mouse embryos grown in the presence of high concentrations of 5-HT or serotonin uptake inhibitors develop craniofacial and cardiac abnormalities of the 3rd to 5th brachial arches.[179] Similar abnormalities have been seen in rat and chick embryos.[180] Highly regulated mechanisms control the concentration of intrauterine biogenic amines, which are central to fetal growth and development. Administration of uptake inhibitors to mouse dams in early to mid-gestation during placentation and embryogenesis leads to a high incidence of fetal-placental resorption.[181] In survivors, there is a significant reduction in birth weight and delay in maturational milestones (ear opening).[181] The capacity for placental biogenic amine uptake or transport has a significant impact on intrauterine growth and development. Understanding the ontogeny and regulation of placental biogenic amine transport is important in understanding the way in which the intrauterine neuroendocrine milieu programs develop.

Previous studies on the regulation of monoamine transporters suggest that drugs and maternal mood and anxiety are able to alter transporter activity.[182] Male rats exposed to stress in early gestation were shown to have behavioral manifestations similar to major depression, including maladaptive behavioral reactivity and anhedonia with subsequent increased sensitivity to SRI medication. These rats were found to have decreased SERT in the hippocampus. The authors state that a potential mechanism could be increased 5-HT output and decreased reuptake by SERT. This mechanism may explain increased sensitivity to acute postnatal SRI administration.[183]

Other drugs that affect transporters, such as cocaine, given during fetal rat brain development, have been related to increased norepinephrine turnover rate in older animals[184] and altered cerebral glucose uptake.[185,186] Interestingly, the cocaine-treated animals had enhanced acoustic startle responses to selective serotonin agonists, which were attenuated by the fluoxetine exposure.[186] This finding is consistent with the authors' observations on the effects of antenatal cocaine exposure on auditory brainstem responses, newborn cry, fetal heart rate, and arousal responses.[67,187] In other work, the authors showed that disorders linked to chronic intrauterine stress, including cocaine exposure or intrauterine growth retardation, are associated with decreased placental NET expression, directly proportional to the elevation in umbilical arterial plasma norepinephrine concentrations.[59] The decreased placental NET gene expression the authors have observed, and resultant increases in circulating catecholamines, may explain the adverse effects on the fetus of such drugs as cocaine and MA, which block catecholamine transport and render the fetus more vulnerable to other physiologic derangements.

11β-HSD is expressed in the placenta and converts biologically active cortisol to cortisone.[188,189] 11β-HSD-2 expression in the placenta is widely considered to protect the fetus from maternal hypercortisolism during pregnancy. It is also known that placental 11β-HSD-2 is downregulated by norepinephrine and that chronic intrauterine stress leads to downregulation of placental NET gene expression and increased circulating catecholamine levels in the fetus and the placental microenvironment. Dysregulation of norepinephrine levels in the placental microenvironment in turn leads to alterations in the placental neuroendocrine milieu. One potential mechanism for neurobehavioral effects of drugs, such as cocaine, MA, and SRIs, involves the alteration of fetal placental monoamine transporter expression and the resulting alterations in neuroendocrine and neurotransmitter system development. As an example of how placental gene expression may be related to substance exposure and maternal health conditions, **Fig. 5** shows placental SERT data from 33 mothers. These data demonstrate an interaction for major depressive disorder–SRI use on SERT expression in the placenta. The major depressive disorder–exposed fetuses (no SRI exposure) had lower SERT levels than controls and major depressive disorder plus SRI–exposed fetuses, but were not different from those of SRI-exposed fetuses whose mothers no longer met criteria for major depressive disorder. These data highlight how maternal diagnosis might change substance exposure–related outcomes. The authors have also shown this same type of alteration in neurobehavioral outcomes in cocaine-exposed infants whose mothers were depressed in the first month of pregnancy.[190]

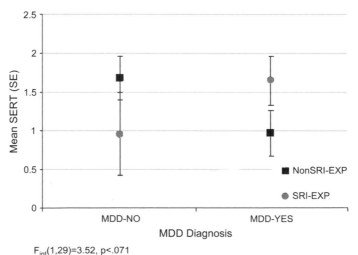

$F_{int}(1,29)=3.52$, p<.071

**Fig. 5.** Placental SERT levels.

## SUMMARY

The developmental trajectories of fetuses exposed to psychoactive substances may be altered by multiple factors. Such drugs as cocaine, MA, and SRIs, however, can be stressors that affect fetal development at multiple levels of the system, including disruptions in fetal placental monoamine transporter expression and altered neuroendocrine and neurotransmitter system development. Stress hormones, such as catecholamines and glucocorticoids, can alter regulation of the neuroendocrine environment by acting on the hypothalamic-pituitary-adrenal axis, which results in an altered set-point for physiologic, metabolic, and behavioral outcomes.[191] Because they are an important feature of the stress response, glucocorticoids have become prominent candidates as mediators of the effects of fetal programming. Another level of effect is potentially through the effects on gene expression through epigenetic mechanisms such as DNA methylation or chromatin remodeling which could also result in altered developmental trajectories.

## REFERENCES

1. Wilson JG. Current status of teratology: general principles and mechanisms derived from animal studies. In: Wilson JG, Fraser FC, editors. Handbook of teratology, general principles and etiology, vol. 1. New York: Plenum Press; 1977. p. 47–74.
2. Wisner KL, Zarin DA, Holmboe ES, et al. Risk-benefit decision making for treatment of depression during pregnancy. Am J Psychiatry 2000;157(12):1933–40.
3. Yonkers KA, Wisner KL, Stowe Z, et al. Management of bipolar disorder during pregnancy and the postpartum period. Am J Psychiatry 2004;161(4):608–20.
4. Lester B, Kosofsky B. Neurobiology of mental illness. In: Charney D, Nestler E, editors. Effects of drugs of abuse on brain development. London: Oxford University Press; 2009. p. 801–27.
5. Bertalanffy LV. General systems theory. New York: Brazilier; 1968.
6. Gottlieb G. Experiential canalization of behavioral development: results. Dev Psychobiol 1991;27:35–9.
7. Barker D. Fetal programming of coronary heart disease. Trends Endocrinol Metab 2002;13(9):364–8.
8. McMillen IC, Robinson JS. Developmental origins of the metabolic syndrome: prediction, plasticity, and programming. Physiol Rev 2005;85(2):571–633.
9. Barker DJ. The fetal origins of adult hypertension. J Hypertens Suppl 1992;10(7): S39–44.
10. Barker DJ, Osmond C, Golding J, et al. Growth in utero, blood pressure in childhood and adult life, and mortality from cardiovascular disease. BMJ 1989; 298(6673):564–7.
11. Falkner B. Birth weight as a predictor of future hypertension. Am J Hypertens 2002;15(2 Pt 2):43S–5S.
12. Rich-Edwards JW, Colditz GA, Stampfer MJ, et al. Birthweight and the risk for type 2 diabetes mellitus in adult women. Ann Intern Med 1999;130(4 Pt 1): 278–84.
13. Stein CE, Fall CH, Kumaran K, et al. Fetal growth and coronary heart disease in south India. Lancet 1996;348(9037):1269–73.
14. Sallout B, Walker M. The fetal origin of adult diseases. J Obstet Gynaecol 2003; 23(5):555–60.
15. Phillips D, Barker D, Hales C, et al. Thinness at birth and insulin resistance in adult life. Diabetologia 1994;37(2):150–4.

16. Ong KK, Dunger DB. Birth weight, infant growth and insulin resistance. Eur J Endocrinol 2004;151(Suppl 3):U131–9.

17. Hales CN, Barker DJ, Clark PM, et al. Fetal and infant growth and impaired glucose tolerance at age 64. BMJ 1991;303(6809):1019–22.

18. Wals M, Reichart CG, Hillegers MH, et al. Impact of birth weight and genetic liability on psychopathology in children of bipolar parents. J Am Acad Child Adolesc Psychiatry 2003;42(9):1116–21.

19. Allin M, Rooney M, Cuddy M, et al. Personality in young adults who are born preterm. Pediatrics 2006;117(2):309–16.

20. Thompson C, Syddall H, Rodin I, et al. Birth weight and the risk of depressive disorder in late life. Br J Psychiatry 2001;179:450–5.

21. Gale CR, Martyn CN. Birth weight and later risk of depression in a national birth cohort. Br J Psychiatry 2004;184:28–33.

22. Welberg LA, Seckl JR. Prenatal stress, glucocorticoids and the programming of the brain. J Neuroendocrinol 2001;13(2):113–28.

23. Gluckman PD, Hanson MA. Living with the past: evolution, development, and patterns of disease. Science 2004;305(5691):1733–6.

24. Lester BM, LaGasse LL, Seifer R. Cocaine exposure and children: the meaning of subtle effects. Science 1998;282(5389):633–4.

25. Gawin FH, Ellinwood EH Jr. Cocaine and other stimulants: actions, abuse, and treatment. N Engl J Med 1988;318(18):1173–82.

26. Wise R. Neural mechanisms of the reinforcing action of cocaine. NIDA Res Monogr 1984;50:15–33.

27. Goodman L. The pharmacological basis of therapeutics. New York: MacMillan Publishing Company; 1985.

28. Bzoskie L, Blount L, Kashiwai K, et al. The contribution of transporter-dependent uptake to fetal catecholamine clearance. Biol Neonate 1997;71(2):102–10.

29. Lau C, Burke S, Slotkin T. Maturation of sympathetic neurotransmission in the rat heart. IX. Development of transsynaptic regulation of cardiac adrenergic sensitivity. J Pharmacol Exp Ther 1982;223:675–80.

30. Padbury JF, Ludlow JK, Humme JA, et al. Metabolic clearance and plasma appearance rates of catecholamines in preterm and term fetal sheep. Pediatr Res 1986;20(10):992–5.

31. Stein H, Oyama K, Martinez A, et al. Plasma epinephrine appearance and clearance rates in fetal and newborn sheep. Am J Physiol 1993;265(4 Pt 2):R756–60.

32. Garg UC, Turndorf H, Bansinath M. Effect of cocaine on macromolecular syntheses and cell proliferation in cultured glial cells. Neuroscience 1993; 57(2):467–72.

33. Nassogne MC, Evrard P, Courtoy PJ. Selective neuronal toxicity of cocaine in embryonic mouse brain cocultures. Proc Natl Acad Sci U S A 1995;92(24): 11029–33.

34. Nassogne MC, Evrard P, Courtoy PJ. Selective direct toxicity of cocaine on fetal mouse neurons: teratogenic implications of neurite and apoptotic neuronal loss. Ann N Y Acad Sci 1998;846:51–68.

35. Akbari HM, Whitaker-Azmitia PM, Azmitia EC. Prenatal cocaine decreases the trophic factor S-100 beta and induced microcephaly: reversal by postnatal 5-HT1A receptor agonist. Neurosci Lett 1994;170(1):141–4.

36. Gressens P, Gofflot F, Van Maele-Fabry G, et al. Early neurogenesis and teratogenesis in whole mouse embryo cultures: histochemical, immunocytological and ultrastructural study of the premigratory neuronal-glial units in normal mouse

embryo and in mouse embryos influenced by cocaine and retinoic acid. J Neuropathol Exp Neurol 1992;51(2):206–19.

37. Gressens P, Kosofsky BE, Evrard P. Cocaine-induced disturbances of corticogenesis in the developing murine brain. Neurosci Lett 1992;140(1):113–6.

38. Yablonsky-Alter E, Gleser I, Carter C, et al. Effects of prenatal cocaine treatment on postnatal development of neocortex in white mice: immunocytochemistry of calbindin- and paralbumin-positive populations of gabaergic neurons. Soc Neurosci Abstr 1992;18:367.

39. Steiner H, Gerfen CR. Dynorphin opioid inhibition of cocaine-induced, D1 dopamine receptor-mediated immediate-early gene expression in the striatum. J Comp Neurol 1995;353(2):200–12.

40. Steiner H, Gerfen CR. Cocaine-induced c-fos messenger RNA is inversely related to dynorphin expression in striatum. J Neurosci 1993;13(12):5066–81.

41. Bhat RV, Baraban JM. Activation of transcription factor genes in striatum by cocaine: role of both serotonin and dopamine systems. J Pharmacol Exp Ther 1993;267(1):496–505.

42. Levitt P, Harvey JA, Friedman E, et al. New evidence for neurotransmitter influences on brain development. Trends Neurosci 1997;20(6):269–74.

43. Mayes LC. Developing brain and in utero cocaine exposure: effects on neural ontogeny. Dev Psychopathol 1999;11(4):685–714.

44. Malanga CJ III, Kosofsky BE. Mechanisms of action of drugs of abuse on the developing fetal brain. Clin Perinatol 1999;26(1):17–37, v–vi.

45. Meier E, Schousboe A. Neurotransmitters as developmental signals. Neurochem Int 1991;19(1–2):1–15.

46. Bzoskie L, Blount L, Kashiwai K, et al. Placental norepinephrine transporter development in the ovine fetus. Placenta 1997;18:65–70.

47. Koegler SM, Seidler FJ, Spencer JR, et al. Ischemia contributes to adverse effects of cocaine on brain development: suppression of ornithine decarboxylase activity in neonatal rat. Brain Res Bull 1991;27(6):829–34.

48. Woods JR Jr, Plessinger MA, Clark KE. Effect of cocaine on uterine blood flow and fetal oxygenation. JAMA 1987;257(7):957–61.

49. Reviriego J, Fernandez-Alfonso MS, Marin J. Actions of vasoactive drugs on human placental vascular smooth muscle. Gen Pharmacol 1990;21(5):719–27.

50. Zhang L, Dyer DC. Characterization of alpha-adrenoceptors mediating contraction in isolated ovine umbilical vein. Eur J Pharmacol 1991;197(1):63–7.

51. Dyer DC. An investigation of the mechanism of potentiation by cocaine of responses to serotonin in sheep umbilical blood vessels. J Pharmacol Exp Ther 1970;175(3):571–6.

52. Nair X, Dyer DC. Responses of guinea pig umbilical vasculature to vasoactive drugs. Eur J Pharmacol 1974;27(3):294–304.

53. Bauer CR, Langer JC, Shankaran S, et al. Acute neonatal effects of cocaine exposure during pregnancy. Arch Pediatr Adolesc Med 2005; 159(9):824–34.

54. Lester B, Padbury J. The third pathophysiology of prenatal cocaine exposure. Dev Neurosci 2009;31:23–35.

55. Nguyen TT, Tseng YT, McGonnigal B, et al. Placental biogenic amine transporters: in vivo function, regulation and pathobiological significance. Placenta 1999;20(1):3–11.

56. Meyer JS. Biochemical effects of corticosteroids on neural tissues. Physiol Rev 1985;65(4):946–1020.

57. Lopez-Bernal A, Craft IL. Corticosteroid metabolism in vitro by human placenta, fetal membranes and decidua in early and late gestation. Placenta 1981;2(4): 279–85.

58. Sarkar S, Tsai SW, Nguyen TT, et al. Inhibition of placental 11beta-hydroxysteroid dehydrogenase type 2 by catecholamines via alpha-adrenergic signaling. Am J Physiol Regul Integr Comp Physiol 2001;281(6):R1966–74.

59. Bzoskie L, Yen J, Tseng YT, et al. Human placental norepinephrine transporter mRNA: expression and correlation with fetal condition at birth. Placenta 1997; 18(2–3):205–10.

60. Bottalico B, Larsson I, Brodszki J. Norepinephrine transporter (NET), serotonin transporter (SERT), vesicular monoamine transporter (VMAT2) and organic cation transporters (OCT1, 2 and EMT) in human placenta from pre-eclamptic and normotensive pregnancies. Placenta 2004;25(6):518–29.

61. Gunnar M, Prudhomme-White B. Salivary cortisol measures in infant and child assessment. In: Twarog-Singer L, Zeskind PS, editors. Biobehavioral assessment of the infant. New York: The Guilford Press; 2001. p. 167–89.

62. Magnano CL, Gardner JM, Karmel BZ. Differences in salivary cortisol levels in cocaine-exposed and noncocaine-exposed NICU infants. Dev Psychobiol 1992;25(2):93–103.

63. Jacobson SW, Bihun JT, Chiodo LM. Effects of prenatal alcohol and cocaine exposure on infant cortisol levels. Dev Psychopathol 1999;11(2):195–208.

64. Scafidi FA, Field TM, Wheeden A, et al. Cocaine-exposed preterm neonates show behavioral and hormonal differences. Pediatrics 1996;97(6 Pt 1):851–5.

65. Harvey JA. Cocaine effects on the developing brain: current status. Neurosci Biobehav Rev 2004;27(8):751–64.

66. Lester BM, Tronick EZ, LaGasse L, et al. The maternal lifestyle study: effects of substance exposure during pregnancy on neurodevelopmental outcome in 1-month-old infants. Pediatrics 2002;110(6):1182–92.

67. Lester BM, Lagasse L, Seifer R, et al. The Maternal lifestyle study (MLS): effects of prenatal cocaine and/or opiate exposure on auditory brain response at one month. J Pediatr 2003;142(3):279–85.

68. Bada HS, Das A, Bauer CR, et al. Impact of prenatal cocaine exposure on child behavior problems through school age. Pediatrics 2007;119(2):e348–59.

69. Levine T, Liu J, Das A, et al. Effects of prenatal cocaine exposure on special education in school age children. Pediatrics 2008;122(1):e83–91.

70. Sheinkopf SJ, Lester BM, Sanes JN, et al. Functional MRI and response inhibition in children exposed to cocaine in utero: preliminary findings. Dev Neurosci 2009;31(1–2):159–66.

71. Lester B, LaGasse L. Children of addicted women. J Addict Dis, in press.

72. US Drug Enforcement Administration. Methamphetamine. Available at: http://www.usdoj.gov/dea/concern/meth.html. Accessed March 11, 2009.

73. Rawson R, Huber A, Brethen P, et al. Cocaine users: differences in characteristics and treatment retention. J Psychoactive Drugs 2000;32(2):233–8.

74. United Nations Office on Drugs and Crime. World Drug Report, analysis, vol. 1. Vienna: United Nations Publication; 2004.

75. Substance Abuse and Mental Health Services Administration (SAMSA). Office of Applied Studies, National Survey on Drug Use and Health, 2004, 2005, 2006 and 2007. Available at: http://www.oas.samhsa.gov/nsduh/2k7nsduh/2k7Results.pdf. Accessed August 5, 2009.

76. Arria AM, Derauf C, Lagasse LL, et al. Methamphetamine and other substance use during pregnancy: preliminary estimates from the Infant Development,

Environment, and Lifestyle (IDEAL) study. Matern Child Health J 2006;10(3): 293–302.
77. Substance Abuse and Mental Health Services Administration (SAMSA). Preliminary results from the 1997 National Household Survey on Drug Abuse 1998. Available at: http://www.oas.samhsa.gov/nhsda/nhsda97/toc.htm. Accessed August 5, 2009.
78. Substance Abuse and Mental Health Services Administration (SAMSA). National Household Survey on Drug Abuse (NHSDA), National Institute on Drug Abuse, 1999. Available at: http://www.oas.samhsa.gov/nhsda/2kdetailedtabs/Preface.htm. Accessed August 5, 2009.
79. King RS. The next big thing: methamphetamine in the United States. Washington, DC: The Sentencing Project: Research and Advocacy for Reform; 2006.
80. Heller A. Neurotoxicology and developmental effects of meth and MDMA: effects of in utero exposure to methamphetamines. Bethesda (MD): National Institute on Drug Abuse; 2000.
81. Karch S. The pathology of drug abuse. Boca Raton (FL): CRC Press; 1993.
82. Catanzarite VA, Stein DA. Crystal and pregnancy: methamphetamine-associated maternal deaths. West J Med 1995;162(5):454–8.
83. Bennett BA, Hyde CE, Pecora JR, et al. Differing neurotoxic potencies of methamphetamine, mazindol, and cocaine in mesencephalic cultures. J Neurochem 1993;60(4):1444–52.
84. Jones SR, Gainetdinov RR, Wightman RM, et al. Mechanisms of amphetamine action revealed in mice lacking the dopamine transporter. J Neurosci 1998; 18(6):1979–86.
85. Ricaurte GA, Schuster CR, Seiden LS. Long-term effects of repeated methylamphetamine administration on dopamine and serotonin neurons in the rat brain: a regional study. Brain Res 1980;193(1):153–63.
86. McCann UD, Ricaurte GA. Amphetamine neurotoxicity: accomplishments and remaining challenges. Neurosci Biobehav Rev 2004;27(8):821–6.
87. Frost DO, Cadet JL. Effects of methamphetamine-induced neurotoxicity on the development of neural circuitry: a hypothesis. Brain Res Brain Res Rev 2000; 34(3):103–18.
88. Quinton MS, Yamamoto BK. Causes and consequences of methamphetamine and MDMA toxicity. AAPS J 2006;8(2):E337–47.
89. Plessinger MA. Prenatal exposure to amphetamines: risks and adverse outcomes in pregnancy. Obstet Gynecol Clin North Am 1998;25(1):119–38.
90. Stek A, Fisher BK, Baker RS, et al. Maternal and fetal cardiovascular responses to methamphetamine in the pregnant sheep. Am J Obstet Gynecol 1993;169(4): 888–97.
91. Stek AM, Baker RS, Fisher BK, et al. Fetal responses to maternal and fetal methamphetamine administration in sheep. Am J Obstet Gynecol 1995;173(5): 1592–8.
92. Wouldes T, LaGasse L, Sheridan J, et al. Maternal methamphetamine use during pregnancy and child outcome: what do we know? N Z Med J 2004;114(1206): 1–10.
93. Smith LM, LaGasse LL, Derauf C, et al. The infant development, environment, and lifestyle study: effects of prenatal methamphetamine exposure, polydrug exposure, and poverty on intrauterine growth. Pediatrics 2006;118(3): 1149–56.
94. Smith LM, Lagasse LL, Derauf C, et al. Prenatal methamphetamine use and neonatal neurobehavioral outcome. Neurotoxicol Teratol 2008;30(1):20–8.

95. Burchfield DJ, Lucas VW, Abrams RM, et al. Disposition and pharmacodynamics of methamphetamine in pregnant sheep. JAMA 1991;265(15):1968–73.

96. Fuller R, Hemrick-Luecke S. Further studies on the long-term depletion of striatal dopamine in iprindole-treated rats by amphetamine. Neuropharmacology 1992; 21(5):433–8.

97. Pu C, Vorhees CV. Developmental dissociation of astrocyte reaction in rat striatum. Brain Res Dev Brain Res 1993;72(2):325–8.

98. Seiden LS, Sabol KE. Methamphetamine and methylenedioxymethamphetamine neurotoxicity: possible mechanisms of cell destruction. NIDA Res Monogr 1996; 163:251–76.

99. Gibb JW, Johnson M, Elayan I, et al. Neurotoxicity of amphetamines and their metabolites. NIDA Res Monogr 1997;173:128–45.

100. Ricaurte GA, McCann UD. Neurotoxic amphetamine analogues: effects in monkeys and implications for humans. Ann N Y Acad Sci 1992;648:371–82.

101. Volkow ND, Chang L, Wang GJ, et al. Association of dopamine transporter reduction with psychomotor impairment in methamphetamine abusers. Am J Psychiatry 2001;158(3):377–82.

102. Cabrera TM, Levy AD, Li Q, et al. Prenatal methamphetamine attenuates serotonin mediated renin secretion in male and female rat progeny: evidence for selective long-term dysfunction of serotonin pathways in brain. Synapse 1993; 15(3):198–208.

103. Weissman AD, Caldecott-Hazard S. Developmental neurotoxicity to methamphetamines. Clin Exp Pharmacol Physiol 1995;22(5):372–4.

104. Acuff-Smith KD, George M, Lorens SA, et al. Preliminary evidence for methamphetamine-induced behavioral and ocular effects in rat offspring following exposure during early organogenesis. Psychopharmacology 1992;109(3):255–63.

105. Cho DH, Lyu HM, Lee HB, et al. Behavioral teratogenicity of methamphetamine. J Toxicol Sci 1991;16(Suppl 1):37–49.

106. Slamberova R, Pometlova M, Charousova P. Postnatal development of rat pups is altered by prenatal methamphetamine exposure. Prog Neuropsychopharmacol Biol Psychiatry 2006;30(1):82–8.

107. Woolverton WL, Ricaurte GA, Forno LS, et al. Long-term effects of chronic methamphetamine administration in rhesus monkeys. Brain Res 1989;486(1):73–8.

108. Wallace TL, Gudelsky GA, Vorhees CV. Methamphetamine-induced neurotoxicity alters locomotor activity, stereotypic behavior, and stimulated dopamine release in the rat. J Neurosci 1999;19:9141–8.

109. Itoh J, Nabeshima T, Kameyama T. Utility of an elevated plusmaze for dissociation of amnesic and behavioral effects of drugs in mice. Eur J Pharmacol 1991; 194:71–6.

110. Acuff-Smith KD, Schilling MA, Fisher JE, et al. Stage-specific effects of prenatal d-methamphetamine exposure on behavioral and eye development in rats. Neurotoxicol Teratol 1996;18(2):199–215.

111. Yamamoto Y, Yamanoto K, Fukui Y, et al. Teratogenic effects of methamphetamine in mice. Nihon Hoigaku Zasshi 1992;46(2):126–31.

112. Williams MT, Blankenmeyer IL, Schaefer TL, et al. Long-term effects of neonatal methamphetamine exposure in rats on spatial learning in the Barnes maze and on cliff avoidance, corticosterone release, and neurotoxicity in adulthood. Brain Res Dev Brain Res 2003;147(1–2):163–75.

113. Jeng W, Wong AW, Ting AKR, et al. Methamphetamine-enhanced embryonic oxidative DNA damage and neurodevelopmental deficits. Free Radic Biol Med 2005;39(3):317–26.

114. Ramamoorthy JD, Ramamoorthy S, Leibach FH, et al. Human placental mono-amine transporters as targets for amphetamines. Am J Obstet Gynecol 1995; 173:1782–7.
115. Altshuler LL, Cohen LS, Moline ML, et al. Treatment of depression in women. Post-graduate Medicine. March 2001;Special report (The Expert Consensus Guideline Series):1–28. Available at: http://www.psychguides.com/Depression%20in%20Women%20contents.pdf. Accessed August 5, 2009.
116. Swinkels JA, de Jonghe F. Safety of antidepressants. Int Clin Psychopharmacol 1995;9(Suppl 4):19–25.
117. Stafford RS, MacDonald EA, Finkelstein SN. National patterns of medication treatment for depression, 1987 to 2001. Prim Care Companion J Clin Psychiatry 2001;3(6):232–5.
118. Pirraglia PA, Stafford RS, Singer DE. Trends in prescribing of selective serotonin reuptake inhibitors and other newer antidepressant agents in adult primary care. Prim Care Companion J Clin Psychiatry 2003;5(4):153–7.
119. Marcus SM, Flynn HA, Blow F, et al. A screening study of antidepressant treat-ment rates and mood symptoms in pregnancy. Arch Womens Ment Health 2005; 8(1):25–7.
120. Andrade SE, Raebel MA, Brown J, et al. Use of antidepressant medica-tions during pregnancy: a multisite study. Am J Obstet Gynecol 2008; 198:194.
121. Shelton R. The dual-action hypothesis: does pharmacology matter? J Clin Psychiatry 2004;65(Suppl 17):5–10.
122. Hendrick V, Stowe ZN, Altshuler LL, et al. Placental passage of antidepressant medications. Am J Psychiatry 2003;160(5):993–6.
123. Rampono J, Proud S, Hackett LP, et al. A pilot study of newer antidepressant concentrations in cord and maternal serum and possible effects in the neonate. Int J Neuropsychopharmacol 2004;7(3):329–34.
124. Loughhead AM, Fisher AD, Newport DJ, et al. Antidepressants in amniotic fluid: another route of fetal exposure. Am J Psychiatry 2006;163(1):145–7.
125. Morrison JL, Chien C, Riggs KW, et al. Effect of maternal fluoxetine administra-tion on uterine blood flow, fetal blood gas status, and growth. Pediatr Res 2002; 51(4):433–42.
126. Sodhi MS, Sanders-Bush E. Serotonin and brain development. Int Rev Neurobiol 2004;59:111–74.
127. Lesch KP. Serotonergic gene expression and depression: implications for devel-oping novel antidepressants. J Affect Disord 2001;62(1–2):57–76.
128. Herlenius E, Lagercrantz H. Neurotransmitters and neuromodulators during early human development. Early Hum Dev 2001;65(1):21–37.
129. Gingrich JA, Ansorge MS, Merker R, et al. New lessons from knockout mice: the role of serotonin during development and its possible contribution to the origins of neuropsychiatric disorders. CNS Spectr 2003;8(8):572–7.
130. Wurtman RJ. Genes, stress, and depression. Metabolism 2005;54(5 Suppl 1): 16–9.
131. Lesch KP, Mossner R. Genetically driven variation in serotonin uptake: is there a link to affective spectrum, neurodevelopmental, and neurodegenerative disor-ders? Biol Psychiatry 1998;44(3):179–92.
132. Hamet P, Tremblay J. Genetics and genomics of depression. Metabolism 2005; 54(5 Suppl 1):10–5.
133. Heils A, Teufel A, Petri S, et al. Allelic variation of human serotonin transporter gene expression. J Neurochem 1996;66(6):2621–4.

134. Lesch KP, Bengel D, Heils A, et al. Association of anxiety-related traits with a polymorphism in the serotonin transporter gene regulatory region. Science 1996;274(5292):1527–31.

135. Caspi A, Sugden K, Moffitt TE, et al. Influence of life stress on depression: moderation by a polymorphism in the 5-HTT gene. Science 2003;301(5631): 386–9.

136. Serretti A, Benedetti F, Zanardi R, et al. The influence of serotonin transporter promoter polymorphism (SERTPR) and other polymorphisms of the serotonin pathway on the efficacy of antidepressant treatments. Prog Neuropsychopharmacol Biol Psychiatry 2005;29(6):1074–84.

137. Rahimi R, Nikfar S, Abdollahi M. Pregnancy outcomes following exposure to serotonin reuptake inhibitors: a meta-analysis of clinical trials. Reprod Toxicol 2006;4:571–5.

138. Chambers CD, Johnson KA, Dick LM, et al. Birth outcomes in pregnant women taking fluoxetine. N Engl J Med 1996;335(14):1010–5.

139. Einarson TR, Einarson A. Newer antidepressants in pregnancy and rates of major malformations: a meta-analysis of prospective comparative studies. Pharmacoepidemiol Drug Saf 2005;14(12):823–7.

140. GlaxoSmithKline. 2005 Safety alerts for drugs, biologics, medical devices, and dietary supplements: Paxil (paroxetine HCL) and Paxil CR (Posted 09/27/2005) In: MedWatch F, Editor. 2005. Available at: http://www.fda.gov/Safety/MedWatch/SafetyInformation/SafetyAlertsforHumanMedicalProducts/ucm152310.htm.

141. Chambers CD, Hernandez-Diaz S, Van Marter LJ, et al. Selective serotonin-reuptake inhibitors and risk of persistent pulmonary hypertension of the newborn. N Engl J Med 2006;354(6):579–87.

142. Simon GE, Cunningham ML, Davis RL. Outcomes of prenatal antidepressant exposure. Am J Psychiatry 2002;159(12):2055–61.

143. Hendrick V, Smith LM, Suri R, et al. Birth outcomes after prenatal exposure to antidepressant medication. Am J Obstet Gynecol 2003;188(3):812–5.

144. Cohen LS, Heller VL, Bailey JW, et al. Birth outcomes following prenatal exposure to fluoxetine. Biol Psychiatry 2000;48(10):996–1000.

145. Kulin NA, Pastuszak A, Sage SR, et al. Pregnancy outcome following maternal use of the new selective serotonin reuptake inhibitors: a prospective controlled multicenter study [see comment]. J Am Med Assoc 1998;279(8):609–10.

146. Suri R, Altshuler L, Hendrick V, et al. The impact of depression and fluoxetine treatment on obstetrical outcome. Arch Womens Ment Health 2004;7(3): 193–200.

147. Lattimore KA, Donn SM, Kaciroti N, et al. Selective serotonin reuptake inhibitor (SSRI) use during pregnancy and effects on the fetus and newborn: a meta-analysis. J Perinatol 2005;25(9):595–604.

148. Gentile S. The safety of newer antidepressants in pregnancy and breastfeeding. Drug Saf 2005;28(2):137–52.

149. Moses-Kolko EL, Bogen D, Perel J, et al. Neonatal signs after late in utero exposure to serotonin reuptake inhibitors: literature review and implications for clinical applications. JAMA 2005;293(19):2372–83.

150. Nordeng H, Spigset O. Treatment with selective serotonin reuptake inhibitors in the third trimester of pregnancy: effects on the infant. Drug Saf 2005;28(7): 565–81.

151. Kallen B. Neonate characteristics after maternal use of antidepressants in late pregnancy. Arch Pediatr Adolesc Med 2004;158(4):312–6.

152. Sanz EJ, De-las-Cuevas C, Kiuru A, et al. Selective serotonin reuptake inhibitors in pregnant women and neonatal withdrawal syndrome: a database analysis. Lancet 2005;365(9458):482–7.
153. Levinson-Castiel R, Merlob P, Linder N, et al. Neonatal abstinence syndrome after in utero exposure to selective serotonin reuptake inhibitors in term infants. Arch Pediatr Adolesc Med 2006;160(2):173–6.
154. Lainwala S, Brown ER, Weinschenk NP, et al. A retrospective study of length of hospital stay in infants treated for neonatal abstinence syndrome with methadone versus oral morphine preparations. Adv Neonatal Care 2005;5(5):265–72.
155. Dean JC, Hailey H, Moore SJ, et al. Long term health and neurodevelopment in children exposed to antiepileptic drugs before birth. J Med Genet 2002;39(4): 251–9.
156. Fulroth R, Phillips B, Durand DJ. Perinatal outcome of infants exposed to cocaine and/or heroin in utero. Am J Dis Child 1989;143(8):905–10.
157. Zeskind PS, Stephens LE. Maternal selective serotonin reuptake inhibitor use during pregnancy and newborn neurobehavior. Obstet Gynecol Surv 2004; 59(8):564–6.
158. Oberlander TF, Eckstein Grunau R, Fitzgerald C, et al. Prolonged prenatal psychotropic medication exposure alters neonatal acute pain response. Pediatr Res 2002;51(4):443–53.
159. Oberlander TF, Grunau RE, Fitzgerald C, et al. Pain reactivity in 2-month-old infants after prenatal and postnatal serotonin reuptake inhibitor medication exposure. Pediatrics 2005;115(2):411–25.
160. Oberlander TF, Grunau R, Mayes L, et al. Hypothalamic-pituitary-adrenal (HPA) axis function in 3-month old infants with prenatal selective serotonin reuptake inhibitor (SSRI) antidepressant exposure. Early Hum Dev 2008;84(10):689–97.
161. Oberlander TF, Weinberg J, Papsdorf M, et al. Prenatal exposure to maternal depression, neonatal methylation of human glucocorticoid receptor gene (NR3C1) and infant cortisol stress responses. Epigenetics 2008;3(2):97–106.
162. Morrison JL, Rurak DW, Chien C, et al. Maternal fluoxetine infusion does not alter fetal endocrine and biophysical circadian rhythms in pregnant sheep. J Soc Gynecol Investig 2005;12(5):356–64.
163. Vogel GW. A review of REM sleep deprivation. Arch Gen Psychiatry 1975;32(6): 749–61.
164. Portas CM, Bjorvatn B, Ursin R. Serotonin and the sleep/wake cycle: special emphasis on microdialysis studies. Prog Neurobiol 2000;60(1):13–35.
165. Maeda K, Tatsumura M, Utsu M. Analysis of fetal movements by Doppler actocardiogram and fetal B-mode imaging. Clin Perinatol 1999;26(4):829–51.
166. Maeda K. Computerized analysis of cardiotocograms and fetal movements. Baillieres Clin Obstet Gynaecol 1990;4(4):797–813.
167. DiPietro JA, Costigan KA, Pressman EK. Fetal movement detection: comparison of the Toitu actograph with ultrasound from 20 weeks gestation. J Matern Fetal Med 1999;8(6):237–42.
168. de Vries JIP, Visser GHA, Prechtl HFR. The emergence of fetal behavior, I. Qualitative aspects. Early Human Development 1982;7:301–22.
169. Salisbury AL, Fallone MD, Lester B. Neurobehavioral assessment from fetus to infant: the NICU network neurobehavioral scale and the fetal neurobehavior coding scale. Ment Retard Dev Disabil Res Rev 2005;11(1):14–20.
170. Pillai M, James DK, Parker M. The development of ultradian rhythms in the human fetus. Am J Obstet Gynecol 1992;167(1):172–7.

171. DiPietro JA, Hodgson DM, Costigan KA, et al. Development of fetal movement–fetal heart rate coupling from 20 weeks through term. Early Hum Dev 1996; 44(2):139–51.

172. Fox SB, Khong TY. Lack of innervation of human umbilical cord: an immunohistological and histochemical study. Placenta 1990;11(1):59–62.

173. Walker DW, McLean JR. Absence of adrenergic nerves in the human placenta. Nature 1971;229(5283):344–5.

174. Kobayashi K, Morita S, Sawada H, et al. Targeted disruption of the tyrosine hydroxylase locus results in severe catecholamine depletion and perinatal lethality in mice. J Biol Chem 1995;270(45):27235–43.

175. Zhou QY, Quaife CJ, Palmiter RD. Targeted disruption of the tyrosine hydroxylase gene reveals that catecholamines are required for mouse fetal development. Nature 1995;374(6523):640–3.

176. Thomas SA, Matsumoto AM, Palmiter RD. Noradrenaline is essential for mouse fetal development. Nature 1995;374(6523):643–6.

177. Thomas SA, Palmiter RD. Examining adrenergic roles in development, physiology, and behavior through targeted disruption of the mouse dopamine beta-hydroxylase gene. Adv Pharmacol 1998;42:57–60.

178. Yavarone MS, Shuey DL, Tamir H, et al. Serotonin and cardiac morphogenesis in the mouse embryo. Teratology 1993;47(6):573–84.

179. Shuey D, Sadler T, Tamir H, et al. Transient expression of serotonin uptake and binding protein during craniofacial morphogenesis in the mouse. Anat Embryol (Berl) 1993;187(1):75–85.

180. Choi D, Ward S, Messaddeq N, et al. 5-HT2B receptor-mediated serotonin morphogenetic functions in mouse cranial neural crest and myocardiac cells. Development 1997;124:1745–55.

181. Church MW, Rauch HC. Prenatal cocaine exposure in the laboratory mouse: effects on maternal water consumption and offspring outcome. Neurotoxicol Teratol 1992;14(5):313–9.

182. Jayanthi LD, Ramamoorthy S. Regulation of monoamine transporters: influence of psychostimulants and therapeutic antidepressants. AAPS J 2005;7(3): E728–38.

183. Mueller BR, Bale TL. Sex-specific programming of offspring emotionality after stress early in pregnancy. J Neurosci 2008;28(36):9055–65.

184. Seidler FJ, Slotkin TA. Fetal cocaine exposure causes persistent noradrenergic hyperactivity in rat brain regions: effects on neurotransmitter turnover and receptors. J Pharmacol Exp Ther 1992;263(2):413–21.

185. Dow-Edwards DL, Freed-Malen LA, Gerkin LM, et al. Sexual dimorphism in the brain metabolic response to prenatal cocaine exposure. Developmental Brain Research 2001;129(1):73–9.

186. Dow-Edwards DL. Preweaning cocaine administration alters the adult response to quipazine: comparison with fluoxetine. Neurotoxicology and Teratology 1998; 20(2):133–42.

187. Lester BM, Boukydis CF, Garcia-Coll CT, et al. Developmental outcome as a function of the goodness of fit between the infant's cry characteristics and the mother's perception of her infant's cry. Pediatrics 1995;95(4):516–21.

188. Peters DA. Prenatal stress: effects on brain biogenic amine and plasma corticosterone levels. Pharmacol Biochem Behav 1982;17(4):721–5.

189. Lakshmi V, Nath N, Muneyyirci-Delale O. Characterization of 11 beta-hydroxysteroid dehydrogenase of human placenta: evidence for the existence of two

species of 11 beta-hydroxysteroid dehydrogenase. J Steroid Biochem Mol Biol 1993;45(5):391–7.

190. Salisbury AL, Lester BM, Seifer R, et al. Prenatal cocaine use and maternal depression: effects on infant neurobehavior. Neurotoxicol Teratol 2007;29(3): 331–40.

191. Matthews SG. Antenatal glucocorticoids and the developing brain: mechanisms of action. Semin Neonatol 2001;6(4):309–17.

# Primary Disorders of Metabolism and Disturbed Fetal Brain Development

Asuri N. Prasad, MBBS, FRCPC, FRCPE[a,b], Gustavo Malinger, MD[c],
Tally Lerman-Sagie, MD[d,e],*

**KEYWORDS**

- Inborn errors of metabolism • Fetal brain
- Cerebral dysmorphogenesis • Prenatal diagnosis
- Neurosonography • Ultrasound

The interaction between embryogenesis and the in utero environment is a dynamic and complex process. The metabolic microenvironment during embryogenesis (fetal metabolome) profoundly influences the entire gamut of developmental processes leading to organogenesis. This process spans a time window from the third week postfertilization into the postnatal period well beyond the first 2 years of life.[1,2]

The composition of the fetal metabolome is dependent on the state of maternal health and disease; maternal nutrition; placental integrity and function; and genetic factors affecting the mother, the fetus, or both. The effects of nutrient deficiency (macronutrients or micronutrients) and maternal exposures to neurotoxins and teratogens are difficult to assess and quantify in humans. The effects occur at a cellular or subcellular level, and the consequences may be restricted to neurobehavioral effects, cognitive deficits, and learning disabilities.[3] In a few circumstances, the

[a] Section of Clinical Neurosciences, Department of Pediatrics and Child Health, Children's Hospital of Western Ontario, London Health Sciences Centre, University of Western Ontario, B-509, 800 Commissioners Road East, London, Ontario, N6C4G5, Canada
[b] Section of Pediatric Neurology, Department of Clinical Neurosciences, Children's Hospital of Western Ontario, London Health Sciences Centre, University of Western Ontario, B-509, 800 Commissioners Road East, London, Ontario, N6C4G5, Canada
[c] Prenatal Diagnosis Unit, Department of Obstetrics and Gynecology, Wolfson Medical Center, POB 5, Holon, 58100 Sackler School of Medicine, Tel Aviv University, Halohamim Street, Tel Aviv, Israel
[d] Pediatric Neurology Unit, Wolfson Medical Center, POB 5, Holon, 58100 Sackler School of Medicine, Tel Aviv University, Halohamim Street, Tel Aviv, Israel
[e] Metabolic Neurogenetic Service, Wolfson Medical Center, POB 5, Holon, 58100 Sackler School of Medicine, Tel Aviv University, Halohamim Street, Tel Aviv, Israel
* Corresponding author. Pediatric Neurology Unit, Wolfson Medical Center, POB 5, Holon, 58100 Sackler School of Medicine, Tel Aviv University, Halohamim Street, Tel Aviv, Israel.
*E-mail address:* asagie@post.tau.ac.il (T. Lerman-Sagie).

Clin Perinatol 36 (2009) 621–638
doi:10.1016/j.clp.2009.06.004
0095-5108/09/$ – see front matter © 2009 Elsevier Inc. All rights reserved.

perinatology.theclinics.com

effects may indeed be detectable prenatally: for instance, the occurrence of neural tube defects in association with folate deficiency, or the occurrence of microcephaly associated with fetal alcohol exposure.

Inborn errors of metabolism (IEM) caused by single gene defects result in enzymatic blocks within biochemical pathways, often caused by the deficiency of an enzyme or cofactor. These blocks usually lead to accumulation of potentially toxic intermediate compounds that are accompanied by the deficiency of critical end products necessary for cell function. The resulting changes from metabolite-metabolite interactions influence the internal and external microenvironment and cellular homeostatic mechanisms.[3]

The association of IEM with developmental malformations has long been recognized. Following initial reports of association of callosal dysgenesis,[4] widespread developmental abnormalities in the brain have been recognized with IEM.[5] A logical extension of these observed associations is the exploration of the possibilities of detection and diagnosis during the prenatal period. The detection of developmental malformations of the fetal brain using ultrasonography is limited only by the degree of resolution that can be obtained. Current advances in fetal ultrasonography and MRI permit visualization of the fetal brain in considerably greater detail than was previously possible. Furthermore, these techniques permit the monitoring of serial changes over time. Recognition of specific patterns and associations with IEMs serves to guide the neurologist and the metabolic specialist in targeting appropriate investigations critical for diagnosis, treatment, and counseling.

## CEREBRAL DYSMORPHOGENESIS IN INBORN ERRORS OF METABOLISM

There are excellent reviews summarizing the wide variation in the nature of malformations of the central nervous system in a variety of IEMs.[3–6] These can be categorized into two groups: those resulting from interference in the early processes of neurulation in the first trimester, and those associated with abnormalities of neuronal migration and subsequent processes in the second and third trimesters.[5] Although a specific correlation between the metabolic phenotype and the nature of malformation may not always exist, the following discussion provides specific examples where the combination of malformations may be sufficient to point the experienced pediatric neurologist and a metabolic geneticist toward appropriate diagnostic considerations.

## INBORN ERRORS OF METABOLISM AND CEREBRAL DYSMORPHOGENESIS

Interference with formation of the telencephalic vesicles (holoprosencephaly), dysgenesis of the corpus callosum, absence of the septi pellucidi, cerebellar dysgenesis, and abnormalities in ventricular shape (colpocephaly, single ventricle) may be visualized in early fetal life. Later, as the brain grows in complexity, abnormalities may extend to involve the gray matter (atrophy of the cortical ribbon, atrophy of the basal ganglia); white matter (thinning out or loss of volume, demyelination, or dysmyelination of white matter); encephaloclastic lesions (porencephalic cysts); and neuronal migration defects (pachygyria) may appear.

IEMs affect different biochemical and metabolic pathways, which involve different substrates, intermediary compounds, and end products. How can one explain the association of such abnormalities with diverse and unrelated defects in biochemical pathways? The anomalies observed vary from neural tube defects (folate deficiency); to agenesis of the corpus callosum (nonketotic hyperglycinemia [NKH]); to holoprosencephaly (Smith-Lemli-Opitz syndrome [SLOS]). Changes within the brain that can account for these observed abnormalities include neuronal loss or cell death (neurotoxic or apoptotic) and secondary axonal degeneration, leading to atrophy and volume loss in the gray matter and white matter, respectively. Encephaloclastic lesions, such as porencephalic cysts, are seen secondary to ischemic injury following vascular occlusion and focal neuronal necrosis. Interference with key processes that involve neuronal proliferation, neuronal differentiation, migration, and determination of cell fate are also likely to occur in IEM. Secondary processes, such as laying down of myelin by glial cells, can be affected, giving rise to delayed effects on the developing nervous system extending well into postnatal life.[6] There may also be a selective regional vulnerability within the nervous system; for example, the cerebellum is often affected in primary disorders of energy metabolism, such as pyruvate dehydrogenase (PDH) deficiency and mitochondrial disorders.[5]

## POTENTIAL MECHANISMS LINKING BIOCHEMICAL PATHWAYS TO MORPHOGENESIS
### Accumulation of Neurotoxic Intermediaries

The intracellular accumulation of metabolites, such as glycine (NKH) and sulfites (sulfite oxidase deficiency), can produce direct neurotoxic effects.[7] In sulfite oxidase deficiency, disruption of mitochondrial energy production by sulfite accumulation inhibits glutamate dehydrogenase,[8] and is accompanied by sulfate deficiency and impaired production of sulfatides in neural tissue, factors that adversely affect brain development. Pockets of neuronal cell death or focal ischemia may lead to encephaloclastic lesions, such as porencephalic cysts.[9–11]

### Defective Cell Respiration and Energy Metabolism

Aerobic metabolism in the brain tends to increase during periods of rapid neuronal proliferation, differentiation, and neuronal migration. PDH deficiency (discussed later) is often associated with severe malformations.[5,12] Similarly, disorders of the respiratory chain are also associated with multiple developmental defects in the nervous system.[13–16]

### Defects Within Cellular Signaling Pathways

Deficiency of the enzyme 7-dehydrocholesterol reductase results in low serum cholesterol levels in SLOS.[17] Cholesterol is involved in the posttranslation modification of the Sonic hedgehog gene product.[18] It is well known that signaling molecules are also reused at different phases of embryonic development[19]; the failure of posttranslational modification of the Sonic hedgehog protein in SLOS leads to a variety of craniofacial and brain abnormalities, the most severe of which is holoprosencephaly.[17,20–22]

### Alterations in the Biophysical Properties of Cell Membranes

Emerging evidence supports an important role for the cell membrane and its physical properties, such as rigidity in the maintenance of concentration gradients necessary for chemotropic signaling.[23,24] Membrane clustering of receptors and ligands form concentration gradients critical to axonal guidance. Deficient cholesterol within membranes affects fluidity,[24] potentially interfering with efficient anchoring of tyrosine kinase receptors and diffusibility of signaling molecules, resulting in disrupted signaling gradients.

### Interrelationships in Subcellular Organelle Function

The cholesterol biosynthetic pathway, for instance, involves the participation of several subcellular organelles: cytosol, mitochondria, and the peroxisomes. Sequential steps in the pathway are compartmentalized and distributed in these organelles.[25,26] Disturbance in peroxisomal function affects cholesterol biosynthesis in the mitochondria and vice versa. Intrinsic genetic factors less well understood may also contribute to the central nervous system anomalies seen in peroxisomal disorders, such as Zellweger syndrome.[27]

### Neuroplasticity Modifies Final Expression of Disturbance in Development

The concept of neuroplasticity in the developing nervous system dates back to the work of Cajal.[28] Although the timing of an insult is critical for the initiation or triggering of an abnormal developmental sequence, adaptive changes in the nervous system are also responsible for the final appearance of the nervous system and neuronal connectivity at both the microscopic and macroscopic level.[29,30]

### THE VALUE OF FETAL ULTRASONOGRAPHY WITH PARTICULAR RELEVANCE TO INBORN ERRORS OF METABOLISM

The broad processes of morphogenesis can be followed by the use of current two-dimensional, three-dimensional, and transvaginal fetal ultrasonography.[31–33] The use of these complementary techniques provides the unique ability to detect cerebral malformations in the prenatal period. The cranial end of the embryo can be discerned by the seventh postmenstrual week, and the principle divisions of the fetal brain can be distinguished by the following week. By the ninth week, the falx cerebri and choroid plexuses can be identified. The second trimester is a period of rapid increase in brain volume, increasing complexity of cortical organization and connectivity, the union of cerebellar hemispheres, and the development of the corpus callosum. These changes are further accompanied by development of gyri and sulci, and formation of the occipital horns and the occipital lobes.[34] Of particular interest to ultrasonographers, obstetricians, and pediatric neurologists are changes occurring in the midline structures: the corpus callosum, the septi pellucidi, the ventricular system, the cerebellar vermis, and the retrocerebellar spaces in the posterior fossa.[35,36]

**Table 1** provides a list of abnormalities that are likely to guide the perinatologist in search of potential genetic and metabolic etiologies. The reader is referred to other sections that deal with the details in the techniques for acquisition and display of the relevant images.

The following discusses selected disorders associated with developmental malformations of the fetal brain and nervous system that may be detected by ultrasonic examination during pregnancy. The recognition of a pattern provides the initial clues to the obstetrician or perinatologist to prompt consultation with a pediatric neurologist and a metabolic specialist. Further imaging studies and the use of advanced ultrasound and MRI should lead to greater precision in defining the abnormalities. Metabolic investigations can be commenced in the prenatal period through biochemical analysis of amniotic fluid, and through enzymatic studies on cultured cells following amniocentesis.

### INBORN ERRORS OF METABOLISM FREQUENTLY AFFECTING THE FETAL NERVOUS SYSTEM
### Pyruvate Dehydrogenase Deficiency

One of the commonest causes of congenital lactic acidosis, this disorder is well known to be associated with central nervous system malformations in the prenatal period.[37,38]

#### Biochemistry and genetics
Genetic mutations involving the PDH complex (OMIM *300,502 E1; EC 4.1.1.1) lead to primary lactic acidosis. The enzyme is a multienzyme complex with three components: PDH (E1), dihydrolipoamide acetyltransferase (E2), and lipoamide dehydrogenase (E3).

**Table 1**
**Abnormalities likely to point to potential metabolic etiologies**

| Fetal Ultrasonographic Features | Comments on Significance in Relationship to Inborn Errors of Metabolism |
| --- | --- |
| Intrauterine growth retardation | Nonspecific, wide differential, represents global effects of metabolic perturbation on the fetus, frequently seen in disorders of energy metabolism |
| Fetal akinesia/hypokinesia | Indicative of hypotonia, weakness in utero described in peroxisomal biogenesis disorders |
| Anomalies in head size: microcephaly and macrocephaly | Indicates poor cerebral growth, can be severe in Amish microcephaly, macrocrania a feature of glutaric aciduria type I and hydroxyglutaric aciduria |
| Forebrain development differentiation, midline anomalies | Holoprosencephaly is a feature of Smith-Lemli-Opitz syndrome |
| Ventriculomegaly | Nonspecific feature; may reflect brain anoxic damage, seen in mitochondrial disorders |
| Callosal abnormalities | Callosal dysgenesis is a marker for almost all inborn errors of metabolism: nonketotic hyperglycinemia, pyruvate dehydrogenase deficiency, mitochondrial disorders, maternal phenylketonuria, peroxisomal disorders, organic acidurias |
| Posterior fossa abnormalities | Cerebellar atrophy that is progressive is a feature of defects in energy metabolism, cerebellar hypoplasia is associated with congenital disorders of glycosylation type 1a |
| Neural tube segmentation | Disorders of folate metabolism |
| Association of dysplastic and disruptive lesions | Reflects abnormal energy supply occurring at different stages of pregnancy, mitochondrial disorders, pyruvate dehydrogenase deficiency |
| Cerebral atrophy and calcifications | Nonspecific, indicates progressive disease as a consequence of neuronal loss/drop out, mitochondrial disorders |
| Intracranial hemorrhage, effusions | Subdural hemorrhages and effusions associated with organic acidemias, such as glutaric aciduria type 1 |
| Stroke/encephaloclastic lesions (porencephaly) | Nonspecific association with defects in energy metabolism, sulfite oxidase deficiency |
| Malformations of cortical development | These are more difficult to detect on ultrasound alone; may need fetal MRI and follow-up postnatal imaging studies; most frequent in peroxisomal disorders, fumarase deficiency, Smith-Lemli-Opitz syndrome |
| Periventricular pseudocysts | Germinolytic cysts can be seen in defects of energy metabolism and peroxisomal biogenesis disorders |

The complex catalyzes the first step involved in the conversion of pyruvate to acetyl CoA. De novo mutations in the gene coding for the alpha subunit of the PDHE1 component lead to an X-linked form of PDH deficiency.[39–43] Both males and heterozygous females carrying one copy of the defective gene tend to be symptomatic.

### Clinical features and pathology

Infants present either with severe lactic acidosis and encephalopathy at birth, or in a neurologic form that may be detected prenatally on account of the associated anomalies. The neuropathologic features associated include cerebral atrophy, cavitating lesions in the white matter and deep gray nuclei, callosal dysgenesis of varying severity, absence of the pyramids, heterotopias of the olive, and abnormalities of the dentate nuclei.[44]

### Prenatal diagnosis

Prenatal ultrasound examination could be useful in identification of cortical atrophy, the cavitating and necrotic lesions of the white matter, and callosal and posterior fossa abnormalities. Fetal MRI may bring a higher level of resolution to the abnormalities involving the brainstem and cerebellum. Lactate elevation in the brain can be demonstrated on magnetic resonance spectroscopy.[45] Although enzyme activity in cultured fibroblasts is typically low, in heterozygous females activity levels may be normal, and hence a reliable diagnosis requires a search of mutations in the gene coding for the PDHE1-alpha subunit through molecular DNA diagnostics.[46]

### Treatment

Some forms of PDH deficiency are thiamine responsive, and thiamine supplements are helpful, whereas the lactic acidosis may be treated with the introduction of a ketogenic diet and the concomitant use of dichloroacetate. The ketogenic diet has been used successfully in the rescue of a zebrafish model for PDH deficiency.[47]

### Smith-Lemli-Opitz Syndrome

SLOS (OMIM#270,400) is a common birth defect (1:20,000–1:40,000) associated with malformations within multiple systems; craniofacial dysmorphic features; limb defects; and abnormalities of the heart, lungs, kidney, and genitalia.[48–50] Although two forms of the disorder are described (a severe form with neonatal presentation and a milder form), these likely represent two ends of a pathologic spectrum.

### Biochemistry and genetics

SLOS is caused by a defect in the enzyme 7-dehydrocholesterol reductase (OMIM *602,858, EC 1.3.1.21) involved in the pathway for cholesterol biosynthesis. Plasma cholesterol levels are typically low, whereas the levels of the precursor 7-dehydrocholesterol are elevated.[51] Maternal serum and urinary dihydroxysteroid ratios in combination with fetal anomalies detectable on ultrasound greatly enhance the likelihood of establishing a prenatal diagnosis.[52,53] The disorder is autosomal-recessive in its inheritance with mutations in the gene encoding the enzyme sterol delta-7-reductase, and common mutations can be identified through a polymerase chain reaction assay.[54,55]

### Clinical features

The occurrence of multiple malformations involving the face, limbs (polydactyly, syndactyly), genital abnormalities (hypospadias, ambiguous genitalia, micropenis, hypoplastic scrotum, bifid scrotum), and renal anomalies (agenesis, renal cysts, hydronephrosis), along with central nervous system abnormalities (microcephaly, hypoplasia of the frontal lobes, holoprosencephaly, callosal dysgenesis, cerebellar hypoplasia) is typical of the severe forms of the disorder. Considerable clinical heterogeneity exists, however, and milder forms can be more difficult to diagnose prenatally.[56]

### Prenatal diagnosis
Several reports have emphasized the clinical significance of the association of intrauterine growth retardation and nuchal edema on ultrasound examinations prenatally to be highly suggestive of SLOS.[52]

### Glutaric aciduria type I
Glutaric aciduria type I (OMIM#231,670) is an autosomal-recessive disorder resulting from an inherited defect in the glutaryl-CoA dehydrogenase enzyme (enzyme commission number, EC 1.3.99.7; OMIM*231,670). Glutaryl-CoA dehydrogenase is involved in the degradative pathway of the amino acids L-tryptophan, L-lysine, and L-hydroxylysine.[57] The metabolic block leads to accumulation of glutaric acid, 3- hydroxyglutaric acid, and glutaconic acid in urine and blood and the cerebrospinal fluid. Urine organic acid analysis shows excretion of variable amounts of glutaric acid and 3-hydroxyglutaric acid. Mutations in the gene at the glutaryl-CoA dehydrogenase locus (19p13.2) are diagnostic. There is considerable locus heterogeneity and a lack of genotype-phenotype correlations in this disorder.

### Clinical features
The disorder causes an acute devastating neurologic syndrome in infants that is characterized by sudden onset hypotonia, dystonia, and encephalopathy, often in conjunction with a febrile illness. Survivors often have dystonic movements, seizures, and developmental delay. Early diagnosis carries a significant impact on both survival and timely interventions to prevent and mitigate complications of the acute encephalopathic crisis.[58] Neuropathologic features are fairly characteristic for this disorder and include macrocrania and increased brain size and weight, subdural effusions and hematomas, a pattern of frontotemporal atrophy associated with incomplete opercularization, and atrophy of the caudate and putamina bilaterally.[59]

### Prenatal diagnosis
Although the neuropathologic findings are easily detected in the postnatal period on MRI, ultrasonographic studies during the prenatal period seem to suggest that the combination of macrocrania, abnormal opercularization of the sylvian fissure, ventriculomegaly, and subdural effusions may be highly suggestive.[60–62] This combination should definitely prompt a thorough search for glutaryl-CoA dehydrogenase mutations using DNA from chorionic villus biopsy or cultured amniocytes.[63] Biochemical confirmation through assays of glutarylcarnitine in dried blood spots from the newborn using tandem mass spectrometry is an alternative.[64]

### Congenital Disorders of Glycosylation

The congenital disorders of glycosylation (CDG) are a group of recessively inherited disorders resulting from enzyme defects in the glycosylation pathways (pregolgi, endoplasmic reticulum, and golgi complex). These disorders present with multisystem involvement, particularly the central and peripheral nervous systems and coagulation and endocrine systems.[65,66] There are two types of glycosylation reactions: N-glycosylation and O-glycosylation. The first disorder in the glycosylation pathway was described in 1980 and was named the "carbohydrate deficient glycoprotein syndrome." The last decade has seen the identification of several subtypes and the original syndromic term has been replaced by the term "congenital disorders of glycosylation." Of the more than 10 subtypes known currently, CDG type 1a is the most frequently encountered and is the one that has severe enough manifestations that can be detected by ultrasound.[67] The discussion is restricted to this subtype.

### Biochemistry and genetics

CDG1a (#212,065) results from mutations in the PMM2 gene coding for the enzyme phosphomannomutase (OMIM*601,785, EC 5.4.2.8). The resulting deficiency leads to reduced availability of GDP-mannose required for the assembly of the dolicholpyrophosphate-linked oligosaccharide in the endoplasmic reticulum.[67] The diagnosis relies on the demonstration of hypoglycosylation of serum proteins using isoelectric focusing of transferrin, which shows a cathodal shift in the presence of partial sialyl groups.[68] Although the enzyme assay can be performed on cultured fibroblasts and amniocytes, the results are not considered uniformly reliable, because low values have been reported in the presence of a normal genotype. Molecular diagnostic studies leading to prenatal diagnosis are possible in the presence of an affected proband.[67]

### Clinical features and pathology

The initial descriptions of this condition included facial dysmorphic features, inverted nipples, abnormal distribution of fat pads, mental retardation, hypotonia, and cerebellar hypoplasia.[65] Cerebellar hypoplasia and hypotonia are, however, consistently noted features in this disorder. There is considerable heterogeneity in the presentation of this condition; it is likely that prenatal ultrasound may be useful only if the abnormalities are severe and above the threshold sensitivity for detection.

### Prenatal ultrasound diagnosis

Current neurosonographic techniques are sophisticated enough to permit detection of posterior fossa abnormalities in the right hands on serial imaging. There are diagnostic pitfalls that need to be considered, however, which have been described in detail.[69] If the combination of cerebellar hypoplasia and fetal akinesia is detected, CDG1a should be a consideration. Other features, such as presentation with nonimmune hydrops fetalis, hyperechoic kidneys, and cardiomyopathy, have also been detected in prenatal studies leading to a diagnosis of CDG1a.[70–72]

## Mitochondrial Disorders

Mitochondrial disorders are disorders of the respiratory chain that cause defective oxidative phosphorylation resulting in energy deficiency of any organ or tissue. The decrease in energy supply may manifest any time, from prenatal to postnatal life. The most affected organs are those that require the largest amount of energy (brain, muscle, and heart).

### Biochemistry and genetics

The mitochondrial respiratory chain catalyzes the oxidation of fuel molecules and the concomitant energy transduction into ATP by five complexes, which are embedded in the inner mitochondrial membrane. Complex I (NADH–coenzyme Q reductase) carries reducing equivalents from NADH to coenzyme Q (ubiquinone) and consists of 40 different polypeptides. Complex II (succinate–coenzyme Q reductase) carries reducing equivalents from $FADH_2$ to coenzyme Q and contains four polypeptides, including the FAD-dependent succinate dehydrogenase and iron-sulfur proteins. Complex III (reduced coenzyme Q–cytochrome-c reductase) carries electrons from coenzyme Q to cytochrome c; it contains 11 subunits. Complex IV (cytochrome-c oxidase), the terminal oxidase of the respiratory chain, catalyzes the transfer of reducing equivalents from cytochrome c to molecular oxygen. It is composed of two cytochromes (cytochromes $a$ and $a_3$); two copper atoms; and 13 different protein subunits. During the oxidation process, electrons are transferred to oxygen by the energy-transducing complexes of the respiratory chain. The free energy generated from the redox reactions is converted into a transmembrane proton gradient. Complex V (ATP synthase) allows protons to flow back into the mitochondrial matrix and uses the released energy to synthesize ATP. Three ATP molecules are produced for each NADH molecule oxidized.[73]

The mitochondrial respiratory chain is composed of approximately 100 different proteins. Only 13 of the proteins are encoded by mitochondrial genes; the others are encoded by nuclear genes. All complexes of the respiratory chain except complex II have a double genetic origin. Disorders of the respiratory chain may be inherited in all modes of inheritance: maternal, autosomal-recessive, autosomal-dominant, and X-linked.

### Clinical features

Mitochondrial disorders can present at any age and affect all organs. They rarely present in utero. When they do, however, the postnatal presentation is usually early (neonatal period to infancy) and the course fatal.[74] The presentation may be fulminant, with lactic acidosis and multiorgan failure culminating in early demise.

von Kleist-Retzow and colleagues[74] reviewed 300 cases of proved respiratory chain enzyme deficiency for fetal development. Twenty patients had an antenatal presentation, the most common being intrauterine growth retardation and multiple anomalies of organs sharing no common function or embryologic origin. The brain was involved in three patients: ventriculomegaly and porencephalic cysts, Dandy-Walker malformation, and agenesis of corpus callosum. In two additional children, the hypoplasia of the cerebellum and corpus callosum were not identified in utero, and in one case ventriculomegaly and porencephalic germinal matrix cysts were found at 22 weeks of gestation and later resolved. Periventricular pseudocysts in a fetus that later developed a Leigh disease presentation has also been described.

Cerebellar involvement has also been described in two previous articles, manifesting either as cerebellar hypoplasia[75] or pontocerebellar hypoplasia.[14]

Gire and coworkers[76] described the neuroradiologic features of six neonates with mitochondrial disorders. Five had antenatal involvement. A prenatal MRI in one demonstrated ventricular and parenchymal hemorrhages.

Samson and colleagues[77] described ventriculomegaly and intracerebral calcifications in two fetuses with a familial mitochondrial encephalopathy. An autopsy showed extensive encephalopathy with cavitation and calcification in the cerebral hemispheres, polymicrogyria, multiple neuronal heterotopia, partial callosal dysgenesis, and severe Leigh syndrome. White matter calcifications in two consecutive pregnancies of fetuses with multiple mtDNA deletions have also been observed.

### Prenatal diagnosis

Abnormalities of the respiratory chain may cause both brain dysplasia and disruption. There is a continuum of early and late brain involvement that can be identified by ultrasound at different stages of gestation. The ultrasound may identify agenesis of corpus callosum as early as mid pregnancy, and later in the third trimester identify cerebellar hypoplasia and malformations of cortical development.[78] Ventriculomegaly and periventricular pseudocysts may prove to be a relatively common presentation of in utero energy deficiency.

When a fetus presents with an association of multiorgan malformations without a common embryologic origin, intrauterine growth retardation, and brain dysplasia or disruption, a mitochondrial disorder should be suspected. When there is no family history, however, prenatal diagnosis cannot be offered.

When the disease-causing mutation in the nuclear DNA is known, prenatal diagnosis is available. When the mutation is in the mtDNA very little information is available, because the ratio of mutant versus wild-type mtDNA (heteroplasmy) in fetal DNA is considered to be a poor indicator of postnatal outcome. Nevertheless, prenatal diagnosis has been attempted in MELAS (myopathy, encephalopathy, lactic acidosis, and stroke-like) syndrome due to the 3243 mtDNA[79] mutation, and in maternally inherited Leigh syndrome due to the 8993 mtDNA mutation.[80]

Assessment of the respiratory chain in amniotic cells is not reliable because the abnormal enzyme activity may be tissue specific and not involve amniotic cells, and the expression of respiratory chain deficiency during fetal life is time dependent because of differential expression or regulation of the mutant proteins.[81]

## Maternal Phenylketonuria

The maternal phenylketonuria (PKU) syndrome refers to the teratogenic effects of phenylalanine during pregnancy. These effects include mental retardation, microcephaly, congenital heart disease, and intrauterine growth retardation.[82]

### Biochemistry and genetics

PKU (OMIM #261,600) is an autosomal-recessive inborn error of metabolism resulting from a deficiency of phenylalanine hydroxylase (EC 1.14.16.1), an enzyme that catalyzes the hydroxylation of phenylalanine to tyrosine, the rate-limiting step in phenylalanine catabolism.

When the mother has classic PKU with a blood phenylalanine level greater than or equal to 1200 $\mu$M (20 mg/dL), there is a high frequency of teratogenicity in the offspring, with microcephaly and mental retardation in 75% to 90%, and congenital heart disease in 15%. There is a dose-response relationship with progressively lower frequencies of these abnormalities at lower phenylalanine levels.

The pathogenesis may be related to inhibition by phenylalanine of large neutral amino acid transport across the placenta or to direct toxicity of phenylalanine, a phenylalanine metabolite, or both in certain fetal organs. Although phenylalanine hydroxylase is expressed in the fetus as early as the sixth week of gestation, the large load of toxic phenylalanine from the mother overwhelms the limited hydroxylating capacity of the fetus.[83] The oligodendroglia switch to a nonmyelinating phenotype that expresses an astrocyte marker, glial fibrillary acidic protein. The impairment of intrauterine myelination could explain the hypoplastic corpus callosum.

The treatment of maternal PKU consists of biochemical control through a phenylalanine-restricted diet during pregnancy. The best results are obtained with diet initiation before conception or no later than the earliest weeks of pregnancy.

### Clinical picture

Because the fetus does not have PKU, the effect of the increased phenylalanine levels in utero is nonprogressive. The child may be born microcephalic with a congenital heart defect and then show a picture of static developmental delay. Brain MRI may demonstrate a dysgenetic corpus callosum and delayed myelination.[83]

### Prenatal ultrasound diagnosis

When the mother has PKU, she should be monitored for phenylalanine levels even before conception and her diet should be strictly adjusted. A fetal ultrasound should be obtained serially throughout pregnancy. It can demonstrate progressive microcephaly and dysgenesis of the corpus callosum associated with a congenital heart defect.

## Peroxisomal Biogenesis Disorders

The peroxisomal biogenesis disorders (MIM# 601,539) are autosomal-recessive disorders of peroxisome assembly that lead to deficiency of multiple peroxisomal enzymes. They have overlapping phenotypic features and various genetic causes (defects in over 25 PEX genes). Because of their heterogeneity, peroxisomal biogenesis disorders had been divided into four groups: (1) Zellweger syndrome (MIM# 214,100); (2) neonatal adrenoleukodystrophy (MIM# 202,370); (3) infantile Refsum disease (MIM# 266,510); and (4) rhizomelic chondrodysplasia punctata (MIM# 215,100).[84]

### Biochemistry and genetics

Peroxisomes are organelles present in almost all eukaryotic cells. They are essential for the metabolism of branched chain and very long chain fatty acids, ether lipids, polyamines, amino acids, and glyoxylate. During some of these metabolic processes, peroxisomes generate and subsequently inactivate reactive oxygen species.[84] It has been estimated that at least 85 proteins are associated with peroxisome structure and function in humans. Peroxisome matrix proteins are synthesized in the cytosol before import into the peroxisome. Peroxins, encoded by a family PEX genes, are involved in peroxisome biogenesis, with functions ranging from membrane synthesis and matrix protein import to organelle division.[84]

Biochemical studies performed in blood and urine are used to screen for peroxisomal biogenesis disorders. They include elevated plasma very long chain fatty acids, bile acids, phytanic, pristanic, and pipecolic acids contrasting with low plasma plasmalogens. Impaired enzymatic activity of dihydroacetone-phosphate acyltransferase deficiency can be detected in fibroblasts.

### Clinical features

Zellweger syndrome, also known as "cerebrohepatorenal syndrome," is the classic and most severe peroxisomal biogenesis disorder. Inheritance is autosomal-recessive, and affected individuals can be recognized at birth because of prominent hypotonia; hyporeflexia; seizures; craniofacial dysmorphism (prominent forehead, large anterior fontanelle, hypoplastic supraorbital ridges, broad nasal bridge, hypertelorism, and deformed ear lobes); limb anomalies; liver dysfunction; optic atrophy; glaucoma; cataract; failure to thrive; renal cysts; stippled epiphyses; and prominent mental retardation. Accumulation of phytanic acid, very long chain fatty acids, pipecolic acid, and abnormal bile acids in multiple organs are thought to be the underlying mechanism of this fatal condition. Death usually occurs within the first year of life. There is a clinical overlap with neonatal adrenoleukodystrophy and infantile Refsum disease.

Migration anomalies are well documented in peroxisomal disorders. In the Zellweger syndrome spectrum, these anomalies consist of lissencephaly, perirolandic and occipital pachygyria, frontal and perisylvian polymicrogyria, periventricular heterotopias, band heterotopias, hypoplastic corpus callosum, abnormal layering of the cerebellum, and dysplasia of the inferior olivary nuclei and olfactory bulb.[85-94]

Rhizomelic chondrodysplasia punctata is associated with a mutation in the PEX 7 gene and a defect in plasmalogen synthesis. It is characterized clinically by shortening of the proximal limbs, cataracts, a characteristic facial appearance, failure to thrive, and psychomotor retardation.

Malformations of cortical development are less frequent in rhizomelic chondrodysplasia punctata, but there has been a report of pachygyria-polymicrogyria in this syndrome.[95]

### Prenatal diagnosis

The first sign of fetal Zellweger syndrome is increased nuchal translucency.[95] Later, suspicion should be raised in a fetus with hypokinesia, cerebral ventricular enlargement, renal hyperechogenicity, and hepatosplenomegaly. Prenatal ultrasound supplemented with MRI can identify abnormal cortical development in the third trimester. Mochel and colleagues[96] described the fetal MRI features in two fetuses with Zellweger syndrome: one depicted asymmetric ventriculomegaly, abnormally small cerebral convolutions, mostly in the frontal and in the perisylvian cortex, periventricular leukodystrophy predominating in the frontal area, and germinolytic cysts in the subependymal areas; the other depicted bilateral ventricular enlargement associated with a large cavum, abnormal gyration pattern mostly in the frontal and in the perisylvian cortex, and periventricular leukodystrophy, mainly in the frontal area and irregular ventricular walls revealing bilateral subependymal pseudocysts. The combination of cortical malformations of the perisylvian and perirolandic regions, hypomyelination, and germinolytic cysts seems specific for Zellweger syndrome.

When there is a family history and both disease-causing alleles of the affected family member have been identified, a molecular diagnosis can be made. When the suspicion is raised because of the association of the typical brain anomalies with kidney and liver abnormalities, however, the prenatal diagnosis can be made by very long chain fatty acids content and plasmalogen synthesis measured in cultured chorionic villus sampling or amniocytes.[97]

## Nonketotic Hyperglycinemia

NKH (OMIM #605,899) (also known as "glycine encephalopathy") is an inborn error of glycine metabolism in which large quantities of glycine accumulate in all body tissues, including the brain.

### Biochemistry and genetics

NKH is an autosomal-recessive disorder. NKH is caused by a defect in the glycine cleavage system (EC 2.1.2.10), which is confined to the mitochondria, and composed of four protein components: (1) P protein (a pyridoxal phosphate–dependent glycine decarboxylase); (2) H protein (a lipoic acid–containing protein); (3) T protein (a tetrahydrofolate-requiring enzyme); and (4) L protein (a lipoamide dehydrogenase). NKH may be caused by a defect in any one of these enzymes.

Glycine encephalopathy is suspected in individuals with elevated glycine concentration in urine, plasma, and cerebrospinal fluid. Simultaneous cerebrospinal fluid and plasma samples are required to establish the diagnosis of glycine encephalopathy. An abnormal cerebrospinal fluid/plasma glycine ratio suggests the diagnosis of glycine encephalopathy.

### Clinical features

Most patients with NKH have the neonatal phenotype, presenting in the first few days of life with lethargy, hypotonia, and myoclonic jerks, and progressing to apnea and often to death. Those who regain spontaneous respiration develop intractable seizures and profound mental retardation. In the infantile form of glycine encephalopathy, patients present with seizures and have various degrees of mental retardation after a symptom-free interval and seemingly normal development for up to 6 months.

MRI demonstrates agenesis or thinning of the corpus callosum, dysmyelination, and gyral abnormalities.[98–101]

### Prenatal diagnosis

Paupe and colleagues[102] reported the prenatal diagnosis of hypoplasia of the corpus callosum in a fetus that was diagnosed with NKH. The differential diagnosis on prenatal diagnosis of agenesis of the corpus callosum with or without associated cortical malformations should include NKH.

Prenatal diagnosis for pregnancies at increased risk is possible by analysis of DNA extracted from fetal cells obtained by amniocentesis. Prenatal testing using measurement of amniotic fluid glycine concentration and the glycine/serine ratio are unreliable because normal and affected values overlap.

## SUMMARY

Brain development is a time-locked process orchestrated by complex neurobiologic processes. Organogenesis involves processes beginning with neurulation, formation of the craniocaudal axis, morphologic differentiation, neuronal proliferation, migration, and the development of neural connectivity. IEM can lead to disturbances in brain development through multiple mechanisms that include critical nutrient deficiency, accumulation of neurotoxic substrates, deficits in energy metabolism, abnormality in cell membrane constituents, and interference in cell-to-cell signaling pathways. There is a temporal relationship between exposure to metabolic perturbation and its consequence, followed by adaptive changes through neuroplasticity, which determine the final appearance of a developmental malformation. The anomalies observed vary from neural tube defects and agenesis of the corpus callosum to holoprosencephaly and cortical migration disorders. The cerebellum is also often affected.

Most of these brain abnormalities can be identified in utero by serial neurosonography supplemented by fetal MRI. The differential diagnosis in these cases should include IEM. Early diagnosis is critical for institution of treatment, which may positively influence the final outcome, and for the purpose of genetic counseling.

## ACKNOWLEDGMENT

The authors acknowledge C. Prasad, MD, FRCPC, FCCMG, Associate Professor, Genetics Program of South-Western Ontario, Children's Hospital, for her useful comments and suggestions.

## REFERENCES

1. Volpe JJ. Overview: normal and abnormal human brain development. Ment Retard Dev Disabil Res Rev 2000;6(1):1–5.
2. O'Rahilly R, Müller F. The embryonic human brainan atlas of developmental stages. 3rd edition. Hoboken (NJ): Wiley-Liss; 2006.
3. Graf W. Cerebral dysgenesis secondary to metabolic diseases in fetal life. In: Aminoff MJ, Boller F, Swaab DF, editors. Handbook of clinical neurology. Amsterdam: Handb Clin Neurol 2007;87:459–76.
4. Bamforth F, Bamforth S, Poskitt K, et al. Abnormalities of corpus callosum in patients with inherited metabolic diseases [letter]. Lancet 1988;2(8608):451.
5. Nissenkorn A, Michelson M, Ben-Zeev B, et al. Inborn errors of metabolism: a cause of abnormal brain development. Neurology 2001;56(10):1265–72.

6. Prasad A, Rupar C, Prasad C, et al. Cellular bioenergetics and cerebral dysmorphogenesis: lessons from Amish microcephaly. Neuropediatrics 2006;37(S1). Available at: http://www.thieme-connect.com/ejournals/abstract/neuropediatrics/doi/10.1055/s-2006-945606. Accessed June 28, 2009.

7. Dobyns WB. Agenesis of the corpus callosum and gyral malformations are frequent manifestations of nonketotic hyperglycinemia. Neurology 1989;39(6): 817–20.

8. Zhang X, Vincent AS, Halliwell B, et al. A mechanism of sulfite neurotoxicity: direct inhibition of glutamate dehydrogenase. J Biol Chem 2004;279(41):43035–45.

9. Schiaffino MC, Fantasia AR, Minniti G, et al. Isolated sulphite oxidase deficiency: clinical and biochemical features in an Italian patient. J Inherit Metab Dis 2004; 27(1):101–2.

10. Rupar CA, Gillett J, Gordon BA, et al. Isolated sulfite oxidase deficiency. Neuropediatrics 1996;27(6):299–304.

11. Roth A, Nogues C, Monnet JP, et al. Anatomo-pathological findings in a case of combined deficiency of sulphite oxidase and xanthine oxidase with a defect of molybdenum cofactor. Virchows Arch A Pathol Anat Histopathol 1985;405(3): 379–86.

12. van Straaten HL, van Tintelen JP, Trijbels JM, et al. Neonatal lactic acidosis, complex I/IV deficiency, and fetal cerebral disruption. Neuropediatrics 2005; 36(3):193–9.

13. Chow CW, Thorburn DR. Morphological correlates of mitochondrial dysfunction in children. Hum Reprod 2000;15(Suppl 2):68–78.

14. de Koning TJ, de Vries LS, Groenendaal F, et al. Pontocerebellar hypoplasia associated with respiratory-chain defects. Neuropediatrics 1999;30(2):93–5.

15. Sarnat HB, Marin-Garcia J. Pathology of mitochondrial encephalomyopathies. Can J Neurol Sci 2005;32(2):152–66.

16. Shevell MI, Matthews PM, Scriver CR, et al. Cerebral dysgenesis and lactic acidemia: an MRI/MRS phenotype associated with pyruvate dehydrogenase deficiency. Pediatr Neurol 1994;11(3):224–9.

17. Porter FD. Human malformation syndromes due to inborn errors of cholesterol synthesis. Curr Opin Pediatr 2003;15(6):607–13.

18. Ingham PW. Hedgehog signaling: a tale of two lipids. Science 2001;294(5548): 1879–81.

19. Ahlgren S, Bronner-Fraser M. Recycling signaling molecules during development. Nat Neurosci 2002;5(2):87–8.

20. Caruso PA, Poussaint TY, Tzika AA, et al. MRI and 1H MRS findings in Smith-Lemli-Opitz syndrome. Neuroradiology 2004;46(1):3–14.

21. Johnson JA, Aughton DJ, Comstock CH, et al. Prenatal diagnosis of Smith-Lemli-Opitz syndrome, type II. Am J Med Genet 1994;49(2):240–3.

22. Lanoue L, Dehart DB, Hinsdale ME, et al. Limb, genital, CNS, and facial malformations result from gene/environment-induced cholesterol deficiency: further evidence for a link to sonic hedgehog. Am J Med Genet 1997;73(1): 24–31.

23. Guirland C, Suzuki S, Kojima M, et al. Lipid rafts mediate chemotropic guidance of nerve growth cones. Neuron 2004;42(1):51–62.

24. Simons K, Ehehalt R. Cholesterol, lipid rafts, and disease. J Clin Invest 2002; 110(5):597–603.

25. Baumgart E, Vanhorebeek I, Grabenbauer M, et al. Mitochondrial alterations caused by defective peroxisomal biogenesis in a mouse model for Zellweger syndrome (PEX5 knockout mouse). Am J Pathol 2001;159(4):1477–94.

26. Kovacs WJ, Olivier LM, Krisans SK. Central role of peroxisomes in isoprenoid biosynthesis. Prog Lipid Res 2002;41(5):369–91.
27. Faust PL, Banka D, Siriratsivawong R, et al. Peroxisome biogenesis disorders: the role of peroxisomes and metabolic dysfunction in developing brain. J Inherit Metab Dis 2005;28(3):369–83.
28. Stahnisch FW, Nitsch R. Santiago Ramon y Cajal's concept of neuronal plasticity: the ambiguity lives on. Trends Neurosci 2002;25(11):589–91.
29. Johnston MV, Nishimura A, Harum K, et al. Sculpting the developing brain. Adv Pediatr 2001;48:1–38.
30. Johnston MV. Injury and plasticity in the developing brain. Exp Neurol 2003; 184(Suppl 1):S37–41.
31. Pooh RK, Pooh K. Transvaginal 3D and Doppler ultrasonography of the fetal brain. Semin Perinatol 2001;25(1):38–43.
32. Pooh RK, Pooh K, Nakagawa Y, et al. Clinical application of three-dimensional ultrasound in fetal brain assessment. Croat Med J 2000;41(3):245–51.
33. Timor-Tritsch IE, Monteagudo A, Mayberry P. Three-dimensional ultrasound evaluation of the fetal brain: the three horn view. Ultrasound Obstet Gynecol 2000; 16(4):302–6.
34. Monteagudo A, Timor-Tritsch IE. Normal sonographic development of the central nervous system from the second trimester onwards using 2D, 3D and transvaginal sonography. Prenat Diagn 2009;29:326–39.
35. Monteagudo A, Timor-Tritsch IE, Mayberry P. Three-dimensional transvaginal neurosonography of the fetal brain: navigating in the volume scan. Ultrasound Obstet Gynecol 2000;16(4):307–13.
36. Pilu G, Segata M, Ghi T, et al. Diagnosis of midline anomalies of the fetal brain with the three-dimensional median view. Ultrasound Obstet Gynecol 2006;27(5): 522–9.
37. Israels S, Haworth JC, Dunn HG, et al. Lactic acidosis in childhood. Adv Pediatr 1976;22:267–303.
38. Aleck KA, Kaplan AM, Sherwood WG, et al. In utero central nervous system damage in pyruvate dehydrogenase deficiency. Arch Neurol 1988;45(9): 987–9.
39. de Meirleir LJ, Lissens W, Vamos E, et al. Pyruvate dehydrogenase deficiency due to a mutation of the E1 alpha subunit. J Inherit Metab Dis 1991;14(3):301–4.
40. De Meirleir L, Lissens W, Vamos E, et al. Pyruvate dehydrogenase (PDH) deficiency caused by a 21-base pair insertion mutation in the E1 alpha subunit. Hum Genet 1992;88(6):649–52.
41. Chun K, MacKay N, Petrova-Benedict R, et al. Mutations in the X-linked E1 alpha subunit of pyruvate dehydrogenase leading to deficiency of the pyruvate dehydrogenase complex. Hum Mol Genet 1993;2(4):449–54.
42. Hansen LL, Brown GK, Brown RM, et al. Pyruvate dehydrogenase deficiency caused by a 5 base pair duplication in the E1 alpha subunit. Hum Mol Genet 1993;2(6):805–7.
43. Otero LJ, Brown RM, Brown GK. Arginine 302 mutations in the pyruvate dehydrogenase E1alpha subunit gene: identification of further patients and in vitro demonstration of pathogenicity. Hum Mutat 1998;12(2):114–21.
44. Chow CW, Anderson RM, Kenny GC. Neuropathology in cerebral lactic acidosis. Acta Neuropathol 1987;74(4):393–6.
45. Zand DJ, Simon EM, Pulitzer SB, et al. In vivo pyruvate detected by MR spectroscopy in neonatal pyruvate dehydrogenase deficiency. AJNR Am J Neuroradiol 2003;24(7):1471–4.

46. Brown RM, Brown GK. Prenatal diagnosis of pyruvate dehydrogenase E1 alpha subunit deficiency. Prenat Diagn 1994;14(6):435–41.
47. Taylor MR, Hurley JB, Van Epps HA, et al. A zebrafish model for pyruvate dehydrogenase deficiency: rescue of neurological dysfunction and embryonic lethality using a ketogenic diet. Proc Natl Acad Sci U S A 2004;101(13):4584–9.
48. Opitz JM, Penchaszadeh VB, Holt MC, et al. Smith-Lemli-Opitz (RSH) syndrome bibliography. Am J Med Genet 1987;28(3):745–50.
49. Penchaszadeh VB. The nosology of the Smith-Lemli-Opitz syndrome. Am J Med Genet 1987;28(3):719–21.
50. Porter FD. Smith-Lemli-Opitz syndrome: pathogenesis, diagnosis and management. Eur J Hum Genet 2008;16(5):535–41.
51. Irons M, Elias ER, Tint GS, et al. Abnormal cholesterol metabolism in the Smith-Lemli-Opitz syndrome: report of clinical and biochemical findings in four patients and treatment in one patient. Am J Med Genet 1994;50(4):347–52.
52. Goldenberg A, Wolf C, Chevy F, et al. Antenatal manifestations of Smith-Lemli-Opitz (RSH) syndrome: a retrospective survey of 30 cases. Am J Med Genet A 2004;124(4):423–6.
53. Shinawi M, Szabo S, Popek E, et al. Recognition of Smith-Lemli-Opitz syndrome (RSH) in the fetus: utility of ultrasonography and biochemical analysis in pregnancies with low maternal serum estriol. Am J Med Genet A 2005;138(1):56–60.
54. Battaile KP, Maslen CL, Wassif CA, et al. A simple PCR-based assay allows detection of a common mutation, IVS8-1G→C, in DHCR7 in Smith-Lemli-Opitz syndrome. Genet Test 1999;3(4):361–3.
55. Wassif CA, Maslen C, Kachilele-Linjewile S, et al. Mutations in the human sterol delta7-reductase gene at 11q12-13 cause Smith-Lemli-Opitz syndrome. Am J Hum Genet 1998;63(1):55–62.
56. Nowaczyk MJ, Heshka T, Kratz LE, et al. Difficult prenatal diagnosis in mild Smith-Lemli-Opitz syndrome. Am J Med Genet 2000;95(4):396–8.
57. Goodman SI, Kohlhoff JG. Glutaric aciduria: inherited deficiency of glutaryl-CoA dehydrogenase activity. Biochem Med 1975;13(2):138–40.
58. Superti-Furga A, Hoffmann GF. Glutaric aciduria type 1 (glutaryl-CoA-dehydrogenase deficiency): advances and unanswered questions. Report from an international meeting. Eur J Pediatr 1997;156(11):821–8.
59. Funk CB, Prasad AN, Frosk P, et al. Neuropathological, biochemical and molecular findings in a glutaric acidemia type 1 cohort. Brain 2005;128(Pt 4):711–22.
60. Forstner R, Hoffmann GF, Gassner I, et al. Glutaric aciduria type I: ultrasonographic demonstration of early signs. Pediatr Radiol 1999;29(2):138–43.
61. Lin SK, Hsu SG, Ho ES, et al. Glutaric aciduria (type I): prenatal ultrasonographic findings. Ultrasound Obstet Gynecol 2002;20(3):305–7.
62. Lin SK, Hsu SG, Ho ES, et al. Novel mutation and prenatal sonographic findings of glutaric aciduria (type I) in two Taiwanese families. Prenat Diagn 2002;22(8):725–9.
63. Busquets C, Coll MJ, Merinero B, et al. Prenatal molecular diagnosis of glutaric aciduria type I by direct mutation analysis. Prenat Diagn 2000;20(9):761–4.
64. Baric I, Zschocke J, Christensen E, et al. Diagnosis and management of glutaric aciduria type I. J Inherit Metab Dis 1998;21(4):326–40.
65. Jaeken J, Carchon H. The carbohydrate-deficient glycoprotein syndromes: an overview. J Inherit Metab Dis 1993;16(5):813–20.
66. Krasnewich D, Gahl WA. Carbohydrate-deficient glycoprotein syndrome. Adv Pediatr 1997;44:109–40.

67. Matthijs G, Schollen E, Van Schaftingen E. The prenatal diagnosis of congenital disorders of glycosylation (CDG). Prenat Diagn 2004;24(2):114–6.
68. Jaeken J, Carchon H, Stibler H. The carbohydrate-deficient glycoprotein syndromes: pre-Golgi and Golgi disorders? Glycobiology 1993;3(5):423–8.
69. Malinger G, Lev D, Lerman-Sagie T. The fetal cerebellum: pitfalls in diagnosis and management. Prenat Diagn 2009;29(4):372–80.
70. Hertz-Pannier L, Dechaux M, Sinico M, et al. Congenital disorders of glycosylation type I: a rare but new cause of hyperechoic kidneys in infants and children due to early microcystic changes. Pediatr Radiol 2006;36(2):108–14.
71. Malhotra A, Pateman A, Chalmers R, et al. Prenatal cardiac ultrasound finding in congenital disorder of glycosylation type 1a. Fetal Diagn Ther 2009;25(1):54–7.
72. van de Kamp JM, Lefeber DJ, Ruijter GJ, et al. Congenital disorder of glycosylation type Ia presenting with hydrops fetalis. J Med Genet 2007;44(4): 277–80.
73. Rötig A, Munnich A. Genetic features of mitochondrial respiratory chain disorders. J Am Soc Nephrol 2003;14(12):2995–3007.
74. von Kleist-Retzow JC, Cormier-Daire V, Viot G, et al. Antenatal manifestations of mitochondrial respiratory chain deficiency. J Pediatr 2003;143(2):208–12.
75. Lincke CR, van den Bogert C, Nijtmans LG, et al. Cerebellar hypoplasia in respiratory chain dysfunction. Neuropediatrics 1996;27:216–8.
76. Gire C, Girard N, Nicaise C, et al. Clinical features and neuroradiological findings of mitochondrial pathology in six neonates. Childs Nerv Syst 2002;18(11): 621–8.
77. Samson JF, Barth PG, de Vries JI, et al. Familial mitochondrial encephalopathy with fetal ultrasonographic ventriculomegaly and intracerebral calcifications. Eur J Pediatr 1994;153(7):510–6.
78. Malinger G, Kidron D, Schreiber L, et al. Prenatal diagnosis of malformations of cortical development by dedicated neurosonography. Ultrasound Obstet Gynecol 2007;29(2):178–91.
79. Bouchet C, Steffann J, Corcos J, et al. Prenatal diagnosis of myopathy, encephalopathy, lactic acidosis, and stroke-like syndrome: contribution to understanding mitochondrial DNA segregation during human embryofetal development. J Med Genet 2006;43(10):788–92.
80. Dahl HH, Thorburn DR, White SL. Towards reliable prenatal diagnosis of mtDNA point mutations: studies of nt8993mutations in oocytes, fetal tissues, children and adults. Hum Reprod 2000;15(Suppl 2):246–55.
81. Minai L, Martinovic J, Chretien D, et al. Mitochondrial respiratory chain complex assembly and function during human fetal development. Mol Genet Metab 2008; 94(1):120–6.
82. Levy HL, Ghavami M. Maternal phenylketonuria: a metabolic teratogen. Teratology 1996;53(3):176–84.
83. Levy HL, Lobbregt D, Barnes PD, et al. Maternal phenylketonuria: magnetic resonance imaging in offspring. J Pediatr 1996;128:770–5.
84. Yik WY, Steinberg SJ, Moser AB, et al. Identification of novel mutations and sequence variation in the Zellweger syndrome spectrum of peroxisome biogenesis disorders. Hum Mutat 2009;30(3):E467–80.
85. Volpe JJ, Adams RD. Cerebro-hepato-renal syndrome of Zellweger: an inherited disorder of neuronal migration. Acta Neuropathol 1972;20:175–98.
86. Liu MH, Bangaru BS, Kidd J, et al. Neuropathological considerations in cerebro-hepato-renal syndrome (Zellweger's syndrome). Acta Neuropathol 1976;34: 115–23.

87. Gichrist KW, Gilbert EF, Goldfarb S, et al. Studies of malformation syndromes of man XIB: the cerebro-hepato-renal syndrome of Zellweger: comparative pathology. Eur J Pediatr 1976;121:99–118.
88. Evrard P, Caviness VS, Prats–Vinas J, et al. The mechanism of arrest of neuronal migration in the Zellweger malformation: an hypothesis based upon cytoarchitectonic analysis. Acta Neuropathol 1978;41:109–17.
89. Sarnat HB, Treven CL, Darwish HS. Ependymal abnormalities in cerebro-hepato-renal disease of Zellweger. Brain Dev 1993;15:270–7.
90. Van der Knaap MS, Valk J. The MR spectrum of peroxisomal disorders. Neuroradiology 1991;33:30–7.
91. Barkovich AJ, Peck WW. MR of Zellweger syndrome. AJNR Am J Neuroradiol 1997;18:1163–70.
92. Torvik A, Torp S, Kase BF, et al. Infantile Refsum disease: a generalized peroxisomal disorder. Case report with postmortem examination. J Neurol Sci 1988; 85:39–53.
93. Kyllerman M, Blomstrand S, Mansson JE, et al. Central nervous system malformations and white matter changes in pseudo-neonatal adrenoleukodystrophy. Neuropediatrics 1990;21:199–201.
94. Young S, Rabi Y, Lodha AK. Band heterotopia in Zellweger syndrome (cerebro-hepato-renal syndrome). Neurol India 2007;55(1):93.
95. Goh S. Neuroimaging features in a neonate with rhizomelic chondrodysplasia punctata. Pediatr Neurol 2007;37(5):382–4.
96. Mochel F, Grébille AG, Benachi A, et al. Contribution of fetal MR imaging in the prenatal diagnosis of Zellweger syndrome. AJNR Am J Neuroradiol 2006;27(2): 333–6.
97. Steinberg SJ, Dodt G, Raymond GV, et al. Peroxisome biogenesis disorders. Biochim Biophys Acta 2006;1763(12):1733–48.
98. Press G, Barshop BA, Haas RH, et al. Abnormalities of the brain in nonketotic hyperglycinemia: MR manifestations. AJNR Am J Neuroradiol 1989;10:315–21.
99. Fletcher JM, Bye AME, Naynar V, et al. Non-ketotic hyperglycinemia presenting as pachygyria. J Inherit Metab Dis 1995;18:665–8.
100. Alejo J, Rincon P, Vaquerizo J, et al. Transient non-ketotic hyperglycinemia: ultrasound, CT and MRI: case report. Neuroradiology 1997;39:658–60.
101. Scher MS, Bergman I. Neurophysiological and anatomical correlations in neonatal nonketotic hyperglycinemia. Neuropediatrics 1986;17:137–43.
102. Paupe A, Bidat L, Sonigo P, et al. Prenatal diagnosis of hypoplasia of the corpus callosum in association with non-ketotic hyperglycinemia. Ultrasound Obstet Gynecol 2002;20(6):616–9.

# Fetal Infections and Brain Development

James F. Bale, Jr, MD[a,b],*

**KEYWORDS**

- Congenital infection • Cytomegalovirus • Rubella
- Lymphocytic choriomeningitis virus • Toxoplasmosis

Nearly four decades ago TORCH, an acronym signifying *Toxoplasma gondii*, *R*ubella, *C*ytomegalovirus (CMV), and *H*erpesviruses, emerged as a unifying concept that underscored the importance of intrauterine infections in humans.[1] This acronym reminds clinicians that several infectious agents can produce similar and potentially devastating effects on the fetus and developing nervous system. Although rubella has since disappeared in nations with compulsory immunization against this agent and some have questioned the use of the TORCH concept, the pathogens signified by TORCH, and more recently recognized agents, including lymphocytic choriomeningitis (LCM virus), remain major causes of deafness, blindness, and permanent neurodevelopmental disabilities among children born in both developed and developing nations.

This article summarizes current knowledge regarding the clinical manifestations, pathogenesis, treatment, and prevention of congenital infections with these agents. In particular, this material updates readers regarding the encouraging results of treatment trials for congenital toxoplasmosis and CMV disease. The article concludes with a brief section describing perinatal parechovirus and herpes simplex virus (HSV) infections, additional disorders that can damage the developing nervous system during the immediate postnatal period.

## EPIDEMIOLOGY

Before widespread immunization against rubella virus, epidemics of rubella (German measles), once the most common cause of congenital infection in humans, occurred worldwide at 6- to 9-year intervals. Humans represent the only reservoir of rubella virus; transmission results from contact with infected respiratory secretions. During the 1962 to 1965 pandemic, the last major outbreak of rubella in the United States,

a Division of Pediatric Neurology, Departments of Pediatrics and Neurology, The University of Utah School of Medicine, Salt Lake City, UT 84158, USA
b Pediatric Residency Office, Third Floor, Primary Children's Medical Center, 100 North Mario Capecchi Drive, PO Box 581289, Salt Lake City, UT 84113, USA
* Pediatric Residency Office, Third Floor, Primary Children's Medical Center, 100 North Mario Capecchi Drive, Salt Lake City, UT 84113.
*E-mail address:* james.bale@hsc.utah.edu

Clin Perinatol 36 (2009) 639–653
doi:10.1016/j.clp.2009.06.005
0095-5108/09/$ – see front matter © 2009 Published by Elsevier Inc.

approximately 20,000 infants were affected by congenital rubella syndrome (CRS). In addition, there were more than 10,000 fetal deaths and 2000 neonatal deaths[2] during the pandemic. By the late 1980s, CRS had largely disappeared from the United States and other developed nations because of compulsory immunization programs.[3,4] A comprehensive French study identified an incidence of 28 cases per 100,000 live births during the 1970s and 1980s and a 10-fold reduction by 2002 after aggressive immunization of young children.[5] CRS remains a major health concern in developing nations, however, and as recently as 2006, more than 100,000 cases of CRS were estimated to occur worldwide annually. Moreover, CRS still appears sporadically in the United States and other developed nations as the result of immunization noncompliance and importation of cases from countries without immunization programs. Eliminating CRS remains a major goal of the World Health Organization.[6]

With the near-elimination of rubella in developed nations, congenital CMV infection emerged as the most commonly recognized congenital or intrauterine viral infection in many regions. United States studies indicate that 0.25% to 1% of infants shed CMV at birth, and because 5% to 10% of these have symptomatic infections, approximately 4000 infants are born annually in the United States with congenital CMV disease.[7] CMV resides in human populations with transmission resulting from direct human-to-human contact with infected saliva, urine, semen, or cervical secretions. Maternal risk factors for delivering a congenitally infected infant include young maternal age; multiple sexual partners; and contact with young children, a major reservoir of CMV in human populations.

Congenital toxoplasmosis currently represents the second most commonly recognized congenital infection. *T gondii*, a ubiquitous parasite, infects birds and many mammals, especially felines, worldwide. Domestic cats, a major source of human infection, excrete vast quantities of oocysts, and the resulting sporozoites remain viable in soils for extended periods. Human infection results from ingestion of meats containing viable *T gondii* tissue cysts or foods contaminated with oocysts. The seroprevalence rates of toxoplasmosis are highest in France; intermediate in Latin American, sub-Saharan Africa, and central Europe; and lowest in North America, South-East Asia, and Oceana.[8] Rates of congenital infection range from less than 0.1 to approximately 1 per 1000 live births.

Each year as many as 2 million pregnant women worldwide acquire syphilis, the consequence of infection with the spirochete *Treponema pallidum*. Infection results from direct contact with infected human secretions by oral, anal, or vaginal intercourse. Fomites do not participate in the transmission of *T pallidum*. Transmission of the spirochete to the fetus occurs in as many as 50% of the maternal infections, leading to fetal death, stillbirth, and congenital infection. Rare in most developed countries, congenital syphilis affects several hundred infants annually in the United States, especially in densely populated urban areas or in the rural South.[9]

Congenital infections with other pathogens occur less frequently. The incidence of neonatal HSV infections ranges from 0.025 to 0.3 per 1000 live births, but only 5% to 10% of these represent congenital infections.[10] The rates of varicella in pregnant women range from less than 1 to 3 per 1000, and very few of the infected women (< 2%) deliver infants with congenital infections. Infections with LCM virus, a rodent-borne arenavirus, have been reported from the United States and Eastern Europe,[11–14] but the incidence of congenital infection, although presumed to be very low, is unknown. Humans become infected with LCM virus through contact with infected aerosols or fomites. Current data regarding the incidence of congenital Chagas disease, caused by maternal infection with the parasite *Trypanosoma cruzi*, although imprecise, suggest that as many as 10,000 infants are infected with this agent annually in the Americas.[15] Finally, despite considerable concern about the public health consequences of West Nile virus infection of pregnant women, only a single case of congenital West Nile virus infection has been reported to date.[16,17] The current annual incidence of these selected intrauterine and perinatal infections is presented in **Table 1**.

## CLINICAL MANIFESTATIONS
### Early

Most of the pathogens associated with intrauterine infections can produce systemic and neurologic features that appear in the neonatal period. Clinicians should suspect intrauterine infections when infants display jaundice, hepatomegaly, splenomegaly, rash, intrauterine growth retardation, microcephaly, hydrocephalus, or chorioretinitis. Although the TORCH paradigm reminds clinicians of the manifestations potentially shared by these agents, some pathogens have unique clinical characteristics. Rubella virus, as an example, is the only agent causing congenital heart lesions, characteristically patent ductus arteriosus, and varicella zoster virus (VZV) is the only agent causing a unique pattern of skin scarring known as a "cicatrix." Prominent osteopathy suggests congenital syphilis or CRS, whereas isolated chorioretinitis is compatible with either congenital toxoplasmosis or LCM virus infection. LCM virus affects only the brain and eye of congenitally infected infants, causing microcephaly, hydrocephalus, and chorioretinitis.[12,14]

Jaundice, hepatomegaly, and splenomegaly are the most frequently encountered systemic manifestations of intrauterine infections. Of symptomatic infants with congenital CMV infection, jaundice and hepatosplenomegaly are each exhibited in approximately 70% or more,[18] and more than 75% of the infants with congenital toxoplasmosis also have jaundice and hepatosplenomegaly. Approximately 50% of the infants with congenital Chagas disease or congenital syphilis have these abnormalities. By contrast, infants with CRS have relatively low rates of jaundice or hepatosplenomegaly, on the order of 20%, and such features are distinctly unusual in congenital infections with varicella and LCM virus.

Purpuric or petechial rash should suggest congenital CMV disease, toxoplasmosis, syphilis, or CRS, whereas vesicular rash can suggest congenital varicella syndrome or

**Table 1**
**The incidence of selected intrauterine and perinatal infections**

| Agent | Annual Incidence (Per 1000 Live Births) |
|---|---|
| Cytomegalovirus | 2.9–10[a] |
| Herpes simplex virus (congenital) | < 0.01–0.33 |
| Lymphocytic choriomeningitis virus | Unknown, but presumed rare |
| Rubella virus[b] | 0–>1 |
| Toxoplasma gondii | < 0.1–1 |
| Treponema pallidum | 0.1 |
| Trypanosoma cruzi | 0.01–0.7 |
| Varicella zoster virus | < 0.01 |
| West Nile virus | Very rare |
| Human parechovirus | Unknown |

Estimated from various sources.
[a] Approximately 90% are asymptomatic.
[b] Congenital rubella syndrome.

congenitally or perinatally acquired HSV infections. As many as 30% of the infants with disseminated or encephalitic perinatal HSV infections, however, lack vesicular rash. Petechiae or purpura are present in 70% of CMV-infected infants and in 20% to 25% of the infants affected by congenital toxoplasmosis or syphilis. The classic "blueberry muffin" rash, a sign indicating extramedullary hematopoiesis, can be observed in congenital rubella virus or CMV infections. Zigzag skin lesions (cicatrix) conforming to a dermatomal distribution suggest congenital varicella syndrome; rarely, bullous lesions can be observed in congenital infections with HSV or LCM virus. Infants with congenital syphilis can exhibit maculopapular or bullous rashes of the palms; mucous patches; or condyloma lata, raised wartlike lesions.

The neonatal neurologic manifestations of congenital infections consist of microcephaly, hydrocephalus, seizures, meningoencephalitis, and abnormalities of muscle tone. Microcephaly commonly accompanies infections with congenital CMV, rubella virus, HSV, and VZV, whereas macrocephaly, usually indicating hydrocephalus, commonly accompanies congenital toxoplasmosis. Microcephaly or hydrocephalus can be observed in congenital LCM virus infections, and hydrocephalus and macrocephaly can develop postnatally as a result of obstructive hydrocephalus in infants who were initially microcephalic.[19] Seizures, focal or generalized, can be an early or late manifestation of congenital infection with several agents. Features of meningoencephalitis caused by CMV, rubella, or HSV can include lethargy, irritability, and full or bulging fontanels.

Ophthalmologic features in congenital infections include chorioretinitis, cataract, pigmentary retinopathy, optic atrophy, and microphthalmia. Chorioretinitis occurs in greater than 90% of the infants with congenital LCM virus infection, 75% of the infants with congenital toxoplasmosis, approximately 50% of the infants with congenital varicella syndrome, and 10% to 20% of the infants with congenital CMV disease. Approximately 80% or more of the infants with CRS have cataracts, and a substantial number also have pigmentary retinopathy or microphthalmia. Cataracts can be observed in congenital infections with VZV, HSV, and LCM virus, but are distinctly uncommon in congenital infections with CMV and T gondii. Cortical visual impairment, reflecting damage to the occipital cortex or optic pathway, can be a complication of virtually all of these infections.

Sensorineural hearing loss is a prominent manifestation of CRS and congenital CMV disease. During the 1962 to 1965 United States epidemic of German measles, more than 20,000 infants were born with CRS, and nearly 90% had sensorineural hearing loss.[3] In many, deafness was the only manifestation of CRS. CMV currently represents the most common nongenetic cause of permanent hearing loss among children living in the United States. Sensorineural hearing loss affects 50% of the infants with congenital CMV disease and approximately 8% of the so-called "asymptomatically infected infants."[20,21] The latter infants lack clinical or laboratory manifestations of congenital infection at birth, but exhibit sensorineural hearing loss that can appear during childhood and fluctuate or progress. Sensorineural hearing loss in congenitally infected infants can be unilateral or bilateral and ranges from mild to profound. Approximately 10% of the infants with congenital toxoplasmosis have sensorineural hearing loss;[22] deafness is an infrequent complication of infections with T pallidum, T cruzi, varicella, LCM virus, or HSV.

### Late

Certain neurologic or systemic manifestations of congenital infections may not appear for months or years after intrauterine infection. Classic examples of this phenomenon are the immune-mediated endocrinologic abnormalities, diabetes mellitus, and hypothyroidism, which appear in the teens or early 20s in patients with CRS.[23,24] Late-onset sensorineural hearing loss in children with congenital CMV disease can be progressive or fluctuating, even among infants without signs of CMV infection during the neonatal period.[20,21] Infants with congenital syphilis can have a constellation of late findings that includes saber shins; saddlenose deformity; mulberry molars; frontal bossing; rhagades; and Hutchinson's triad (sensorineural deafness, interstitial keratitis, and Hutchinson teeth [peg-shaped upper incisors]). Obstructive hydrocephalus can occur postnatally in infants with congenital LCM virus infections.[19] Infantile spasms can appear during the first year of life in infants with congenital CMV infection, congenital toxoplasmosis, CRS, or perinatal HSV infection.[25] Infants with CRS are a risk of postrubella panencephalitis, a rare, fatal neurodegenerative disorder that can appear years after CRS.[26]

## LABORATORY FEATURES AND MICROBIAL DIAGNOSIS
### Laboratory Features

Laboratory abnormalities suggesting intrauterine infection include direct hyperbilirubinemia, hemolytic anemia, thrombocytopenia, and elevations of the serum transaminases alanine aminotransferase and aspartate aminotransferase. Approximately 70% of the infants with congenital CMV disease have mild to moderate elevations of the serum transaminases;[16] occasional infants have severe hepatitis that leads to cirrhosis and liver failure. These features reflect viral replication in hepatocytes and virus-induced hepatic dysfunction. Transient hepatic dysfunction commonly occurs also in congenital toxoplasmosis, CRS, and congenital syphilis.

Thrombocytopenia, often in the range of 15,000 to 50,000/μL, can be seen in infections with CMV, *T gondii*, and rubella virus. Approximately 50% or more of the infants with congenital CMV disease have thrombocytopenia, and about one third of these have platelet counts lower than 50,000/μL.[16] Most infants with symptomatic CRS have thrombocytopenia;[27,28] nearly 20% of such infants have platelet counts less than 20,000/μL. Thrombocytopenia in congenital CMV disease and other congenital infections results from a combination of virus-induced marrow dysfunction, consumption of platelets by disseminated intravascular coagulopathy or hypersplenism, and autoimmune destruction of mature platelets.

Anemia, resulting from marrow dysfunction or hemolysis, commonly accompanies congenital syphilis, toxoplasmosis, CMV disease, Chagas disease, and CRS. Hemolytic anemia is suggested by an increased reticulocyte count and peripheral smears showing polychromasia, nucleated red blood cells, and abnormalities of erythrocyte morphology. Examination of bone marrow aspirates may show an increased erythroid/myeloid ratio in cases of hemolysis or decreased erythrocyte precursors in cases of virus-induced marrow suppression. Cerebrospinal fluid features of congenital infection can consist of protein elevation and lymphocytic pleocytosis.[16] Normal cerebrospinal fluid results, however, do not eliminate congenital infection from consideration.

### Microbial Diagnosis

The diagnosis of congenital infections relies on serologic, molecular, or culture methods, depending on the pathogen (**Table 2**). Serologic methods remain the most useful strategy when infections caused by *T gondii* or LCM virus are suspected. Because IgM and IgA do not cross the placenta, detection of *T gondii*–specific IgM or IgA in the infant's serum strongly suggests congenital toxoplasmosis. By contrast, absence of *T gondii*–specific IgG or IgM in the infant's serum and IgG in maternal

**Table 2**
**Methods to detect selected pathogens associated with congenital and perinatal infection**

| Agent | Preferred Diagnostic Method |
|---|---|
| Cytomegalovirus | Urine PCR or culture |
| Herpes simplex viruses | CSF, serum, vesicle fluid PCR |
| Lymphocytic choriomeningitis virus | Serum lymphocytic choriomeningitis virus–specific IgM |
| Rubella virus | Serum rubella-specific IgM; RT-PCR |
| Toxoplasma gondii | T gondii-specific IgM |
| Treponema pallidum | CSF, serum VDRL |
| Varicella-zoster virus | Varicella-zoster virus–specific IgM; CSF PCR |
| West Nile virus | CSF, serum West Nile virus–specific IgM |
| Human parechovirus | CSF PCR |

Abbreviations: CSF, cerebrospinal fluid; PCR, polymerase chain reaction; RT-PCR, reverse transcriptase polymerase chain reaction; VDRL, Venereal Disease Research Laboratories.

serum virtually eliminates this disorder. Congenital LCM virus infection is supported by detection of LCM virus–specific IgM in the infant's serum using ELISA.

Although culture of CMV from an infant's saliva or urine during the first 3 weeks of life remains the gold standard for the diagnosis of congenital CMV disease, congenital infection is established by detection of CMV-specific IgM in the infant's serum or CMV nucleic acids in urine or saliva using the polymerase chain reaction. Because CMV is commonly acquired by nursing infants, congenital infection cannot be confirmed by culture or polymerase chain reaction detection of CMV in urine samples obtained after 4 weeks of age. Polymerase chain reaction detection of CMV in neonatal blood spots using Guthrie cards represents an important breakthrough in the ability retrospectively to establish congenital CMV infection.[29,30] Virus culture or polymerase chain reaction can be used to establish the diagnosis of intrauterine or perinatally acquired HSV infections; HSV DNA can be detected in the cerebrospinal fluid of approximately 70% of the infants with perinatal HSV meningoencephalitis.[10] The diagnosis of congenital varicella syndrome can be made by detection of VZV-specific DNA in tissues or fluids, detection of VZV-specific IgM in neonatal serum, or persistence of VZV-specific IgG beyond 7 months of age.[31]

### NEUROIMAGING FEATURES

CT and MRI have major roles in evaluating infants with suspected or proved congenital or perinatal infections; neuroimaging features, such as intracranial calcifications, may be the initial clue to the presence of a congenital infection. Ultrasonography remains a useful imaging modality for studying unstable infants who cannot be transported to an imaging suite, but cranial ultrasound lacks the sensitivity to characterize adequately the central nervous system effects of intrauterine infections. Features common to congenital infections include periventricular hyperechogenicities, intracranial calcifications, cystic encephalomalacia, atrophic ventriculomegaly, and periventricular leukomalacia.

Approximately 50% of the infants with congenital CMV disease have intracranial calcifications (**Fig. 1**), usually in a periventricular distribution, and periventricular calcifications can also be observed in infants with CRS, LCM virus infections, and congenital toxoplasmosis. In the latter disease intracranial calcifications tend to be scattered diffusely throughout the brain parenchyma (**Fig. 2**), but some infants with

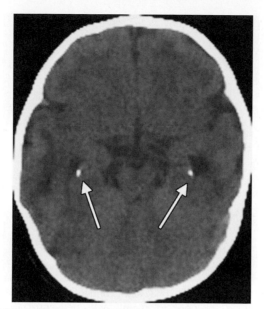

**Fig. 1.** Unenhanced head CT of a child with suspected congenital CMV infection shows bilateral periventricular calcifications (*arrows*).

CMV or LCM virus infections can also have a parenchymal pattern of calcifications (**Fig. 3**).[14,32] Calcifications in infants with congenital HSV infections distinctively involve the thalamus and basal ganglia.[33] Infants with CRS have periventricular or parenchymal calcifications, but because CRS largely disappeared in developed

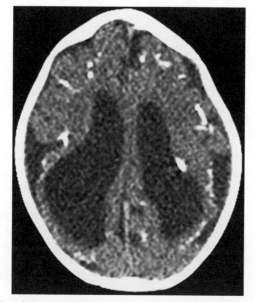

**Fig. 2.** Unenhanced head CT of a child with congenital toxoplasmosis shows passive ventriculomegaly, cortical dysplasia, and calcifications scattered throughout both cerebral hemispheres.

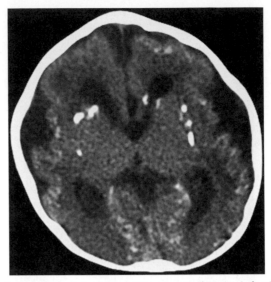

**Fig. 3.** Unenhanced head CT of a child with congenital CMV infection shows cortical dysplasia, compatible with polymicrogyria, and periventricular and parenchymal calcifications.

nations before major advances in neuroimaging, the neuroradiographic descriptions of CRS are quite sparse.[34]

Various abnormalities of the cerebral cortex, including polymicrogyria, schizencephaly, pachygyria-lissencephaly, hydranencephaly, and cleft cortical dysplasia, can be observed in infants with congenital HSV, CMV, LCM virus, and VZV infections.[12,14,32–36] CMV commonly causes polymicrogyria (see **Fig. 3**) and can also produce lissencephaly, schizencephaly, and various patterns of cortical dysplasia (**Fig. 4**). Cerebellar hypoplasia can occur in infants with congenital CMV (**Fig. 5**) or LCM virus infections.[14] These imaging features, influenced primarily by the timing of fetal infection, provide important insights into the pathogenesis of intrauterine infections.

## THE PATHOGENESIS OF BRAIN ABNORMALITIES ASSOCIATED WITH CONGENITAL INFECTION

The neurodevelopmental consequences of congenital infection reflect several factors, including maternal immunity, the infectious agent, the cellular tropism of the infectious agent, and the timing of maternal infection. Less well understood are the genetically regulated factors that may determine susceptibility to infection or the severity of maternal or fetal infection. Because congenital infections must begin with maternal infection, maternal immune status is an important factor. The fetuses of rubella-immune women, as indicated by the presence of rubella-virus specific IgG in mothers preconceptually, are protected from CRS,[2,28] and women who are seropositive for CMV preconceptually are less likely than seronegative women to give birth to infants with congenital CMV disease.[37]

The timing of maternal infection has a major influence on the outcome of fetal infection and the pathogenesis of the central nervous system abnormalities associated with congenital infection. This paradigm is illustrated best by the pathogenesis of CRS

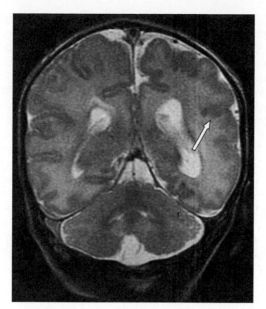

**Fig. 4.** T2-weighted, coronal MRI of an infant with congenital CMV infection showing dysplastic cortex (*arrow*).

following maternal rubella virus infection.[27,28] Maternal rubella during the initial 8 to 12 weeks of pregnancy in nonimmune women can lead to ophthalmologic abnormalities and congenital heart disease, and infection during the initial 16 weeks can cause sensorineural hearing loss. Intracranial abnormalities, particularly periventricular or

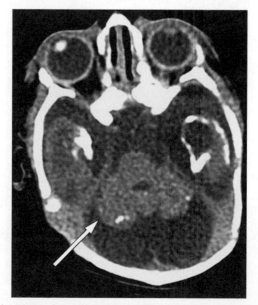

**Fig. 5.** Unenhanced head CT of another child with congenital CMV infection shows marked hypoplasia of the cerebellum (*arrow*) and cerebellar and cerebral calcifications.

parenchymal calcifications, can appear during this time. By contrast, infections after the twentieth week, although producing sensorineural hearing loss in some infants, are usually silent and unassociated with permanent neurodevelopmental disabilities. Overall, 20% to 50% of first-trimester rubella virus infections result in CRS.[27]

Although the relationship between the timing of maternal infection and outcome in congenital CMV infections is less clearly established than in CRS, CMV-induced defects of neuronal migration, such as lissencephaly, schizencephaly, polymicrogyria, and cortical dysplasia (**Fig. 6**), suggest that infections before the twentieth week of gestation produce more severe neurodevelopmental abnormalities. Early infections with the parasite *T gondii* also seem to be associated with more severe outcome.[22] The outcome of LCM virus infections is tightly linked to the timing of maternal infection, a conclusion supported by studies of LCM virus infection of experimental animals.[38] Finally, congenital varicella syndrome rarely, if ever, happens when maternal infection occurs before the fifth week or after the twenty-fourth week of gestation.[31]

The pathogenesis of CRS begins with maternal infection and viremia and continues when the placenta becomes infected.[27] The virus replicates in placental tissues, causing villitis, capillary endothelial necrosis, and cellular viral inclusions, pathologic features indicating active viral replication.[27] The virus then enters the fetal circulation and disseminates hematogenously to target organs, particularly the liver, spleen, heart, brain, cochlea, and eye, where virus replication and cell death lead to tissue damage and congenital defects. Pathologic studies of neural tissues demonstrate leptomeningitis and ischemic necrosis of cerebral parenchyma.[39] The latter leads to dystrophic cerebral calcifications, a feature common in CRS and several other viral or parasitic intrauterine infections, and atrophic ventriculomegaly. Unlike infections with CMV and LCM virus, cortical malformations are unusual features of CRS.

For the most part, other congenital infections, whether viral, spirochetal, or parasitic, begin with maternal and placental infections and culminate in dissemination

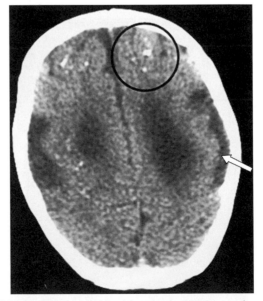

**Fig. 6.** Unenhanced head CT of a child with pseudo-TORCH syndrome shows scattered calcifications, especially frontally (*circle*), and cortical dysplasia reminiscent of cytomegalovirus or LCM virus infection (*arrow*).

of the infectious pathogen to the fetus, replication in target organs, and damage to fetal tissues, including the brain. Although dystrophic calcifications can be attributed to virus-induced necrosis of neuronal tissues, the pathogenesis of other neuropathologic abnormalities, such as CMV-induced lissencephaly, schizencephaly, or cerebellar hypoplasia, is not readily explained by direct viral replication in neural tissues. Placental inflammation can lead to vasculitis and placental insufficiency, causing fetal death, miscarriage, stillbirth, intrauterine growth retardation, and impaired brain growth and development.

Studies of murine CMV infection suggest that virus-induced inflammatory responses participate in the pathogenesis of CMV-induced cerebellar hypoplasia (see **Fig. 5**).[40] Whether this or other mechanisms, such as virus-induced vasculitis or inactivation of genes critical to brain development, cause cortical dysplasia, schizencephaly, or polymicrogyria in congenital infections, is unknown. Schizencephaly, for example, can result from mutations in EMX2, and perisylvian polymicrogyria is associated with mutations in several genes, including SRPX2, PAX6, TBR2, KIAA1279, RAB3GAP1, and COL18A1.[41] The intriguing similarities between the imaging and the neuropathologic features of congenital viral infections, especially CMV and LCM virus, and rare familial disorders, such as pseudo-TORCH syndrome (see **Fig. 6**),[42,43] suggest that much remains to be learned about the interplay of virus infections and the genes that determine the complex patterns of neural development.

## PREVENTION AND TREATMENT OF CONGENITAL INFECTIONS

As illustrated by the remarkable success in eradicating CRS from developed nations, immunization of susceptible women before conception remains the most effective means to eliminate the neurologic morbidity associated with many congenital infections. By September 2008, 65% of the world's countries incorporated rubella vaccine into their national immunization schedule;[6] eliminating CRS remains a major goal of the World Health Organization. Widespread use of VZV vaccine will likely have comparable effects in eliminating the congenital varicella syndrome. Despite the obvious success of the rubella vaccine campaign and the potential benefits of VZV immunization, progress in eliminating congenital CMV disease by vaccine has been remarkably slow.

Public health measures can have a beneficial impact by diminishing the burden of disease caused by several congenital infections. Congenital syphilis, for example, can be prevented by identifying women infected with *T pallidum* and treating them with penicillin. Cases of congenital toxoplasmosis can be prevented by recommending that pregnant women not clean cat litter boxes and avoid undercooked meats, and some cases of congenital LCM virus infection could theoretically be prevented by recommending that women avoid contact with mice, hamsters, or their excreta during pregnancy. Transmission of *T cruzi*, the cause of Chagas disease, can be interrupted by screening blood products and controlling triatominae insects, the principal vectors for human infection in endemic areas of Latin America.[44] Prevention of congenital or perinatal HSV infections remains problematic, however, given that most infected women are unaware of their HSV infections.

Postnatal treatment of certain congenital infections can substantially improve the neurodevelopmental prognosis for infants with congenital toxoplasmosis and the hearing outcomes in infants with congenital CMV disease. Shunting of obstructive hydrocephalus and extended courses of antitoxoplasma therapy using pyrimethamine and sulfadiazine have a remarkably beneficial effect on the outcome of infants with congenital toxoplasmosis.[45,46] Resolution or improvement in intracranial calcifications has been reported in treated children.[47] Postnatal therapy with ganciclovir for 6 weeks is associated with improved hearing outcomes in congenitally infected infants.[48]

Infants who survive congenital infections are at high risk of permanent neurodevelopmental disabilities consisting of cerebral palsy, deafness, visual dysfunction, epilepsy, and developmental delay or mental retardation. Longitudinal studies performed in infants with symptomatic congenital CMV infections before the availability of ganciclovir suggested that approximately 80% had permanent disability attributable to CMV infection.[49] Infants with intracranial calcifications are more likely to have adverse neurodevelopmental sequelae.[50,51] At least 50% of the infants with congenital CMV disease had sensorineural hearing loss; fewer ganciclovir-treated infants likely have permanent deafness. The potential effect of ganciclovir on other neurodevelopmental outcomes is uncertain at this time. Among infants with congenital toxoplasmosis treated with pyrimethamine-sulfadiazine, most have normal outcomes and very few have sensorineural hearing loss or new eye lesions caused by *T gondii* recrudescence.[46] This contrasts with greater than 50% morbidity associated with symptomatic congenital toxoplasmosis in the pretreatment era.[22]

The long-term morbidity associated with congenital syphilis can be prevented by perinatal penicillin therapy.[52] Although the benefit of antiparasitic therapy in infants with congenital Chagas disease has not been established by controlled trials, consensus statements from the Southern Cone of America and the World Health Organization recommend 30 to 60 days of antiparasitic therapy, using benznidazole or nifurtimox.[53,54] Currently, no effective antiviral therapy exists for infants with CRS, and although postnatal therapy with acyclovir seems logical in infants with suspected congenital HSV or VZV infections, there are no studies suggesting that acyclovir improves the outcome of such infants.

## PERINATAL VIRAL INFECTIONS

Neonatal infections with HSV, either type 1 or type 2, affect 500 to 2000 infants annually in the United States, and most occur perinatally.[55] Approximately 2% of women in the United States acquire HSV-2 annually[55] and approximately 80% of these occur without symptoms. Neonatal HSV infections have historically been considered mucocutaneous (skin, eye, mouth, without central nervous system involvement); disseminated (with or without central nervous system involvement); and encephalitic.[10] The latter infants become symptomatic somewhat later than those with mucocutaneous or disseminated infants and present subtly with fussiness, lethargy, or poor feeding or overtly with seizures and coma. Because one third of the infants with perinatal HSV encephalitis lack cutaneous signs of HSV and more than two thirds of the mothers of such infants have no known history of HSV infection, clinicians must maintain a high index of suspicion for this disorder. Management consists of high-dose (60 mg/kg/d) acyclovir for 21 to 28 days.[56] Infants who survive perinatal HSV infections are at high risk for cerebral palsy, epilepsy, and developmental delay despite aggressive acyclovir therapy.[10]

Neonatal infections with parechovirus, a picornavirus with at least 14 types, can be associated with encephalitis and central nervous system injury.[57] Verboon-Maciolek and colleagues[58] recently described 10 infants with this disorder and indicated that 50% had neurodevelopmental sequelae consisting of epilepsy, cerebral palsy, or developmental delays. MRIs showed white matter injury in most of the infants. This disorder should be suspected in infants with fever, rash, and seizures, features that mimic neonatal enterovirus infection; diagnosis can be established by polymerase chain reaction studies of cerebrospinal fluid. At present, no specific antiviral therapy exists for this disorder.

## REFERENCES

1. Nahmias AJ. The TORCH complex. Hosp Pract 1974;9:65–72.
2. Centers for Disease Control and Prevention. Elimination of rubella and congenital rubella syndrome—United States, 1969–2004. MMWR Morb Mortal Wkly Rep 2005 Mar 25;54:279–82
3. CDC. Rubella surveillance report 1. Atlanta (GA): CDC; 1969.
4. Ueda K, Tokugawa K, Nishida Y, et al. Incidence of congenital rubella virus syndrome in Japan (1965–1985). Am J Epidemiol 1986;124:807–15.
5. Robert-Gnansia E. Congenital rubella syndrome. Orphanet Encyclopedia, Nov 2004;1–2.
6. WHO. Available at: http://www.who.int/immunization_monitoring/diseases/Rubella_map_age.jpg; 2007. Accessed June 26, 2009.
7. Istas A, Demmler GJ, Dobbins JG, et al. Surveillance for congenital cytomegalovirus disease: a report from the National Congenital Cytomegalovirus Disease Registry. Clin Infect Dis 1994;20:665–70.
8. Zuber P, Jacquier P. Epidemiology of toxoplasmosis: current worldwide status. Schweiz Med Wochenschr Suppl 1995;65:19S–22S.
9. Centers for Disease Control and Prevention. Sexually transmitted disease surveillance 2007. Available at: http://www.cdc.gov/std/stats07/syphilis.htm.
10. Kimberlin DW. Neonatal herpes simplex infection. Microbiol Rev 2004;17:1–13.
11. Sheinbergas M. Hydrocephalus due to prenatal infection with the lymphocytic choriomeningitis virus. Infection 1976;4:185–91.
12. Wright R, Johnson D, Neumann M, et al. Congenital lymphocytic choriomeningitis virus syndrome: a disease that mimics congenital toxoplasmosis or cytomegalovirus infection. Pediatrics 1997;100(1):E9. Available at: http://www.pediatrics.aappublications.org/cgi/reprint/100/1/e9.pdf. Accessed June 26, 2009.
13. Barton LL, Mets MB. Congenital lymphocytic choriomeningitis virus infection: a decade of rediscovery. Clin Infect Dis 2001;33:370–4.
14. Bonthius DJ, Wright R, Tseng B, et al. Congenital lymphocytic choriomeningitis virus infection: spectrum of disease. Ann Neurol 2007;62:347–55.
15. Yamagata Y, Nakagawa J. Control of chagas disease. Adv Parasitol 2006;61:129–65.
16. Alpert SG, Fergerson J, Noel P. Intrauterine West Nile virus: ocular and systemic findings. Am J Ophthalmol 2003;136:733–5.
17. O'Leary DR, Kuhn S, Kniss L, et al. Birth outcomes following West Nile virus infection of pregnant women in the United States: 2003–2004. Pediatrics 2006;117:e537–45.
18. Boppana SB, Pass RF, Britt WJ, et al. Symptomatic congenital cytomegalovirus infection: neonatal morbidity and mortality. Pediatr Infect Dis J 1992;11:93–9.
19. Larsen PD, Chartrand SA, Tomashek KY, et al. Hydrocephalus complicating lymphocytic choriomeningitis virus infection. Pediatr Infect Dis J 1993;12:528–31.
20. Grosse SD, Ross DS, Dollard SC. Congenital cytomegalovirus (CMV) infection as a cause of permanent bilateral hearing loss: a quantitative assessment. J Clin Virol 2008;41:57–62.
21. Fowler KB, McCollister FP, Dahle AJ, et al. Progressive and fluctuating sensorineural hearing loss in children with asymptomatic congenital cytomegalovirus infection. J Pediatr 1997;130:624–30.

22. Swisher CN, Boyer K, McLeod R, et al. Congenital toxoplasmosis. Semin Pediatr Neurol 1994;1:4–25.
23. Ginsberg-Fellner F, Witt ME, Yagihashi S, et al. Congenital rubella syndrome as a model for type 1 (insulin-dependent) diabetes mellitus: increased prevalence of islet cell surface antibodies. Diabetologia 1984;27(Suppl):87–9.
24. Takasu N, Tomomi Ikema T, Komiya I, et al. Forty-year observation of 280 Japanese patients with congenital rubella syndrome. Diabetes Care 2005;28:2331–2.
25. Dunin-Wasowicz D, Kasprzyk-Obara J, Jurkiewicz E, et al. Infantile spasms and cytomegalovirus infection: antiviral and antiepileptic treatment. Dev Med Child Neurol 2008;49:684–92.
26. Townsend JJ, Baringer RB, Wolinsky JS, et al. Progressive rubella panencephalitis: late onset after congenital rubella. N Engl J Med 1975;292:990–3.
27. Hanshaw JB, Dudgeon JA. Viral diseases of the fetus and newborn. Philadelphia: WB Saunders; 1978.
28. Dudgeon JA. Congenital rubella. J Pediatr 1975;87:1078–86.
29. Barbi M, Binda S, Caroppo S, et al. A wider role for congenital cytomegalovirus infection in sensorineural hearing loss. Pediatr Infect Dis J 2003;22:39–42.
30. Walter S, Atkinson C, Sharland M, et al. Congenital cytomegalovirus: association between dried blood spot viral load and hearing loss. Arch Dis Child Fetal Neonatal Ed 2008;93:F280–5.
31. Sauerbrei A. Varicella-zoster infections during pregnancy. In: Mushahwa IK, editor, Congenital and other related infectious diseases of the newborn: perspectives in medical virology, vol. 13. Amsterdam: Elsevier; 2007. p. 51–73.
32. Bale JF, Bray PF, Bell WE. Neuroradiographic abnormalities in congenital cytomegalovirus infection. Pediatr Neurol 1985;1:42–7.
33. Hutto C, Arvin A, Jacobs RF, et al. Intrauterine herpes simplex virus infections. J Pediatr 1987;110:97–101.
34. Ishikawa A, Murayama T, Sakuma N, et al. Computed cranial tomography in congenital rubella syndrome. Arch Neurol 1982;39:420–1.
35. Hayward JC, Thitelbaum DS, Clancy RR, et al. Lissencephaly-pachygyria associated with congenital cytomegalovirus infection. J Child Neurol 1991;6:109–14.
36. Iannetti P, Nigro G, Spalice A, et al. Cytomegalovirus infection and schizencephaly: case reports. Ann Neurol 1998;43:123–7.
37. Fowler KB, Stagno S, Pass RF. Maternal immunity and prevention of congenital cytomegalovirus infection. J Am Med Assoc 2003;289:1008–11.
38. Bonthius DJ, Nichols B, Harb H, et al. Lymphocytic choriomeningitis virus infection of the developing brain: role of host age. Ann Neurol 2007;62:356–74.
39. Desmond MM, Wilson GS, Melnick JL, et al. Congenital rubella encephalitis. J Pediatr 1967;71:311–31.
40. Koontz T, Bralic M, Tomac J, et al. Altered development of the brain after focal herpesvirus infection of the central nervous system. J Exp Med 2008;205:423–35.
41. Spalice A, Parisi P, Nicita F, et al. Neuronal migration disorders: clinical, neuroradiologic and genetics aspects. Acta Paediatr 2009;98:421–33.
42. Briggs TA, Wolf NI, D'Arrigo S, et al. Band-like intracranial calcification with simplified gyration and polymicrogyria: a distinct pseudo-TORCH phenotype. Am J Med Genet A 2008;146A:3173–80.
43. Abdel-Salam GM, Zaki MS, Saleem SN, et al. Microcephaly, malformation of brain development and intracranial calcification in sibs: pseudo-TORCH or a new syndrome. Am J Med Genet A 2008;146A:2929–36.
44. Rassi A Jr, Dias JC, Marin-Neto JA, et al. Challenges and opportunities for primary, secondary, and tertiary prevention of Chagas' disease. Heart 2009;95:524–34.

45. Guerina NS, Hsu HW, Meissner HC, et al. Neonatal serologic screening and early treatment for congenital *Toxoplasma gondii* infection. The New England Regional Toxoplasma Working Group. N Engl J Med 1994;330:1858–63.

46. McLeod R, Boyer K, Karrison T, et al. Outcome of treatment for congenital toxoplasmosis, 1981–2004: the National Collaborative Chicago-Based, Congenital Toxoplasmosis Study. Clin Infect Dis 2006;42:1383–94.

47. Patel DV, Holfels EM, Vogel NP, et al. Resolution of intracranial calcifications in infants with treated congenital toxoplasmosis. Radiology 1996;199:433–40.

48. Kimberlin DW, Lin CY, Sanchez P, et al. Effect of ganciclovir therapy on hearing in symptomatic congenital cytomegalovirus disease involving the central nervous system: a randomized, controlled trial. J Pediatr 2003;143:16–25.

49. Pass RF, Stagno S, Meyers G, et al. Outcome of symptomatic congenital cytomegalovirus infection. Pediatrics 1980;66:758–62.

50. Boppana SB, Fowler KB, Vaid Y, et al. Neuroradiographic findings in the newborn period and the long term outcome in children with symptomatic congenital cytomegalovirus infection. Pediatrics 1997;99:409–14.

51. Noyola DE, Demmler GJ, Nelson CT, et al. Early predictors of neurodevelopmental outcome in symptomatic congenital cytomegalovirus infection. J Pediatr 2001; 138:325–31.

52. American Academy of Pediatrics. Syphilis. In: Pickering LK, Baker CJ, Long SS, et al, editors. Red book: 2006 report of the committee on infectious diseases. 27th edition. Elk Grove Village (IL): American Academy of Pediatrics; 2006. p. 637–9.

53. WHO. Control of Chagas disease. Technical Report Series No. 905. Geneva: WHO; 2002.

54. Schijman AG. Congenital chagas disease. In: Mushahar IK, editor. Congenital and other related infectious diseases of the newborn. Amsterdam: Elsevier; 2007. p. 223–58.

55. Miner L, Bale JF. Herpes simplex virus infections of the newborn. In: Mushahar IK, editor. Congenital and other related infectious diseases of the newborn. Amsterdam: Elsevier; 2007. p. 21–35.

56. Kimberlin DW, Lin CY, Jacobs RF. Safety and efficacy of high-dose intravenous acyclovir in the management of neonatal herpes simplex virus infections. Pediatrics 2001;108:230–8.

57. Verboon-Maciolek MA, Groenendaal F, Hahn CD, et al. Human parechovirus causes encephalitis with white matter injury in neonates. Ann Neurol 2008;64: 266–73.

58. Verboon-Maciolek MA, Krediet TG, Gerards LJ, et al. Severe neonatal parechovirus infection and similarity with enterovirus infection. Pediatr Infect Dis J 2008;27: 241–5.

# The Fetal Heart Rate Response to Hypoxia: Insights from Animal Models

Laura Bennet, PhD*, Alistair Jan Gunn, MBChB, PhD

**KEYWORDS**

- Fetus • Hypoxia • Heart rate monitoring • Deceleration
- Heart rate variability • Gestational age • Fetal sex

Sir Joseph Barcroft first drew a close analogy between the low partial pressure of oxygen of the fetus in utero and that which would be found in humans at an altitude of 30,000 to 33,000 ft on Mt. Everest when he observed, "The fetus then grows in an environment the oxygen concentration of which is falling all the time—an uphill business you may say. True indeed, for is it not the problem of Everest, the maintenance of the organism in the atmosphere becoming progressively rarer?"[1] He later neatly summarized this concept with the phrase, "Mt. Everest in utero."[2]

We now know that despite an oxygen demand twice that of the adult and far lower absolute partial pressures of oxygen and hemoglobin saturations, the fetus more than adequately compensates and so under normal conditions actually has a surplus of available oxygen.[3,4] Despite this observation, reviews of fetal oxygenation often refer to the fetus as living in a naturally hypoxic environment.[5,6] This concept gives the impression that the fetus lives in a delicate ecosystem where the slightest change in oxygenation will have quick and dramatic consequences. Coupled with the fact that the fetus is, by definition, immature in its development of organs and their functional control, this concept seems to suggest that the fetus should be exquisitely vulnerable to hypoxia and without the necessary physiologic responses to protect itself. This concept has limited clinical development of heart rate monitoring.

In reality, an adult abruptly dropped onto the top of Mt. Everest without the aid of an oxygen bottle would be far more at risk of injury and death than a fetus who experiences a similar relative degree of hypoxia. The combination of remarkable fetal

The authors' work reported in this article has been supported by the Health Research Council of New Zealand, the Lottery Health Board of New Zealand, the Auckland Medical Research Foundation, and the March of Dimes Birth Defects Trust.

Department of Physiology, Faculty of Medical and Health Sciences, The University of Auckland, Private Bag 92019, Auckland, New Zealand
* Corresponding author.
*E-mail address:* l.bennet@auckland.ac.nz (L. Bennet).

Clin Perinatol 36 (2009) 655–672
doi:10.1016/j.clp.2009.06.009
0095-5108/09/$ – see front matter © 2009 Elsevier Inc. All rights reserved.

anaerobic tolerance, plus the capacity of even very young fetuses to mount a coordinated cardiovascular and metabolic defense to hypoxia, means that the fetus can survive profound hypoxia for extraordinary periods of time and often without injury.[4,7,8] This knowledge is cold comfort to the obstetrician faced with the delivery of an infant who develops acute, evolving brain injury after severe hypoxia during labor. The central dilemma is that uterine contractions during labor are associated with a nearly linear fall in maternal uterine artery blood flow[9] and with repeated mild hypoxia even in normal uncomplicated labor.[10–12] It is insufficient to merely identify exposure to hypoxia; the clinician needs to detect adverse progress during labor before injury occurs but without intervening in normal deliveries.

Fetal heart rate (FHR) monitoring is nearly universally available in the developed world and yet remains surrounded by confusion and controversy.[13,14] This review briefly explores our understanding of the physiology behind the essential clinical components of FHR patterns and their changes with hypoxia—decelerations, accelerations, and variability. Other aspects of fetal responses to hypoxia have been reviewed elsewhere.[3,4]

The majority of experimental studies of the pathophysiology of fetal hypoxia have been performed in chronically instrumented fetal sheep in utero. The sheep is a highly precocial species whose neural development at around 0.8 to 0.85 of gestation approximates that of the term human.[15] At this age the baseline fetal sheep FHR is around 20 beats per minute higher than that of the human fetus.

## THE CHEMOREFLEX ARC: THREAT DETECTION, ASSESSMENT, AND RESPONSE

By definition, hypoxia is a threat to cellular oxygen homeostasis and bioenergetics and ultimately, if severe enough, to the organism's survival. Hypoxia must be rapidly detected, assessed, and acted upon. Hypoxia stimulates the peripheral chemoreceptors, which are known to be functional in utero.[4] During moderate hypoxia the aortic chemoreceptors do not appear to have a role in these responses,[16] although they may have a role during profound hypoxia (asphyxia).[17] Unlike the adult, the fetus suppresses rather than increases respiratory drive during hypoxia, and this reaction is mediated by the brain and not by carotid chemoreceptor activation.[18] There is a coordinated cardiovascular response designed to sustain perfusion, initiated by neural chemoreflexes and augmented by slower acting endocrine, endothelial, and behavioral responses.[3,4] Ultimately, experimental studies confirm that hypotension and consequent failure of perfusion is one of the major factors associated with neural injury.[19,20]

This chemoreflex response is not a blunt all-or-nothing response but rather a sensitive and complex balancing of the severity of the insult against the cellular tolerance of the individual. Once triggered, the response is also titrated, producing varied responses. This fact can be seen clinically in the "variable" decelerations in FHR, which represent the majority of decelerations seen in labor,[21] in which abrupt changes in FHR baseline frequently vary in shape, depth, and duration.

This review focuses on acute onset insults. The reader should keep in mind that slower onset insults, which allow the fetus to make homeostatic adaptations to hypoxia, initiate very different FHR patterns.[4] For example, slow onset moderate hypoxia induces only tachycardia;[22] hypoxia that is sufficiently severe to cause neural injury, as seen during progressive partial uterine artery occlusion, can induce a slow fetal metabolic deterioration without the initial fetal cardiovascular responses of bradycardia and hypertension.[23]

The most distinctive feature of FHR recordings in labor is the repetitive falls in FHR. Profound prolonged bradycardia due to sustained profound asphyxia occurs more rarely, is easy to detect, and its diagnostic value clear; unfortunately, such abrupt sustained insults are seldom predictable or preventable.[24] Short and frequent "variable" decelerations are the key feature of interest but also one of the most difficult to interpret.[25]

## DECELERATIONS

The initial mean FHR response of the term or near-term fetus to a rapid onset hypoxic challenge is characterized by a rapid deceleration (**Figs. 1** and **2**).[26,27] The depth to which the FHR falls is broadly related to the severity of the hypoxia.[28] Shallow decelerations indicate a modest reduction in uteroplacental flow, whereas a deep deceleration indicates near total or total reduction (see **Fig. 2**).[29,30] This initial bradycardia is mediated by muscarinic (parasympathetic) pathways and can be abolished by

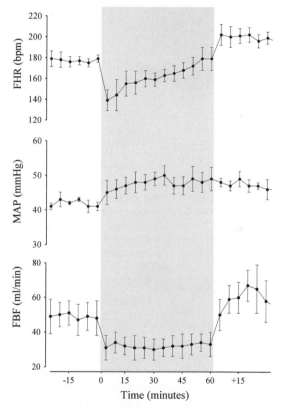

**Fig. 1.** Responses to moderate isocapnic hypoxia in near-term fetal sheep. Time sequence of changes in fetal heart rate (FHR, bpm), mean arterial pressure (MAP, mm Hg), and femoral blood flow (FBF, mL/min) during moderate isocapnic hypoxia induced by a reduction in the maternal fraction of inspired oxygen which reduces the fetal partial pressure of oxygen by 10% (reducing the fetal partial pressure of oxygen by approximately 50%). Data are 5-minute averages ± SEM from 30 minutes before to 30 minutes after 60 minutes of hypoxia (shaded region). Note the transient fall in FHR, followed by a return to baseline as the insult continued. (*Data from* Bennet L, Peebles DM, Edwards AD, et al. The cerebral hemodynamic response to asphyxia and hypoxia in the near-term fetal sheep as measured by near infrared spectroscopy. Pediatr Res 1998;44(6):951–7.)

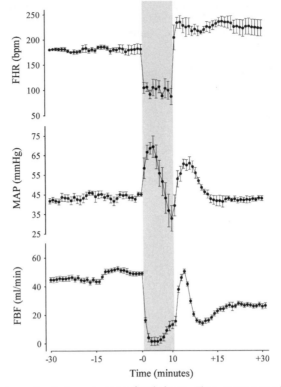

**Fig. 2.** Responses to asphyxia in near-term fetal sheep. Time sequence of changes in fetal heart rate (FHR, bpm), mean arterial blood pressure (MAP, mm Hg), and femoral blood flow (FBF, mL/min) during complete umbilical cord occlusion for 10 minutes. Data are 1-minute averages ± SEM from 30 minutes before umbilical cord occlusion (shaded region) until 30 minutes after occlusion. Note the greater initial bradycardia compared with that seen with moderate hypoxia (see **Fig.1**) and the sustained bradycardia throughout the insult. (*Data from* Bennet L, Peebles DM, Edwards AD, et al. The cerebral hemodynamic response to asphyxia and hypoxia in the near-term fetal sheep as measured by near infrared spectroscopy. Pediatr Res 1998;44(6):951–7.)

vagotomy[2] or by blockade with atropine.[27,31] Bradycardia markedly reduces cardiac work in the face of limited resources, and its role is likely to be a defense mechanism designed to preserve cardiac glycogen and reduce cardiac stress.[32]

A fall in FHR leads to a reduction in combined ventricular output, and blood pressure is then maintained by peripheral vasoconstriction (see **Figs. 1** and **2**).[3,4] The fetus can fully maintain normal oxygen delivery to vital organs during moderate hypoxemia, essentially indefinitely.[33,34] Similar observations have been made based on experiments of brief repeated umbilical cord occlusions lasting 1 minute and repeated every 5 minutes (1:5, consistent with contractions in early labor) (**Fig. 3**A). Each occlusion was accompanied by a variable FHR deceleration with rapid return to baseline levels between occlusions.[35,36] Fetal blood pressure rose at the onset of each occlusion, never fell below baseline levels during the occlusions, and was elevated between occlusions. Acidosis, even by the end of the occlusion series (4 hours), was minor. This experiment demonstrated the remarkable capacity of the healthy fetus to fully adapt to a low frequency of repeated episodes of severe hypoxia.

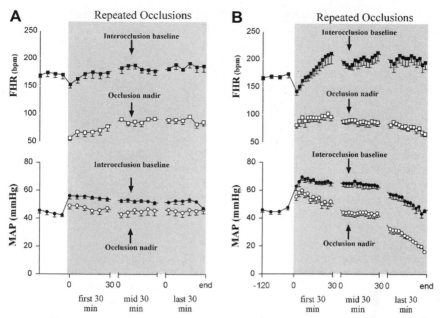

**Fig. 3.** Fetal heart rate (FHR) and mean arterial pressure (MAP) responses to brief repeated umbilical cord occlusion in near-term fetal sheep. (*A*) One-minute umbilical cord occlusion repeated every 5 minutes for 4 hours (1:5 group). (*B*) One-minute occlusions repeated every 2.5 minutes (1:2.5 group) until fetal MAP fell <20 mm Hg. The minimum (ie, nadir of deceleration) FHR and MAP during each occlusion and the interocclusion baseline FHR and MAP are shown. Because the individual experiments in the 1: 2.5 group were of unequal duration, the data are presented for three time intervals: the first 30 minutes, the middle 30 minutes (defined as the median ±15 minutes), and the final 30 minutes of occlusions. In the 1:5 group, there was no significant change in interocclusion baseline FHR, and the MAP was higher during occlusions. The FHR decelerations were uniform in size. In the 1:2.5 group, interocclusion baseline FHR was higher in the first and middle 30 minutes. In the first 30 minutes, minimum MAP transiently rose to greater than baseline values but fell progressively in the last 30 minutes. The FHR decelerations appeared to become much larger due to a small fall in the nadir and a rise in the interocclusion baseline FHR. (*Data from* de Haan HH, Gunn AJ, Gluckman PD. Fetal heart rate changes do not reflect cardiovascular deterioration during brief repeated umbilical cord occlusions in near-term fetal lambs. Am J Obstet Gynecol 1997;176(1 Pt 1):8–17; and Westgate JA, Bennet L, Gunn AJ. Fetal heart rate variability changes during brief repeated umbilical cord occlusion in near term fetal sheep. Br J Obstet Gynaecol 1999;106(7):664–71.)

## FREQUENCY OF INSULTS

Notably, this capacity is challenged when the frequency of the insult is changed from 1:5 to 1 minute every 2.5 minutes (1:2.5, consistent with second stage labor) (see **Fig. 3**B).[37,38] Although this paradigm was also associated with a series of variable decelerations, the outcome in this group was substantially different, with seizures and focal neuronal damage observed, whereas neither were seen in the 1:5 group.[39] These findings are highly consistent with clinical evidence that fetal intracerebral oxygenation is impaired during short labor contraction intervals (<2.3 min).[40] Underpinning these neural findings was the observation of progressive hypotension and metabolic acidosis. The changes in the pattern of the FHR associated with this deterioration were primarily deepening of the decelerations with occlusions and eventual stasis in the rise in interocclusion baseline FHR. These changes developed progressively and surprisingly slowly, even during frequent occlusions. These experimental studies demonstrate that a series of prolonged brief variable decelerations can ultimately lead to severe, repeated hypotension and metabolic acidosis even in healthy singleton fetuses if they are repeated sufficiently frequently for long enough.

## SLOPE OF THE FETAL HEART RATE DECELERATION

Studies in near-term fetal sheep have suggested that during a series of repeated variable decelerations there is a progressive slowing of the initial fall in FHR.[41–43] Whereas Akagi and colleagues[41] found that a reduced slope during complete occlusions corresponded closely with the development of fetal acidosis and hypotension, others have reported a similar attenuation with repeated partial or complete cord occlusions without significant metabolic deterioration, suggesting that this phenomenon might reflect attenuation of the chemoreflex.[42,43]

This finding that repeated episodes of hypoxia seemed to blunt the chemoreflex FHR response is in many ways counterintuitive to our understanding of the importance of the chemoreflex in fetal adaptation to hypoxia,[4] and we might anticipate that its attenuation would compromise adaptation to labor.[42] In a study of repeated complete but brief umbilical cord occlusions, the rate of initial fall in FHR actually increased during an occlusion series associated with severe developing acidosis, indicating sensitization and not attenuation of the vagally mediated chemoreflex (**Fig. 4**).[36] Late recovery from the variable decelerations was seen in a minority of fetuses in association with hypotension, which, in turn, may be related to reversible cardiac injury and associated dysfunction.[36,44]

These findings strongly suggest that attenuation of the chemoreflex occurs only during episodes of relatively mild hypoxia that the fetus has been able to adapt to wholly. Conceptually, it is important to consider that the term *attenuation* should not necessarily be interpreted as meaning *impairment*. This attenuation of the chemoreflex response seems to reflect better compensation for the hypoxic stress such that there is maintenance of adequate homeostasis; therefore, the fetal responses do not need to be as rapid or sustained.

## SECONDARY FETAL HEART RATE RESPONSES

During mild-to-moderate hypoxia without acidemia, bradycardia is followed by progressively developing tachycardia. These responses are primarily mediated by the increase in circulating catecholamines (see **Fig. 1**).[45] Both parasympathetic and sympathetic responses are, in part, modulated by endogenous opiate receptors;[46,47] for example, the opiate receptor blocker naloxone potentiates release of norepinephrine.[48] The effects of labor analgesics and maternal substance abuse or treatment for substance abuse are important factors in FHR analysis. Tachycardia allows the combined ventricular output to contribute to the maintenance of blood pressure, permitting, in turn, a reduction of peripheral vasoconstriction and greater perfusion of peripheral organs. These adaptations may reflect relative reductions in metabolic activity to meet the reduced level of oxygenation.

Tachycardia does not occur if the insult is more severe (uterine blood flow to 25% or less and a fetal arterial oxygen content of less than 1 mmol/L). Instead, bradycardia progressively deepens (see **Fig. 2**). This secondary fall in FHR is likely due in large part to the direct effects of hypoxia on the heart itself. These experimental data are consistent with the clinical observation by Caldeyro-Barcia and colleagues[49] that

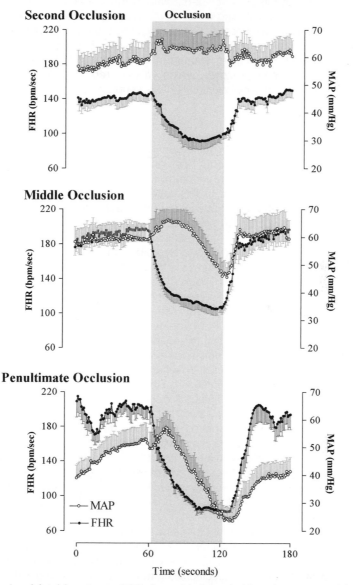

**Fig. 4.** Example of fetal heart rate (FHR, bpm, black symbols) and mean arterial pressure (MAP, mm Hg, white symbols) changes for the second, middle, and penultimate occlusion during 1-minute umbilical cord occlusions repeated every 2.5 minutes (1:2.5). The onset of occlusion was characterized by a rapid fall in FHR followed by a transient increase in MAP. Note the progressively more rapid fall in FHR with later occlusions associated with a progressive baseline tachycardia during occlusions and hypotension. (*Data from* Bennet L, Westgate JA, Lui YC, et al. Fetal acidosis and hypotension during repeated umbilical cord occlusions are associated with enhanced chemoreflex responses in near-term fetal sheep. J Appl Physiol 2005;99(4):1477–82.)

late decelerations during labor are not abolished by atropine. This finding indicates that, in contrast with the initial reflex-mediated bradycardia in the first few minutes of profound asphyxia, continuing bradycardia must be related to severe myocardial hypoxia with depletion of myocardial anaerobic stores such as glycogen.[31] The effect of myocardial hypoxia is a global one. The effect is a global one. Severe hypoxia with increasing acidosis leads to a depletion of myocardial glycogen, creatine phosphate, and adenosine triphosphate stores, which, in turn, reduces the duration of action potentials, and myocardial cell excitability and conductivity.

## "LATE" DECELERATIONS

Fortunately, most episodes of hypoxia during labor are brief, lasting for a minute or less, and are associated with only brief decelerations. Decelerations due to true myocardial hypoxia are extremely uncommon and occur only in the context of pathologically prolonged bradycardia. In this regard, one must consider the concept of "late" decelerations. Shallow late decelerations are those with both a gradual fall to nadir (defined as more than 30 seconds)[50] and with the nadir occurring after the peak of the contraction.[51] They are relatively uncommon in active labor.[21,52] They are associated with markers for chronic hypoxia (reduced variability and fetal movements or growth restriction); therefore, it is frequently assumed that late decelerations must indicate direct myocardial hypoxia. This assumption is not true. Late decelerations can occur for 90 to 100 minutes during labor before acidosis develops[53] and are associated with soft markers of fetal distress (low 1-minute Apgar scores or metabolic acidosis) in only 12% to 50% of cases.[54,55]

The specific mechanisms leading to variable decelerations which are late in timing and to "late" decelerations, as defined previously, remain unclear. Potentially, they may reflect a lag time between insult onset and the actual reduction in fetal oxygenation and, consequently, the chemoreflex-mediated deceleration.[56,57] Repeated partial (50%) reduction of umbilical cord blood flow is associated with a relatively slow onset of bradycardia.[42] It may be speculated that late decelerations may occur in a fetus with limited reserves who is exposed to modest reductions in uterine blood flow that would not cause bradycardia in a healthy fetus. In a study of 5522 low-risk pregnancies, the positive predictive value for low arterial pH (<7.1) rose from circa 12% of 99 patients with recurrent late decelerations to over 50% (9 of 16) in the small subset of patients with recurrent late decelerations plus loss of FHR variability.[55] It is striking that these infants had a high rate of reduced variability on admission, strongly suggesting an element of antenatal hypoxia preceding labor.[21]

Overall, the available evidence suggests that most cases of late decelerations reflect reduced fetal reserve rather than myocardial hypoxia or acidosis. The incidence is low, and it is likely that they are of most value in identifying fetuses at risk of hypoxia when they are accompanied by additional features such as reduced variability. Further research is needed.

## FETAL MATURATION

Perinatal hypoxia with severe metabolic acidosis is more common in infants born prematurely than at term,[58,59] and non-reassuring FHR patterns are associated with greater neurologic depression than seen at term.[59,60] Although understanding the responses of this important perinatal population is critical, current knowledge about how the preterm fetus responds to hypoxia alone and in combination with other conditions such as infection or inflammation is limited.

There are notable age-related differences in fetal responses to hypoxia. A rapid onset moderate hypoxic challenge that elicits bradycardia followed by tachycardia in term fetuses elicits little or no FHR changes in fetuses before 0.7 of gestation and mild tachycardia at 0.7 gestation.[61,62] Even from late gestation to full term, there is a further developmental increase in the magnitude and persistence of fetal brady-cardia to moderate hypoxia in fetal sheep.[32] It has been suggested that fetal autonom-ically mediated responses to hypoxia start to develop at 0.7 of gestation, coincident with maturation of neurohormonal regulators and chemoreceptor function,[45,63] and that this relative immaturity may affect fetal survival.[61,62]

When interpreting these results, it is also important to consider the chemoreflex homeostasis stimulus versus need relationship. As Fletcher and colleagues[32] have demonstrated in near-term and term fetal sheep, as fetuses get older and their aerobic requirements increase, FHR falls faster at the onset of moderate hypoxia, and the bradycardia is of greater magnitude and more sustained. In contrast, the preterm fetus has far greater anaerobic reserves and lower overall aerobic requirements compared with term fetuses.[64,65] Relatively mild hypoxic insults attained in the studies cited previously may not have reduced tissue oxygen availability below the critical homeo-static threshold for this developmental stage. Wassink and colleagues[66] demon-strated that when challenged with a more profound asphyxic insult, the chemoreflex-mediated FHR responses do not substantially differ from 0.6 to 0.85 gestation. In this study, all fetuses had initial bradycardia followed by a progressive fall in FHR, similar to the near-term fetuses shown in **Fig. 2**.

Collectively, these data show that while the preterm fetus does have different autonomic responses, most likely related to maturity, this fact does not prevent the preterm fetus from responding adequately when homeostasis is truly threat-ened. Hypoxia well before birth does occur[67] and may be most frequent earlier in gestation when the fetus has more freedom of movement. A capacity to respond adequately to hypoxia at any gestational age makes teleologic sense for overall species survival.

## FETAL SEX

Male fetuses are at greater risk of perinatal mortality and morbidity, and studies suggest that some male fetuses may be less able to adapt to hypoxic stress.[68] We have shown in preterm fetal sheep that male and female fetuses demonstrate remark-ably similar overall chemoreflex and hemodynamic responses to asphyxia; however, some did have impaired hemodynamic adaptations that were primarily characterized by a greater fall in FHR. This impairment, in turn, mediated earlier and more profound hypotension and hypoperfusion. These fetuses tended to be smaller than those who tolerated asphyxia, but their weight was within the normal range, consistent with clin-ical observations of male mortality and weight.[69] A key observation from this study was that during asphyxia these smaller males were significantly less hypercapnic and had lower plasma lactate levels than fetuses who tolerated asphyxia. This curious observation supports the hypothesis that these smaller males had reduced glycogen stores and reduced anaerobic metabolism, leading to reduced $CO_2$ and lactate production.

Like most fetal monitoring parameters, the acid-base state of the fetus during labor provides good sensitivity (it is indicative of the presence and severity of asphyxia) but low specificity (it is not a fully reliable predictor of outcome). Our study provides an example of why this can happen. The fetuses destined to die or to suffer greater morbidity had blood composition measurements which in many aspects were better than fetuses who tolerated asphyxia. Surprisingly, the validity of the relationship between various FHR patterns and fetal acidemia has not been established in a large unselected series of consecutive pregnancies.[13] Further experimental and clinical studies are required.

## INTERDECELERATION OF FETAL HEART RATE AND VARIABILITY

During repeated cord occlusions, decelerations progressively became deeper as the umbilical cord occlusion was continued. This change was due, in part, to a fall in the nadir but also to the development of interocclusion fetal tachycardia.[36,37] This tachycardia is due to increased catecholamine activity and is not seen in less frequent, well-compensated occlusions.[36]

In addition to the absolute FHR, the FHR variability (FHRV) in the intercontraction period is one of the classic indices of fetal well-being. As recently reviewed, there is good clinical evidence that moderate levels of FHRV are a strong indicator that the fetus is coping well with labor and is unlikely to have significant acidosis (umbilical pH <7.15) or a low Apgar score.[13] A reduction in FHRV, particularly when it is combined with other FHR abnormalities, is reported to be an important indicator of fetal hypoxia and developing acidemia in the term[70] and preterm fetus.[59] A systematic review has suggested that undetectable or minimal FHRV in the presence of late or variable decelerations is the most consistent predictor of newborn acidemia, although the association was relatively low (only 23%).[13]

Perhaps surprisingly, some clinical studies have suggested there is either a weak or no relationship between FHRV and Apgar scores or cord acid-base measures during labor.[71] Indeed, the initial response to acute experimental hypoxemia or repeated asphyxia in the term fetus is an increase in FHRV rather than a decrease;[38,72,73] typically FHRV then becomes suppressed if the insult is chronic or repeated.[38,72,74,75]

Consistent with these data, during repeated brief occlusions in term-equivalent fetal sheep, FHRV increased with the onset of occlusions. Following this transient increase, the onset of severe acidosis and hypotension during repeated umbilical cord occlusions was associated with a fall in FHRV in two thirds of fetuses but by a terminal increase in the remaining third.[38] The significance of this finding of terminal increased FHRV remains unclear. It may be related to the presence of overshoot instability (ie, to a pattern of tachycardia followed by a secondary fall in FHR between decelerations). Clinical examples of this phenomenon can be seen commonly, but further studies are required to demonstrate their significance.

## FETAL HEART RATE OVERSHOOT

It is not unusual to see FHR accelerations or "shoulders" immediately before or after a variable deceleration. A variable FHR deceleration with a transient shoulder only after the deceleration is referred to as an "overshoot" deceleration pattern.[25] Clinically, an overshoot pattern has been observed with fetal hypoxia, newborns requiring resuscitation, and cerebral palsy.[76,77] In fetal sheep, the overshoot pattern after a variable deceleration has been related to the development of fetal acidosis and a fall in the cerebral glucose metabolic rate.[78,79] There is currently no definitive evidence for the prognostic importance of the overshoot FHR pattern in human labor.[76]

We evaluated the relationship between the overshoot pattern and the development of acidosis and hypotension during repeated brief umbilical cord occlusions in near-term fetal sheep.[80] Overshoot accelerations following the decelerations were seen during our 1:2.5 minute repeated occlusion model, but only with developing hypotension and fetal acidosis (pH at the onset of overshoot was 7.17).[80] Overshoot was followed by marked instability of the FHR between occlusions. The accelerations were never seen in the 1:5 minute occlusion group who did not develop hypotension and who had mild acidosis. The mechanisms involved are unclear but may include two factors—reduced myocardial vagal stimulation during the occlusion and beta-adrenergic myocardial stimulation immediately after the occlusion ends.[2,77] Atropine produces overshoot tachycardia in the human[31,81] and fetal sheep[56] and can be abolished by administration of the beta-blocker propranolol.[78] This finding suggests that overshoot is caused by beta-adrenergic stimulation that is unopposed because vagal tone has become relatively attenuated during decelerations.

In contrast to these experiments, overshoot FHR was also seen after the first occlusions of a longer occlusion protocol (2-minute occlusions every 4 minutes), occurring at a time when, by definition, fetuses were neither acidotic nor hypotensive.[80] The data suggest that 2-minute periods of occlusion are sufficient to trigger FHR overshoot from the beginning, because the insult is long enough to result in complete loss of vagal tone by the end of the first occlusion. In contrast, after only 1 minute of occlusion there is likely to be some persisting vagal stimulation combined with markedly less catecholamine release when compared with 2-minute occlusions,[17] preventing subsequent tachycardia. The later development of overshoot with 1-minute occlusions is likely mediated by greater catecholamine release due to worsening systemic compromise.[82]

Collectively these data suggest that, although it is a reflex mechanism, FHR overshoot has been underappreciated as a potential marker of fetal compromise. Further research is needed to determine how its appearance is modulated by other factors such as fetal condition.

## PRE-EXISTING HYPOXIA

The studies addressed thus far have examined the responses of healthy, well-oxygenated fetuses to hypoxia. Naturally the prelabor condition of the fetus, which is seldom easy to ascertain, must have a considerable impact. Cordocentesis has shown that antenatal hypoxia is associated with an increased incidence of stillbirth, metabolic acidosis during labor, and subsequent abnormal neurodevelopment.[83,84] Although this clinical experience strongly suggests that such infants are likely to be compromised by otherwise well-tolerated labor, intriguingly, experimental studies seem to suggest improved or greater cardiovascular adaptation to moderate induced hypoxemia.

When chronically hypoxic fetal sheep were exposed to a further episode of acute hypoxia, they exhibited more pronounced centralization of circulation[85] with enhanced femoral vasoconstriction and greater increases in plasma noradrenalin and vasopressin.[86] These studies used moderate hypoxia rather than laborlike or profound hypoxic insults. It may be speculated that these greater reflex responses reflect reduced fetal reserve that would be exposed during a more severe insult.[85] We tested the response of chronically hypoxic fetuses from multiple pregnancies in our 1:5 minute protocol. Strikingly, the normoxic fetuses were readily able to tolerate this occlusion series, whereas the fetuses with pre-existing hypoxia developed severe, progressive metabolic acidosis and hypotension.[35]

The viability of intrapartum FHR monitoring to improve outcomes is largely based on the concept that fetuses have not experienced prolonged antenatal hypoxia and consequent neuronal damage before labor. Although this assumption is correct for the large majority of fetuses, there is strong evidence that severe hypoxia is not uncommon before labor,[67,87] and that consequent neurologic injury can lead to abnormal FHR patterns in the short and long term. For further discussion on this topic, the reader is referred to other reviews.[25,88]

## INFECTION

Approximately one third of preterm pregnancies are complicated by inflammation and infection, but little is known about the FHR changes related to infection and inflammation alone or in conjunction with hypoxia, and indeed with other clinical treatments such as prepartum steroid administration, which are known to alter many FHR parameters.[89–91] Severe variable decelerations and decreased FHRV at less than 32 weeks' gestation are related to histologic evidence of acute inflammation,[92] but this is not a consistent finding. Tachycardia and elevated basal FHR have also been observed[93,94] without bradycardia or acidemia but associated with an increased risk of cerebral palsy, suggesting different pathophysiology from acute hypoxia-ischemia.[93] Variable heart rate responses are also seen experimentally, and when hypoxia does occur, it is usually not associated with acidosis.[95–98] Preterm fetuses may be more sensitive to inflammation, with preterm but not near-term fetal sheep responding to endotoxin exposure with negative T waves, tachycardia, and increased FHRV.[99]

Currently, FHR monitoring lacks precision in identifying the fetal in utero systemic inflammatory response and neonatal sepsis.[94] This situation can be improved by detailed clinical and experimental studies and appropriate correlations with the type and timing of exposures and their interrelationships with other conditions.

## SUMMARY

Using a physiologic parameter such as FHR, which is controlled by multiple systems, to identify the small minority of infants who become compromised during labor is a formidable challenge. As highlighted in this review, experimental studies have identified subtle but potentially clinically applicable changes in the FHR responses to laborlike insults that correlate with the onset of fetal compromise. Perhaps surprisingly, given how long FHR monitoring has been used in routine practice, large prospective unselected series of consecutive pregnancies are still needed to confirm the predictive value of such FHR changes.[13] Encouragingly, there is already evidence from relatively small cohorts that some FHR patterns are predictive[13] and can be assessed in a standardized way,[100] and that fetal monitoring education can dramatically reduce the incidence of infants born with low Apgar scores and neonatal encephalopathy.[101]

## REFERENCES

1. Barcroft J. The conditions of foetal respiration. Lancet 1933;222(5749):1021–4.
2. Barcroft J. Researches in prenatal life. London: Oxford Blackwell Scientific Publications; 1946.
3. Martin CB Jr. Normal fetal physiology and behavior, and adaptive responses with hypoxemia. Semin Perinatol 2008;32(4):239–42.
4. Bennet L, Westgate J, Gluckman PD, et al. Fetal responses to asphyxia. In: Stevenson DK, Sunshine P, editors. Fetal and neonatal brain injury: mechanisms, management, and the risks of practice. 2nd edition. Cambridge: Cambridge University Press; 2003. p. 83–110.
5. Gagnon R. An obstetric point of view on fetal adaptation and reprogramming. NeoReviews 2006;7(4):e189–94. Available at: http://neoreviews.aappublications.org.
6. Richardson BS, Bocking AD. Metabolic and circulatory adaptations to chronic hypoxia in the fetus. Comp Biochem Physiol A Mol Integr Physiol 1998;119(3): 717–23.

7. Gunn AJ, Quaedackers JS, Guan J, et al. The premature fetus: not as defense-less as we thought, but still paradoxically vulnerable? Dev Neurosci 2001;23(3): 175–9.
8. Gunn AJ, Bennet L. Timing of injury in the fetus and neonate. Curr Opin Obstet Gynecol 2008;20(2):175–81.
9. Janbu T, Nesheim BI. Uterine artery blood velocities during contractions in pregnancy and labour related to intrauterine pressure. Br J Obstet Gynaecol 1987; 94(12):1150–5.
10. Modanlou H, Yeh SY, Hon EH. Fetal and neonatal acid-base balance in normal and high-risk pregnancies: during labor and the first hour of life. Obstet Gynecol 1974;43(3):347–53.
11. Huch A, Huch R, Schneider H, et al. Continuous transcutaneous monitoring of fetal oxygen tension during labour. Br J Obstet Gynaecol 1977;84(Suppl 1): 1–39.
12. Wiberg N, Kallen K, Olofsson P. Physiological development of a mixed metabolic and respiratory umbilical cord blood acidemia with advancing gestational age. Early Hum Dev 2006;82(9):583–9.
13. Parer JT, King T, Flanders S, et al. Fetal acidemia and electronic fetal heart rate patterns: is there evidence of an association? J Matern Fetal Neonatal Med 2006;19(5):289–94.
14. Nelson KB, Dambrosia JM, Ting TY, et al. Uncertain value of electronic fetal monitoring in predicting cerebral palsy. N Engl J Med 1996;334(10):613–8.
15. McIntosh GH, Baghurst KI, Potter BJ, et al. Foetal brain development in the sheep. Neuropathol Appl Neurobiol 1979;5(2):103–14.
16. Bartelds B, van Bel F, Teitel DF, et al. Carotid, not aortic, chemoreceptors mediate the fetal cardiovascular response to acute hypoxemia in lambs. Pediatr Res 1993;34(1):51–5.
17. Jensen A, Hanson MA. Circulatory responses to acute asphyxia in intact and chemodenervated fetal sheep near term. Reprod Fertil Dev 1995;7(5):1351–9.
18. Moore PJ, Parkes MJ, Nijhuis JG, et al. The incidence of breathing movements of fetal sheep in normoxia and hypoxia after peripheral chemodenervation and brain-stem transection. J Dev Physiol 1989;11(3):147–51.
19. Mallard EC, Gunn AJ, Williams CE, et al. Transient umbilical cord occlusion causes hippocampal damage in the fetal sheep. Am J Obstet Gynecol 1992; 167(5):1423–30.
20. Gunn AJ, Parer JT, Mallard EC, et al. Cerebral histologic and electrocortico-graphic changes after asphyxia in fetal sheep. Pediatr Res 1992;31(5):486–91.
21. Sameshima H, Ikenoue T, Ikeda T, et al. Unselected low-risk pregnancies and the effect of continuous intrapartum fetal heart rate monitoring on umbilical blood gases and cerebral palsy. Am J Obstet Gynecol 2004;190(1):118–23.
22. Nijland R, Jongsma HW, Nijhuis JG, et al. Arterial oxygen saturation in relation to metabolic acidosis in fetal lambs. Am J Obstet Gynecol 1995;172(3):810–9.
23. de Haan HH, van Reempts JL, Vles JS, et al. Effects of asphyxia on the fetal lamb brain. Am J Obstet Gynecol 1993;169(6):1493–501.
24. Westgate JA, Gunn AJ, Gunn TR. Antecedents of neonatal encephalopathy with fetal acidaemia at term. Br J Obstet Gynaecol 1999;106(8):774–82.
25. Westgate JA, Wibbens B, Bennet L, et al. The intrapartum deceleration in center stage: a physiological approach to interpretation of fetal heart rate changes in labor. Am J Obstet Gynecol 2007;197(3):e1–11.
26. Itskovitz J, Rudolph AM. Denervation of arterial chemoreceptors and barorecep-tors in fetal lambs in utero. Am J Physiol 1982;242(5):H916–20.

27. Giussani DA, Spencer JA, Moore PJ, et al. Afferent and efferent components of the cardiovascular reflex responses to acute hypoxia in term fetal sheep. J Physiol 1993;461:431–49.

28. Cohn HE, Sacks EJ, Heymann MA, et al. Cardiovascular responses to hypoxemia and acidemia in fetal lambs. Am J Obstet Gynecol 1974;120(6): 817–24.

29. Itskovitz J, LaGamma EF, Rudolph AM. Heart rate and blood pressure responses to umbilical cord compression in fetal lambs with special reference to the mechanism of variable deceleration. Am J Obstet Gynecol 1983;147(4): 451–7.

30. Baan J Jr, Boekkooi PF, Teitel DF, et al. Heart rate fall during acute hypoxemia: a measure of chemoreceptor response in fetal sheep. J Dev Physiol 1993;19(3): 105–11.

31. Caldeyro-Barcia R, Medez-Bauer C, Poseiro J, et al. Control of the human fetal heart rate during labour. In: Cassels D, editor. The heart and circulation in the newborn and infant. New York: Grune & Stratton; 1966. p. 7–36.

32. Fletcher AJ, Gardner DS, Edwards M, et al. Development of the ovine fetal cardiovascular defense to hypoxemia towards term. Am J Physiol Heart Circ Physiol 2006;291(6):H3023–34.

33. Bennet L, Peebles DM, Edwards AD, et al. The cerebral hemodynamic response to asphyxia and hypoxia in the near-term fetal sheep as measured by near infrared spectroscopy. Pediatr Res 1998;44(6):951–7.

34. Richardson BS, Carmichael L, Homan J, et al. Cerebral oxidative metabolism in fetal sheep with prolonged and graded hypoxemia. J Dev Physiol 1993;19(2): 77–83.

35. Westgate J, Wassink G, Bennet L, et al. Spontaneous hypoxia in multiple pregnancy is associated with early fetal decompensation and greater T wave elevation during brief repeated cord occlusion in near-term fetal sheep. Am J Obstet Gynecol 2005;193(4):1526–33.

36. Bennet L, Westgate JA, Lui YC, et al. Fetal acidosis and hypotension during repeated umbilical cord occlusions are associated with enhanced chemoreflex responses in near-term fetal sheep. J Appl Physiol 2005;99(4):1477–82.

37. de Haan HH, Gunn AJ, Gluckman PD. Fetal heart rate changes do not reflect cardiovascular deterioration during brief repeated umbilical cord occlusions in near-term fetal lambs. Am J Obstet Gynecol 1997;176(1 Pt 1):8–17.

38. Westgate JA, Bennet L, Gunn AJ. Fetal heart rate variability changes during brief repeated umbilical cord occlusion in near term fetal sheep. Br J Obstet Gynaecol 1999;106(7):664–71.

39. de Haan HH, Gunn AJ, Williams CE, et al. Brief repeated umbilical cord occlusions cause sustained cytotoxic cerebral edema and focal infarcts in near-term fetal lambs. Pediatr Res 1997;41(1):96–104.

40. Peebles DM, Spencer JA, Edwards AD, et al. Relation between frequency of uterine contractions and human fetal cerebral oxygen saturation studied during labour by near infrared spectroscopy. Br J Obstet Gynaecol 1994; 101(1):44–8.

41. Akagi K, Okamura K, Endo C, et al. The slope of fetal heart rate deceleration is predictive of fetal condition during repeated umbilical cord compression in sheep. Am J Obstet Gynecol 1988;159(2):516–22.

42. Giussani DA, Unno N, Jenkins SL, et al. Dynamics of cardiovascular responses to repeated partial umbilical cord compression in late-gestation sheep fetus. Am J Physiol 1997;273(5 Pt 2):H2351–60.

43. Green LR, Kawagoe Y, Homan J, et al. Adaptation of cardiovascular responses to repetitive umbilical cord occlusion in the late gestation ovine fetus. J Physiol 2001;535(Pt 3):879–88.
44. Gunn AJ, Maxwell L, de Haan HH, et al. Delayed hypotension and subendocardial injury after repeated umbilical cord occlusion in near-term fetal lambs. Am J Obstet Gynecol 2000;183(6):1564–72.
45. Hanson MA. Do we now understand the control of the fetal circulation? Eur J Obstet Gynecol Reprod Biol 1997;75(1):55–61.
46. Lewis AB, Sadeghi M. Naloxone potentiates the plasma catecholamine response to asphyxia in the fetus. Dev Pharmacol Ther 1988;11(4):219–25.
47. LaGamma EF, Itskovitz J, Rudolph AM. Effects of naloxone on fetal circulatory responses to hypoxemia. Am J Obstet Gynecol 1982;143(8):933–40.
48. Martinez A, Padbury J, Shames L, et al. Naloxone potentiates epinephrine release during hypoxia in fetal sheep: dose response and cardiovascular effects. Pediatr Res 1988;23(4):343–7.
49. Mendez-Bauer C, Poseiro JJ, Arellano-Hernandez G, et al. Effects of atropine on the heart rate of the human fetus during labor. Am J Obstet Gynecol 1963;85(8):1033–53.
50. Robinson B, Nelson L. A review of the proceedings from the 2008 NICHD Workshop on Standardized Nomenclature for Cardiotocography: update on definitions, interpretative systems with management strategies, and research priorities in relation to intrapartum electronic fetal monitoring. Rev Obstet Gynecol 2008;1(4):186–92.
51. Visser GH, Redman CW, Huisjes HJ, et al. Nonstressed antepartum heart rate monitoring: implications of decelerations after spontaneous contractions. Am J Obstet Gynecol 1980;138(4):429–35.
52. van Geijn HP, Copray FJ, Donkers DK, et al. Diagnosis and management of intrapartum fetal distress. Eur J Obstet Gynecol Reprod Biol 1991;42:S63–72.
53. Fleischer A, Schulman H, Jagani N, et al. The development of fetal acidosis in the presence of an abnormal fetal heart rate tracing. I. The average for gestational age fetus. Am J Obstet Gynecol 1982;144(1):55–60.
54. Thomas G. The aetiology, characteristics and diagnostic relevance of late deceleration patterns in routine obstetric practice. Br J Obstet Gynaecol 1975;82(2):121–5.
55. Sameshima H, Ikenoue T. Predictive value of late decelerations for fetal acidemia in unselective low-risk pregnancies. Am J Perinatol 2005;22(1):19–23.
56. Harris JL, Krueger TR, Parer JT. Mechanisms of late decelerations of the fetal heart rate during hypoxia. Am J Obstet Gynecol 1982;144(5):491–6.
57. James LS, Yeh MN, Morishima HO, et al. Umbilical vein occlusion and transient acceleration of the fetal heart rate: experimental observations in subhuman primates. Am J Obstet Gynecol 1976;126(2):276–83.
58. Low JA. Determining the contribution of asphyxia to brain damage in the neonate. J Obstet Gynaecol Res 2004;30(4):276–86.
59. Matsuda Y, Maeda T, Kouno S. The critical period of non-reassuring fetal heart rate patterns in preterm gestation. Eur J Obstet Gynecol Reprod Biol 2003;106(1):36–9.
60. Simpson KR. Monitoring the preterm fetus during labor. MCN Am J Matern Child Nurs 2004;29(6):380–8 [quiz: 9–90].
61. Iwamoto HS, Kaufman T, Keil LC, et al. Responses to acute hypoxia in fetal sheep at 0.6-0.7 gestation. Am J Physiol 1989;256(3 Pt 2):H613–20.

62. Matsuda Y, Patrick J, Carmichael L. Effects of sustained hypoxemia on the sheep fetus at midgestation: endocrine, cardiovascular, and biophysical responses. Am J Obstet Gynecol 1992;167(2):531–40.

63. Jensen A. The brain of the asphyxiated fetus: basic research. Eur J Obstet Gynecol Reprod Biol 1996;65(1):19–24.

64. Shelley HJ. Glycogen reserves and their changes at birth and in anoxia. Br Med Bull 1961;17:137–43.

65. Szymonowicz W, Walker AM, Cussen L, et al. Developmental changes in regional cerebral blood flow in fetal and newborn lambs. Am J Physiol 1988; 254(1 Pt 2):H52–8.

66. Wassink G, Bennet L, Booth LC, et al. The ontogeny of hemodynamic responses to prolonged umbilical cord occlusion in fetal sheep. J Appl Physiol 2007;103(4): 1311–7.

67. MacLennan A. A template for defining a causal relation between acute intrapartum events and cerebral palsy: international consensus statement. BMJ 1999; 319(7216):1054–9.

68. Bennet L, Booth LC, Ahmed-Nasef N, et al. Male disadvantage? Fetal sex and cardiovascular responses to asphyxia in preterm fetal sheep. Am J Physiol Regul Integr Comp Physiol 2007;293(3):R1280–6.

69. Joseph KS, Wilkins R, Dodds L, et al. Customized birth weight for gestational age standards: perinatal mortality patterns are consistent with separate standards for males and females but not for blacks and whites. BMC Pregnancy Childbirth 2005;5(1):3.

70. Williams KP, Galerneau F. Comparison of intrapartum fetal heart rate tracings in patients with neonatal seizures vs. no seizures: what are the differences? J Perinat Med 2004;32(5):422–5.

71. Samueloff A, Langer O, Berkus M, et al. Is fetal heart rate variability a good predictor of fetal outcome? Acta Obstet Gynecol Scand 1994;73(1):39–44.

72. Murotsuki J, Bocking AD, Gagnon R. Fetal heart rate patterns in growth-restricted fetal sheep induced by chronic fetal placental embolization. Am J Obstet Gynecol 1997;176(2):282–90.

73. Kozuma S, Watanabe T, Bennet L, et al. The effect of carotid sinus denervation on fetal heart rate variation in normoxia, hypoxia and post-hypoxia in fetal sheep. Br J Obstet Gynaecol 1997;104(4):460–5.

74. Green LR, Homan J, White SE, et al. Cardiovascular and metabolic responses to intermittent umbilical cord occlusion in the preterm ovine fetus. J Soc Gynecol Investig 1999;6(2):56–63.

75. Ikeda T, Murata Y, Quilligan EJ, et al. Fetal heart rate patterns in postasphyxiated fetal lambs with brain damage. Am J Obstet Gynecol 1998;179(5):1329–37.

76. Parer JT. Fetal heart rate patterns basic and variant. In: Schmitt W, editor. Handbook of fetal heart rate monitoring. 2nd edition. Philadelphia: WB Saunders; 1997. p. 145–95.

77. Schifrin BS, Hamilton-Rubinstein T, Shields JR. Fetal heart rate patterns and the timing of fetal injury. J Perinatol 1994;14(3):174–81.

78. Saito J, Okamura K, Akagi K, et al. Alteration of FHR pattern associated with progressively advanced fetal acidemia caused by cord compression. Nippon Sanka Fujinka Gakkai Zasshi 1988;40(6):775–80.

79. Okamura K, Tanigawara S, Shintaku Y, et al. Alteration of FHR pattern and cerebral metabolic rate of glucose of the fetus measured by positron emission tomography during progress of acidemia: the significance of overshoot acceleration in FHR. J Perinat Med 1989;17(4):289–95.

80. Westgate JA, Bennet L, de Haan HH, et al. Fetal heart rate overshoot during repeated umbilical cord occlusion in sheep. Obstet Gynecol 2001;97(3): 454–9.

81. Hon EH, Lee ST. Electronic evaluation of the fetal heart rate. VIII. Patterns preceding fetal death, further observations. Am J Obstet Gynecol 1963;87: 814–26.

82. Rosen KG, Hrbek A, Karlsson K, et al. Fetal cerebral, cardiovascular and meta-bolic reactions to intermittent occlusion of ovine maternal placental blood flow. Acta Physiol Scand 1986;126(2):209–16.

83. Pardi G, Cetin I, Marconi AM, et al. Diagnostic value of blood sampling in fetuses with growth retardation. N Engl J Med 1993;328(10):692–6.

84. Soothill PW, Ajayi RA, Campbell S, et al. Fetal oxygenation at cordocentesis, maternal smoking and childhood neurodevelopment. Eur J Obstet Gynecol Re-prod Biol 1995;59(1):21–4.

85. Block BS, Llanos AJ, Creasy RK. Responses of the growth-retarded fetus to acute hypoxemia. Am J Obstet Gynecol 1984;148(7):878–85.

86. Gardner DS, Fletcher AJ, Bloomfield MR, et al. Effects of prevailing hypoxaemia, acidaemia or hypoglycaemia upon the cardiovascular, endocrine and metabolic responses to acute hypoxaemia in the ovine fetus. J Physiol 2002;540(Pt 1): 351–66.

87. Low JA. Reflections on the occurrence and significance of antepartum fetal asphyxia. Best Pract Res Clin Obstet Gynaecol 2004;18(3):375–82.

88. Phelan JP, Kim JO. Fetal heart rate observations in the brain-damaged infant. Semin Perinatol 2000;24(3):221–9.

89. Quaedackers JS, Roelfsema V, Fraser M, et al. Cardiovascular and endocrine effects of maternal dexamethasone treatment in preterm fetal sheep. Br J Obstet Gynaecol 2005;112(2):182–91.

90. Mulder EJ, de Heus R, Visser GH. Antenatal corticosteroid therapy: short-term effects on fetal behaviour and haemodynamics. Semin Fetal Neonatal Med 2009;14(3):151–6.

91. Hagberg H, Mallard C, Jacobsson B. Role of cytokines in preterm labour and brain injury. BJOG 2005;112(Suppl 1):16–8.

92. Salafia CM, Ghidini A, Sherer DM, et al. Abnormalities of the fetal heart rate in preterm deliveries are associated with acute intra-amniotic infection. J Soc Gynecol Investig 1998;5(4):188–91.

93. Sameshima H, Ikenoue T, Ikeda T, et al. Association of nonreassuring fetal heart rate patterns and subsequent cerebral palsy in pregnancies with intrauterine bacterial infection. Am J Perinatol 2005;22(4):181–7.

94. Aina-Mumuney AJ, Althaus JE, Henderson JL, et al. Intrapartum electronic fetal monitoring and the identification of systemic fetal inflammation. J Reprod Med 2007;52(9):762–8.

95. Garnier Y, Kadyrov M, Gantert M, et al. Proliferative responses in the placenta after endotoxin exposure in preterm fetal sheep. Eur J Obstet Gynecol Reprod Biol 2008;138(2):152–7.

96. Coumans AB, Garnier Y, Supcun S, et al. The effects of low-dose endotoxin on the umbilicoplacental circulation in preterm sheep. J Soc Gynecol Investig 2004; 11(5):289–93.

97. Dalitz P, Harding R, Rees SM, et al. Prolonged reductions in placental blood flow and cerebral oxygen delivery in preterm fetal sheep exposed to endotoxin: possible factors in white matter injury after acute infection. J Soc Gynecol Inves-tig 2003;10(5):283–90.

98. Duncan JR, Cock ML, Scheerlinck JP, et al. White matter injury after repeated endotoxin exposure in the preterm ovine fetus. Pediatr Res 2002;52(6):941–9.
99. Blad S, Welin AK, Kjellmer I, et al. ECG and heart rate variability changes in preterm and near-term fetal lamb following LPS exposure. Reprod Sci 2008; 15(6):572–83.
100. Parer JT, Ikeda T. A framework for standardized management of intrapartum fetal heart rate patterns. Am J Obstet Gynecol 2007;197(1):26, e1–e6.
101. Draycott T, Sibanda T, Owen L, et al. Does training in obstetric emergencies improve neonatal outcome? BJOG 2006;113(2):177–82.

# Probing the Fetal Cardiac Signal for Antecedents of Brain Injury

Adam J. Wolfberg, MD, MPH[a,b,]*, Errol R. Norwitz, MD, PhD[c]

**KEYWORDS**

- Fetal monitoring • Fetal EKG • Cerebral palsy
- Asphyxia • Fetal acidemia

There is no Glasgow Coma Scale for the fetus, nor can the physician interview the in utero patient to assess its neurologic status. As a consequence, clinicians and investigators have long sought an indirect means to assess fetal well-being. Fetal movement is referenced in the Old Testament as a sign of life,[1] and still is an excellent diagnostic test of fetal vitality. In the millennia since Abraham, clinicians have developed a host of sophisticated measures of fetal status. As a consequence, perinatal mortality has declined, particularly in the past 50 years.[2] The ability to diagnose impending fetal neurologic injury has not kept pace, however, with the development of diagnostic technology. This diagnostic dilemma (how to identify the fetus that is at high risk for subsequent or worsening brain injury) is the subject of this article. Although this discussion touches briefly on other technologies used to assess fetal neurologic status, the primary focus is on evaluation of the fetal cardiac signal. This is because fetal heart rate monitoring remains the single most important technology for fetal assessment in clinical obstetrics, in large part because the fetal heart rate is the only continuously available physiologic signal during pregnancy. Although

Adam J. Wolfberg, MD, MPH, is a director and shareholder of MindChild Medical, a company that is developing fetal EKG technology.

[a] Department of Obstetrics and Gynecology, Tufts University School of Medicine, Tufts Medical Center, Tufts Box 360, 800 Washington Street, Boston, MA 02111, USA

[b] Department of Neurology, Children's Hospital Boston and Harvard Medical School, 300 Longwood Avenue, Boston, MA 02115, USA

[c] Division of Maternal-Fetal Medicine, Department of Obstetrics, Gynecology and Reproductive Sciences, Yale University School of Medicine, Yale-New Haven Hospital, 333 Cedar Street, FMB 315A, New Haven, CT 06520–8063, USA

* Corresponding author. Department of Obstetrics and Gynecology, Tufts University School of Medicine, Tufts Medical Center, Tufts Box 360, 800 Washington Street, Boston, MA 02111.

*E-mail address:* awolfberg@tuftsmedicalcenter.org (A.J. Wolfberg).

Clin Perinatol 36 (2009) 673–684
doi:10.1016/j.clp.2009.06.006
0095-5108/09/$ – see front matter © 2009 Elsevier Inc. All rights reserved.

perinatology.theclinics.com

traditional fetal monitoring based on heart rate evaluation is a technology with a dubious record, this article makes the case that the cardiac signal, when analyzed appropriately, provides valuable insight into the health of the fetal brain, insight that will be unlocked in years to come.

Although this article focuses on long-term neurologic outcome, much of the data presented are on short-term measures of newborn well-being. It is extremely difficult to obtain sufficient statistical power for detection of cerebral palsy or newborn brain injury because of the rarity of these events. Rather, research tends to focus on outcome measures that are risk factors for cerebral palsy and long-term neurologic injury, such as inflammation, acidemia, hypoxia, or low 5-minute Apgar score. Although imperfect, this methodologic approach sets the stage for future multicenter clinical trials that evaluate the capacity of vetted diagnostic measures and technology to prevent newborn neurologic injury and cerebral palsy.

The topic of antepartum fetal evaluation with the specific purpose of preventing still-birth overlaps the subject matter of this article. There are many excellent papers evaluating the state of antenatal testing using ultrasound and other technologies, in particular a recent review by Signore and colleagues.[3] This article focuses on use of the fetal cardiac signal during pregnancy and labor to identify fetuses at risk for neurologic injury, particularly cerebral palsy.

## THE EVOLUTION OF APPROACHES TO MONITOR THE FETAL CARDIAC SIGNAL

The fetal heart sound may have been heard as early as 1650, but the routine use of auscultation of the fetal heart to verify fetal viability began in the 1820s with the introduction of the stethoscope.[4] The fetal ECG was first obtained and described by Cremen[5] in 1906 using vaginal leads. It was hoped, in this preultrasound era, that the capacity to identify the fetal ECG noninvasively could confirm fetal life before the point in pregnancy when the fetal heart sounds could be directly auscultated.[6] The technical challenge of measuring the fetal ECG using external sensors placed on the patient's abdomen, a challenge that still exists today, has continued to plague this technology and prevent its introduction into routine clinical practice. Techniques that have remained viable include examination of the fetal heart rate using a fetal scalp electrode[7] and Doppler ultrasound. Research has focused on evaluation of the fetal cardiac signal for two primary reasons. First, it is easily accessible, and second, it was assumed that research in the field of adult electrophysiology could be extended to the fetal cardiac signal.

Obstetric researchers have long understood the interaction between the fetal heart rate and the brain. An intrinsic rate is generated within the heart by pacemaker tissue in the sinoatrial node, the atrioventricular node, and the Purkinje tissues. The direct influence of both the parasympathetic (generally as a depressant) and sympathetic (generally as a stimulant) nervous systems on the fetal heart rate are also well understood, as are the effects of baroreceptors, chemoreceptors, and airway stretch receptors.[8] Early research focused on understanding the development of these different control systems through gestation, and learning how they modulate the influence of external stimuli on the fetal heart rate. Many of these mechanisms were worked out in animal models and in subsequent clinical studies in humans starting in the late 1950s.[9] The fetal heart rate gradually decreases during gestation, and there is a gradual increase in heart rate variability (HRV) with gestational age as the parasympathetic system matures.[10] Variability refers to the variance in the heart rate over a short period of time. Blockade of the parasympathetic system (with atropine) reduces fetal HRV, and this effect becomes more pronounced with increasing gestational age.[11]

Studies in both animals and humans have elucidated the effect of various pathologic conditions on HRV. In animal models, induction of fetal acidosis results in diminished HRV,[12,13] and in humans, HRV has been observed uniformly to be diminished before intrapartum fetal death resulting from a severe hypoxic insult.[14,15]

At the same time that research into HRV was taking place, other investigators were evaluating the response of the fetal heart rate to uterine contractions. The benign "early deceleration," resulting from vagal stimulation, and "variable deceleration," caused by transient cord occlusion, were distinguished from the pathologic "late deceleration" that was thought to result from placental insufficiency (mediated through multiple physiologic mechanisms).[16,17]

The combination of these lines of investigation (HRV and the response of the fetal heart rate to uterine contractions) led to the clinical fetal monitoring system introduced in the 1960s that remains in use today. A 1972 paper by Schifrin and Dame[18] described a scoring system that could be used to predict 5-minute Apgar score, taking into account HRV and fetal heart rate patterns in relation to contractions. Like fetal monitoring today, Schifrin's scoring system reliably predicted Apgar scores of seven and higher, but was quite poor at predicting scores of six or lower (positive predictive value of only 20%).

In spite of consistent evidence that the technology was of limited benefit in identifying fetuses at risk of neurologic injury, clinical fetal heart rate monitoring during labor became the standard of care in the developed world based on the assumption that the technology reduces intrapartum fetal brain injury. In a 1969 interview, Edward Hon claimed that 90% of fetal distress was caused by umbilical cord compression and that continuous fetal heart rate monitoring during labor could save 20,000 babies annually in the United States.[19] Although laudable, this goal has not been realized.

Fetal monitoring today is no better than it was in Schifrin and Dame's 1972 report. A "reassuring" fetal heart rate pattern almost universally predicts a well-oxygenated fetus, whereas the false-positive rate for a concerning finding remains extremely high. A "nonreassuring" fetal heart rate pattern is much more likely to be associated with a well-oxygenated fetus than with a hypoxic or acidotic fetus. A more recent study found that the false-positive rate of fetal monitoring for predicting an umbilical artery pH of less than 7.1 was 89%.[20] Randomized trials comparing continuous fetal heart rate monitoring with intermittent auscultation of the fetal heart rate in labor have generally found the two approaches to be equally good (or bad) at preventing neurologic injury.[21]

## DEFINING THE STANDARD OF CARE FOR FETAL HEART RATE MONITORING

In 1997, the National Institute of Child Health and Human Development convened a workshop to develop a consensus on the interpretation and use of fetal monitoring technology. The subsequent report provided definitions of terms and guidelines for interpretation.[22] This report significantly informed the guidance paper issued as a "Practice Bulletin" by the American College of Obstetricians and Gynecologists in 2005.[23] In this summary describing the role of intrapartum fetal heart rate monitoring, the American College of Obstetricians and Gynecologists reported that the technology is used in at least 85% of labor episodes in the United States, and acknowledged that it results in increased rates of operative deliveries without reducing the incidence of cerebral palsy.[23] It should be noted that reassuring antepartum fetal heart rate monitoring, a "reactive" nonstress test, reliably predicts survival for 2 to 3 days[24] and is useful in the third trimester for high-risk patients.

In response to proposals from national organizations of obstetricians in other countries[25,26] and from American experts,[27] the National Institute of Child Health and

Human Development convened another workshop to re-evaluate the state of fetal monitoring in 2008. The summary statement[28] from this meeting suggested that obstetricians classify fetal heart rate tracings into three groups. Category I tracings are normal and are highly predictive of fetal normoxia. These tracings previously would have been classified as either "reactive" or "reassuring." Category III tracings are "abnormal" and are characterized by absent HRV and either bradycardia or recurrent decelerations in the baseline fetal heart rate. Such tracings are an indication for immediate delivery. Category II tracings are those that fit into neither category I nor III. This system, not yet endorsed by American College of Obstetricians and Gynecologists, simplifies nomenclature but does not change practice. The statement also outlined a modest research agenda focused on observational studies designed to clarify the frequency and meaning of heart rate patterns that fit into category II. The new system can be conceptualized as a simple two-by-two table (**Table 1**).

## ALTERNATIVE APPROACHES TO ANALYSIS OF THE FETAL HEART RATE

Another approach to analysis of the fetal heart rate is the spectral analysis of HRV to quantify the energy in specific frequency components of HRV. This approach was developed in the hope that it would provide further insight into the autonomic nervous system's control of heart rate and possibly into the effects of hypoxia on autonomic nervous system activity.[29] Several reports of spectral analysis during labor suggest that diminished HRV in the low-frequency band (generally in the range of 0.05–0.3 Hz) may be associated with acidosis based on umbilical artery pH at the time of delivery.[30,31] Chung and colleagues[32] reported that a HRV frequency below 0.00013 Hz was both a sensitive and specific test for fetal acidosis. Although these analyses seem promising, they have neither arrived at the bedside nor have they been tested in prospective clinical trials.

Another promising technology is fetal magnetocardiography, an application of magnetobiometry (see the article by Lowery and colleagues elsewhere in this issue) that uses multiple sensors to measure tiny magnetic fields generated by the electrical activity of the fetal heart. These magnetic fields, much smaller than naturally occurring environmental magnetic fields, can be analyzed to provide an extremely accurate measurement of heart rate, more accurate than that measured by extracting the R-R interval using transabdominal Doppler ultrasound.[33] A major problem with this technology is the requirement that recordings be made in magnetically shielded rooms, an expensive and logistically daunting proposition. Further research with this technology is eagerly awaited, however, given preliminary data demonstrating subtle differences in the profile of HRV in normal and at-risk pregnancies[34] and the potential for this technology to be useful in understanding subtle cardiac arrhythmias during the fetal period.[35]

| Table 1 Summary of the 2008 National Institutes for Child Health and Human Development proposed terms for evaluating fetal heart rate tracings | | | |
|---|---|---|---|
| | | **Heart Rate Variability** | |
| | | Present | Absent |
| Repetitive late or variable decelerations | Absent | Category I | Category II |
| | Present | Category II | Category III |

## MOVING BEYOND HEART RATE

Although obstetricians spend considerable time pouring over fetal heart rate tracings and interpreting the shapes drawn by the pen that plots heart rate versus time, all of these analyses, along with spectral analysis of fetal HRV, are analyses of heart rate. Stated differently, the basic unit of analysis for all these tests is the time interval between one heartbeat and the next.

An exciting new era of fetal cardiac analysis involves the analysis of the fetal ECG waveform. This ECG waveform is central to interpretation of adult cardiac function and has been available to the obstetrician since 1958[7] as a single-lead ECG drawn from an electrode attached to the fetal scalp in labor. Because such an ECG is available only from a single lead on the fetal scalp, no analyses are possible that involve transverse vectors relative to the fetal heart, such as aVR or aVL.

The most robust analytic approach to this signal is now included in a commercially available STAN monitor (Neoventa Medical, Goteborg, Sweden). Beginning in the late 1990s, European investigators began using this monitor in routine clinical practice. This system is based on an analysis of the numeric ratio between the amplitude of the fetal T wave and the fetal R wave and on the presence or absence of a biphasic ST segment. The ratio is used clinically either to provide reassurance or raise concern in the event of a nonominous but nonreassuring fetal heart tracing (a category II tracing using the new terminology). The physiologic basis for this test is the observation that repolarization of the adult myocardium is extremely sensitive to hypoxia, resulting in elevation of the ST segment in adults with coronary artery disease. Similar findings have been demonstrated in fetal sheep, with experimental hypoxia leading to elevation in the ST segment and T waves in the fetal ECG.[36] The change in this ratio is thought to represent altered cellular ionic currents during anaerobic cardiac metabolism.[37]

A series of clinical trials were begun that compared use of the STAN monitor algorithm in addition to standard fetal monitoring with fetal monitoring alone. Early results demonstrated that use of the STAN monitor helped to identify cases of intrapartum acidosis.[38–40] Amer-Wahlin and colleagues[39] reported that the use of the STAN technology not only reduced the incidence of umbilical artery acidosis at delivery, but reduced the rate of operative delivery for "fetal distress" compared with those women monitored using standard fetal monitoring technology. In this study, however, newborn outcome based on 5-minute Apgar score was unaffected by the use of the STAN technology. Subsequent observational studies have demonstrated similar performance of the STAN monitor, but without a significant improvement in newborn outcome.[41–43] In contrast, a small Canadian study found that the STAN monitor technology had poor positive predictive value and poor sensitivity for metabolic acidemia at delivery.[44] A recent Cochrane meta-analysis concluded that the use of the STAN monitor modestly reduced the incidence of neonatal encephalopathy and significant metabolic acidosis at birth.[45]

Because of the STAN monitor's modest clinical use over existing technology, the limited clinical circumstances in which it can be used (it requires placement of a fetal scalp electrode), and the significant expense involved in replacing existing monitoring systems with the STAN monitor technology, it has not been widely adopted on clinical units in the United States. It also requires a 20-minute period of normal (category I) fetal heart rate tracing to be used as a baseline for an individual fetus against which to compare subsequent tracings. As such, if the tracing is already abnormal (category II or III) then the STAN monitor cannot be used.

Another analysis of ECG waveform is based on the observation that the PR interval (which represents the atrioventricular conduction time) of fetal sheep subjected to an acute hypoxic insult is shortened, whereas the R-R interval is lengthened (brady-cardia). This finding is in contrast to the general synchronicity of the PR and R-R inter-vals with increasing and decreasing heart rates under conditions of normoxia.[46] The problem with this analysis is that, like analysis of the fetal heart rate, both benign and pathologic conditions can shorten the PR interval.[47,48] As a consequence, perhaps, studies comparing standard fetal monitoring plus PR analysis with fetal monitoring alone demonstrated no significant difference in obstetric or newborn outcomes, although the technology did seem to empower clinicians to perform fewer diagnostic tests, such as scalp blood sampling, to reassure themselves of fetal well-being.[49,50]

These analytic approaches (amplitude-oriented in the case of the commercially available monitor and interval-oriented in the case of PR interval analysis) take advan-tage of ECG waveform parameters that are available using the fetal scalp electrode with its unipolar ECG. A major limitation of this technology is that analyses of vectors are not possible in the fetus as they are in the newborn or adult.

A new analytic approach involves segmenting the ECG waveform into heartbeats, (ie, slicing the continuous ECG signal at points equidistant between one R wave and the next, and treating each heartbeat as a unit of analysis). In this way, sets can be created that contain groups of heartbeats that are similarly shaped (based on quantitative analysis of each beat's shape) and each set can be assigned a symbol.[51] The shape of the heartbeats in relation to clinical events, such as cho-rioamnionitis or maternal fever, can be evaluated by measuring the frequency of the assigned symbols around the clinical event of interest. For example, in a patient who developed chorioamnionitis during labor, it was found that the shape of the ECG waveform changed significantly in the hour before the clinical presentation of intrauterine infection (**Figs. 1** and **2**).[52] These analyses are based on the understanding that the depolarization pathways for signal propagation within the (adult) heart muscle tend to be stable when well oxygenated, but lose this stability in the context of ischemia. This instability is manifest by variability in the propagation pathways that lead, in turn, to variation in the ECG waveform measured at the skin.[53,54]

In this analysis, the segmented beats also can be compared with surrounding beats in terms of heterogeneity of the waveform (essentially, the extent to which beats look different from the ones that come before and after). Analysis of morphologic heteroge-neity has been used to predict death in adults hospitalized following acute coronary events.[55,56] In preliminary studies, the same analyses were applied to fetal ECG wave-forms and a direct association was seen between the degree of ECG heterogeneity and levels of proinflammatory cytokines in umbilical cord serum at delivery (Zeeshan Syed, personal communication.).

These three approaches to analysis of the ECG waveform (ST segment, PR interval, and morphologic analysis), although not practice-changing in their own right, tempt the investigator with a modest gain in sensitivity and specificity compared with exist-ing technology. More research is needed using these technologies, both in isolation and grouped into amalgam measures, to determine whether measures of ECG aber-rations can be crafted into reliable and predictive clinical algorithms.

For future analytic approaches to the fetal cardiac signal, it is useful to look beyond the in utero domain. A growing body of evidence indicates that analyses of HRV can be used postnatal to predict adverse events in hospitalized pediatric[57] and adult popula-tions.[58] Several reports have demonstrated that analysis of HRV in hospitalized premature newborns can reliably predict the onset of urinary tract infections, sepsis, and death.[57,59–62] Beyond the neonatal period, changes in HRV have also been asso-ciated with elevated levels of inflammatory biomarkers in the circulation of adults in the

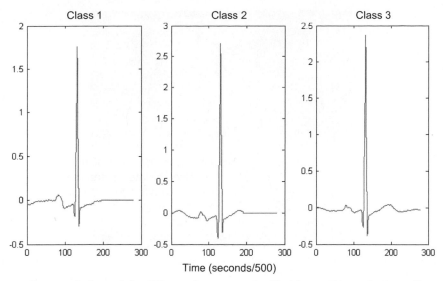

**Fig. 1.** The morphology of the QRS complexes were classified from a 7-hour dataset collected from a woman who developed chorioamnionitis during labor. These are the three most frequent morphologic classes during her labor.

intensive care unit,[63] with adverse outcome in adults with chronic heart failure,[64,65] and with survival in children in septic shock.[66] This heart rate characteristic analysis measures HRV over an extended period of hours to days, and reports data at regular 30-minute epochs. Quantitatively, the heart rate characteristic is able to capture both diminished HRV and decelerations in the heart rate. Because these parameters are central to the subjective interpretation of fetal heart tracings in labor, it is tempting to speculate that a variation on the heart rate characteristic could be used to evaluate quantitatively the fetal cardiac signal during pregnancy before the onset of labor.

## NONINVASIVE INTERROGATION OF THE FETAL ECG

Essentially all of the innovative technologies using the fetal cardiac signal in recent years have used the ECG waveform collected using the fetal scalp electrode. This

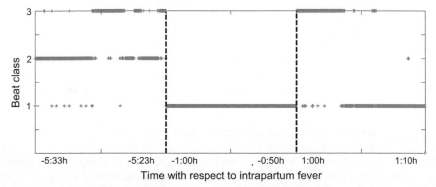

**Fig. 2.** The occurrence of each beat was plotted during 10-minute intervals timed with respect to the onset of maternal fever of the same patient as **Fig. 1**. Note the consistent appearance of class 1 at 1 hour before development of fever.

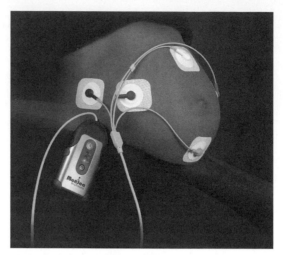

**Fig. 3.** The Monica AN24 (Monica Health care) fetal heart-rate monitor measures the fetal EKG signal at the maternal abdomen.

signal is available only when the patient is in labor with ruptured membranes and a cervix sufficiently dilated to allow placement of this invasive lead. Because the electrodes can cause traumatic or infectious injury to the fetal scalp, its use cannot be justified for research purposes alone. Research can only occur when the electrode is already in place for a clinical indication, a relatively rare event on most labor and delivery suites. Research that depends on the fetal ECG signal collected using a fetal scalp electrode cannot be done before labor.

At the time of this writing, several industry-academic teams are developing technology that can reliably measure the fetal ECG waveform using sensors on the maternal abdomen. Most advanced is Monica Healthcare, Ltd., United Kingdom company that is already marketing a fetal monitoring system using this technology in Europe (**Fig. 3**).[67] Fetal monitoring based on noninvasive recording of the fetal ECG signal holds tremendous promise from a clinical perspective. From a research perspective, this technology opens the door to full analysis of the ECG signal emanating from the fetus. Measures of waveform intervals, morphology, and rhythms will be possible for the first time before labor, and the rich field of quantitative cardiology will be able to step into the domain of obstetric research.

Numerous challenges remain, including but not limited to the development of systems to track the fetal cardiac signal as it moves with the fetus within the uterus. It is also likely that the technical challenges of separating the fetal ECG signal from the ambient electrical noise of the mother, the uterus, and movement artifact will complicate the exploitation of this signal. The emergence of technology that seems to have succeeded at grasping this fetal ECG signal is an exciting development.

## SUMMARY

Quantitative and qualitative analysis of the fetal heart rate tracing have long been used by obstetric care providers to identify fetuses at risk of neurologic injury, with very limited success. Looking toward the future, it is highly unlikely that further analyses based on heart rate alone, either quantitative or subjective, will result in systems that can more accurately predict fetal acidosis or neurologic injury. Head-to-head clinical trials demonstrating that quantitative measures of the fetal ECG signal can reduce the incidence of acidemia or hypoxic injury compared with standard heart rate monitoring are encouraging, even if the clinical improvement is modest. In the authors' view, the future of fetal monitoring is an amalgam measure that combines the features of several quantitative analyses of the fetal ECG. For example, some combination of ST ratio, PR interval, morphologic entropy, and HRV may reliably distinguish hypoxic from normoxic fetuses. Alternatively, the fetal heart rate characteristics along with spectral analysis of one of these basic measures may improve the positive predictive value of the amalgam monitoring analysis.

It will take time to move from a fetal monitoring system that causes at least as much maternal harm as it does newborn benefit, to a better system of in utero fetal assessment. It will also take cooperation and collaboration among investigators in multiple disciplines and competitive for-profit organizations. Indeed, success in every domain, in terms of improved diagnostic accuracy, academic achievement, and profit, depends in large part on the ability of these individuals and organizations to collaborate and work together.

## REFERENCES

1. Exodus. Brenton L. Septuagint LXX in English. London: Bagster and sons; 1851.
2. Data 2010: National Center for Health Statistics; 2009.
3. Signore C, Freeman RK, Spong CY. Antenatal testing: a reevaluation. Executive summary of a Eunice Kennedy Shriver National Institute of Child Health and Human Development workshop. Obstet Gynecol 2009;113(3):687–701.
4. Gunn AL, Wood MC. The amplification and recording of faetal heart sounds. Proc R Soc Med 1953;46(2):85–91.
5. Cremen M. On the direct measurement of the electrical activity of the human heart from the esophagus and the ECG of the fetus. Med Wschr 1906;53:811–3 [in German].
6. Caughey AF Jr. Electronic detection of fetal life: a review. Obstet Gynecol 1961; 17:382–91.
7. Hon EH. The electronic evaluation of the fetal heart rate: preliminary report. Am J Obstet Gynecol 1958;75(6):1215–30.
8. Hainsworth R. The control and physiological importance of heart rate. In: Malik M, Camm A, editors. Heart rate variability. Armonk (NY): Futura Publishing Company; 1995. p. 3–20.
9. Hirsch M, Karin J, Akselrod S. Heart rate variability in the fetus. In: Malik M, Camm A, editors. Heart rate variability. Armonk (NY): Futura Publishing Company; 1995. p. 517–31.
10. Gagnon R, Campbell K, Hunse C, et al. Patterns of human fetal heart rate accelerations from 26 weeks to term. Am J Obstet Gynecol 1987;157(3):743–8.
11. Schifferli P, Caldyero-Barcia R. Effects of atropine and beta-adrenergic drugs on the heart rate of the human fetus. In: Boreus L, editor. Fetal pharmacology. New York: Raven Press; 1973. p. 111–32.
12. Paul RH, Suidan AK, Yeh S, et al. Clinical fetal monitoring. VII. The evaluation and significance of intrapartum baseline FHR variability. Am J Obstet Gynecol 1975; 123(2):206–10.
13. Martin CB Jr. Regulation of the fetal heart rate and genesis of FHR patterns. Semin Perinatol 1978;2(2):131–46.
14. Cetrulo CL, Schifrin BS. Fetal heart rate patterns preceding death in utero. Obstet Gynecol 1976;48(5):521–7.

15. Parer J. Fetal heart rate patterns preceding death in utero. In: Parer J, editor. Handbook of fetal heart rate monitoring. Philadelphia: WB Saunders; 1983. p. 147–56.
16. Hon EH, Yeh SY. Electronic evaluation of fetal heart rate. X. The fetal arrhythmia index. Med Res Eng 1969;8(5):14–9.
17. Kubli FW, Hon EH, Khazin AF, et al. Observations on heart rate and pH in the human fetus during labor. Am J Obstet Gynecol 1969;104(8):1190–206.
18. Schifrin BS, Dame L. Fetal heart rate patterns: prediction of Apgar score. JAMA 1972;219(10):1322–5.
19. Watching the unborn inside the womb: high-risk mothers and the graph that raises their babies' chances. Life 1969;63–5.
20. Sameshima H, Ikenoue T, Ikeda T, et al. Unselected low-risk pregnancies and the effect of continuous intrapartum fetal heart rate monitoring on umbilical blood gases and cerebral palsy. Am J Obstet Gynecol 2004;190(1):118–23.
21. Graham EM, Petersen SM, Christo DK, et al. Intrapartum electronic fetal heart rate monitoring and the prevention of perinatal brain injury. Obstet Gynecol 2006;108(3 Pt 1):656–66.
22. Electronic fetal heart rate monitoring: research guidelines for interpretation. National Institute of Child Health and Human Development Research Planning Workshop. Am J Obstet Gynecol 1997;177(6):1385–90.
23. American College of Obstetricians and Gynecologists. ACOG Practice Bulletin: intrapartum fetal heart rate monitoring. Washington, DC: American College of Obstetricians and Gynecologists; 2005. p. 70.
24. Freeman RK, Anderson G, Dorchester W. A prospective multi-institutional study of antepartum fetal heart rate monitoring. I. Risk of perinatal mortality and morbidity according to antepartum fetal heart rate test results. Am J Obstet Gynecol 1982; 143(7):771–7.
25. Liston R, Sawchuck D, Young D. Fetal health surveillance: antepartum and intrapartum consensus guideline. J Obstet Gynaecol Can 2007;29(9 Suppl 4): S3–56.
26. The use of electronic fetal monitoring: the use and interpretation of cardiotocography in intrapartum fetal surveillance. Evidence-based clinical guideline number 8. Clinical Effectiveness Support Unit 2001. Available at: www.rcog.org. Accessed March 30, 2009.
27. Parer JT, Ikeda T. A framework for standardized management of intrapartum fetal heart rate patterns. Am J Obstet Gynecol 2007;197(1):26.e1–6.
28. Macones GA, Hankins GD, Spong CY, et al. The 2008 National Institute of Child Health and Human Development workshop report on electronic fetal monitoring: update on definitions, interpretation, and research guidelines. Obstet Gynecol 2008; 112(3):661–6.
29. Van Laar JO, Porath MM, Peters CH, et al. Spectral analysis of fetal heart rate variability for fetal surveillance: review of the literature. Acta Obstet Gynecol Scand 2008;87(3):300–6.
30. Siira SM, Ojala TH, Vahlberg TJ, et al. Marked fetal acidosis and specific changes in power spectrum analysis of fetal heart rate variability recorded during the last hour of labour. BJOG 2005;112(4):418–23.
31. Rantonen T, Ekholm E, Siira S, et al. Periodic spectral components of fetal heart rate variability reflect the changes in cord arterial base deficit values: a preliminary report. Early Hum Dev 2001;60(3):233–8.
32. Chung DY, Sim YB, Park KT, et al. Spectral analysis of fetal heart rate variability as a predictor of intrapartum fetal distress. Int J Gynaecol Obstet 2001;73(2): 109–16.

33. Lowery CL, Campbell JQ, Wilson JD, et al. Noninvasive antepartum recording of fetal S-T segment with a newly developed 151-channel magnetic sensor system. Am J Obstet Gynecol 2003;188(6):1491–6 [discussion: 1496–7].

34. Govindan RB, Lowery CL, Campbell JQ, et al. Early maturation of sinus rhythm dynamics in high-risk fetuses. Am J Obstet Gynecol 2007;196(6):572.e1–7 [discussion: 572.e7].

35. Strasburger JF, Cheulkar B, Wakai RT. Magnetocardiography for fetal arrhythmias. Heart Rhythm 2008;5(7):1073–6.

36. Greene KG. The ECG waveform. In: Whittle M, editor. Baillieres clinical obstetrics and gynaecology, vol. 1. London: Bailliere Tindale; 1987. p. 131–55.

37. Greene KR, Rosen KG. Long-term ST waveform changes in the ovine fetal electrocardiogram: the relationship to spontaneous labour and intrauterine death. Clin Phys Physiol Meas 1989;10(Suppl B):33–40.

38. Amer-Wahlin I, Hellsten C, Noren H, et al. Cardiotocography only versus cardiotocography plus ST analysis of fetal electrocardiogram for intrapartum fetal monitoring: a Swedish randomised controlled trial. Lancet 2001;358(9281):534–8.

39. Amer-Wahlin I, Bordahl P, Eikeland T, et al. ST analysis of the fetal electrocardiogram during labor: Nordic observational multicenter study. J Matern Fetal Neonatal Med 2002;12(4):260–6.

40. Luzietti R, Erkkola R, Hasbargen U, et al. European Community multi-Center Trial Fetal ECG Analysis During Labor: ST plus CTG analysis. J Perinat Med 1999; 27(6):431–40.

41. Massoud M, Giannesi A, Amabile N, et al. Fetal electrocardiotocography in labor and neonatal outcome: an observational study in 1889 patients in the French center of Edouard Herriot, Lyon. J Matern Fetal Neonatal Med 2007;20(11): 819–24.

42. Doria V, Papageorghiou AT, Gustafsson A, et al. Review of the first 1502 cases of ECG-ST waveform analysis during labour in a teaching hospital. BJOG 2007; 114(10):1202–7.

43. Noren H, Blad S, Carlsson A, et al. STAN in clinical practice: the outcome of 2 years of regular use in the city of Gothenburg. Am J Obstet Gynecol 2006; 195(1):7–15.

44. Dervaitis KL, Poole M, Schmidt G, et al. ST segment analysis of the fetal electrocardiogram plus electronic fetal heart rate monitoring in labor and its relationship to umbilical cord arterial blood gases. Am J Obstet Gynecol 2004;191(3):879–84.

45. Neilson JP. Fetal electrocardiogram (ECG) for fetal monitoring during labour. Cochrane Database Syst Rev 2009;(3):CD000116.

46. Greene KG. CTG, ECG and fetal blood sampling. In: Rodeck CH, Whittle M, editors. Fetal medicine: basic science and clinical practice. London: Churchill Livingstone; 1999. p. 985–1004.

47. Mohajer MP, Sahota DS, Reed NN, et al. Cumulative changes in the fetal electrocardiogram and biochemical indices of fetal hypoxia. Eur J Obstet Gynecol Reprod Biol 1994;55(1):63–70.

48. Luzietti R, Erkkola R, Hasbargen U, et al. European Community Multicentre Trial Fetal ECG Analysis During Labour: the P-R interval. J Perinat Med 1997;25(1):27–34.

49. Strachan BK, van Wijngaarden WJ, Sahota D, et al. Cardiotocography only versus cardiotocography plus PR-interval analysis in intrapartum surveillance: a randomised, multicentre trial. FECG Study Group. Lancet 2000; 355(9202):456–9.

50. van Wijngaarden WJ, Sahota DS, James DK, et al. Improved intrapartum surveillance with PR interval analysis of the fetal electrocardiogram: a randomized trial

showing a reduction in fetal blood sampling. Am J Obstet Gynecol 1996;174(4): 1295–9.

51. Syed Z, Guttag J, Stultz C. Clustering and symbolic analysis of cardiovascular signals: discovery and visualization of medically relevant patterns in long-term data with limited prior knowledge. EURASIP J Adv Signal Process 2007;2007: 1–24.

52. Wolfberg AJ, Syed Z, Clifford GD, et al. Entropy of fetal EKG associated with intrapartum fever. New England Conference on Perinatal Research. Chatham, Massachusetts, October 1, 2007.

53. Ben-Haim SA, Becker B, Edoute Y, et al. Beat-to-beat electrocardiographic morphology variation in healed myocardial infarction. Am J Cardiol 1991;68(8): 725–8.

54. Josephson ME, Wit AL. Fractionated electrical activity and continuous electrical activity: fact or artifact? Circulation 1984;70(4):529–32.

55. Syed Z, Scirica BM, Mohanavelu S, et al. Relation of death within 90 days of non-ST-elevation acute coronary syndromes to variability in electrocardiographic morphology. Am J Cardiol 2009;103(3):307–11.

56. Syed Z, Sung P, Scirica BM, et al. Spectral energy of ECG morphologic differences to predict death. Cardiovasc Eng 2009;9(1):18–26.

57. Griffin MP, Lake DE, Bissonette EA, et al. Heart rate characteristics: novel physiomarkers to predict neonatal infection and death. Pediatrics 2005;116(5): 1070–4.

58. Chen WL, Chen JH, Huang CC, et al. Heart rate variability measures as predictors of in-hospital mortality in ED patients with sepsis. Am J Emerg Med 2008; 26(4):395–401.

59. Griffin MP, Moorman JR. Toward the early diagnosis of neonatal sepsis and sepsis-like illness using novel heart rate analysis. Pediatrics 2001;107(1):97–104.

60. Griffin MP, O'Shea TM, Bissonette EA, et al. Abnormal heart rate characteristics preceding neonatal sepsis and sepsis-like illness. Pediatr Res 2003;53(6):920–6.

61. Griffin MP, O'Shea TM, Bissonette EA, et al. Abnormal heart rate characteristics are associated with neonatal mortality. Pediatr Res 2004;55(5):782–8.

62. Verklan MT, Padhye NS. Heart rate variability as an indicator of outcome in congenital diaphragmatic hernia with and without ECMO support. J Perinatol 2004;24(4):247–51.

63. Malave HA, Taylor AA, Nattama J, et al. Circulating levels of tumor necrosis factor correlate with indexes of depressed heart rate variability: a study in patients with mild-to-moderate heart failure. Chest 2003;123(3):716–24.

64. Aronson D, Mittleman MA, Burger AJ. Interleukin-6 levels are inversely correlated with heart rate variability in patients with decompensated heart failure. J Cardiovasc Electrophysiol 2001;12(3):294–300.

65. Guzzetta A, Fazzi B, Mercuri E, et al. Visual function in children with hemiplegia in the first years of life. Dev Med Child Neurol 2001;43(5):321–9.

66. Ellenby MS, McNames J, Lai S, et al. Uncoupling and recoupling of autonomic regulation of the heart beat in pediatric septic shock. Shock 2001;16(4):274–7.

67. Graatsma EM, Jacod BC, van Egmond LA, et al. Fetal electrocardiography: feasibility of long-term fetal heart rate recordings. BJOG 2009;116(2):334–7 [discussion: 337–8].

# The Current State and Future of Fetal Imaging

Romy Chung, MD[a], Gregor Kasprian, MD[b,d],
Peter C. Brugger, MD, PhD[c], Daniela Prayer, MD[b,d],*

KEYWORDS

- Fetal • Magnetic resonance • Tractography • Brain
- Morphometry • Volumetry

Fetal magnetic resonance imaging (MRI) has emerged as an essential diagnostic tool in recent years. The excellent soft tissue resolution, and the detailed visualization of fetal and extrafetal structures, may add important diagnostic information to prenatal sonography and has the power to confirm or change decisions at critical points in clinical care. Discussions of fetal surgery or termination of pregnancy may follow fetal MRI evaluation.

Ultrasound is the primary diagnostic tool in pregnancy. Indeed, as most fetal pathologies still initially are detected or suspected by ultrasound, prenatal sonography remains the modality of choice for screening examinations. Ultrasound has some advantages over MRI. It is less expensive, faster, and can be done at the bedside. Ultrasound, however, is user-dependent, and results will vary significantly with the skill and experience of the examiner. Despite being more costly, MRI's high spatial three-dimensional resolution, multiplanar capabilities, large field of view, robust image quality, and its ability to characterize chemical tissue properties are arguments which favor its use as a secondary diagnostic modality in the assessment of fetal pathologies.

MRI has been verified as an important adjunct to ultrasound for clinically serious cases.[1] One study[2] explored the premise that prenatal MRI could provide additional information about fetal sacrococcygeal teratoma (SCT) when compared with prenatal sonography. SCT is seen in 1 in every 35,000 live births, and is the most common

[a] Department of Radiology, University of California, San Diego, School of Medicine, La Jolla, CA 92037, USA
[b] Department of Neuroradiology, Medical University of Vienna, Währingergürtel 18-20, Vienna 1090, Austria
[c] Center of Anatomy and Cell Biology, Medical University of Vienna, Austria Waehringerstrasse 24, Vienna 1090, Austria
[d] Department of Radiology, Medical University of Vienna, Währingergürtel 18-20, Vienna 1090, Austria
* Corresponding author. Department of Radiology, Medical University of Vienna, Währingergürtel 18-20, Vienna 1090, Austria.
*E-mail address:* daniela.prayer@meduniwien.ac.at (D. Prayer).

Clin Perinatol 36 (2009) 685–699
doi:10.1016/j.clp.2009.07.004
0095-5108/09/$ – see front matter
perinatology.theclinics.com

tumor presenting in newborns. Depending on its tissue makeup, SCT can be mistaken on ultrasound for spina bifida (**Fig. 1**). In the study, MRI's characterization of the intra-pelvic and abdominal extent of the tumor was more accurate, and provided more information about its mass effect on adjacent organs, compared with ultrasound. Discrepancies between prenatal MRI and ultrasound occurred in 8 of the 22 fetuses in the cohort. Four fetuses with a type 1 sacrococcygeal teratoma on sonography were assessed as type 2 on MRI; three fetuses diagnosed with type 2 on sonography were type 1 sacrococcygeal teratomas on MRI, and one fetus diagnosed with type 2 on sonography was a type 3 sacrococcygeal teratoma on MRI. Intrapelvic mass effect was seen with MRI in 9 of 22 fetuses (41%), but only three of nine were assessed correctly with ultrasound. The investigators surmised that the additional anatomic resolution afforded by MRI resulted in better prenatal counseling and improved preop-erative planning for surgical resection.[1] This study supports the capacity of MRI to change clinical course.

Until recently, magnetic resonance image acquisition had been lengthy, and its image quality depended on a complete lack of fetal motion. Maternal–fetal sedation was required for coherent images. Ultrafast MRI sequences, however, have proven efficacious at suppressing fetal motion artifacts, and they do not require sedation. In early studies, no statistically significant difference between sonography and ultra-fast MRI was found for the detection of abnormality in any organ system. One study asserts that on occasion, ultrafast MRI was demonstrably superior to sonography in characterizing cerebral abnormalities.[3] Most clinicians, however, still agree that MRI should be limited to clinical situations in which ultrasound findings are ambiguous or impaired.

Relative to ultrasound, MRI has some drawbacks secondary to its recent introduc-tion as an antenatal diagnostic tool. The American College of Obstetrics and Gyne-cology (ACOG)[4] recommends against using MRI in early stages of pregnancy, namely the first trimester, unless specifically indicated. Therefore, fetal MRI usually is performed after 17 gestational weeks (GWs) have passed, ensuring the completion of major organogenesis.[5] The diagnostic window is narrowed further by logistical concerns; in the United States, termination of pregnancy is illegal after 24 GWs,[6] and in addition, most clinics prefer to perform abortions earlier than 22 weeks, because viability is estimated to drop off to 15% in births earlier than 24 GWs.[7]

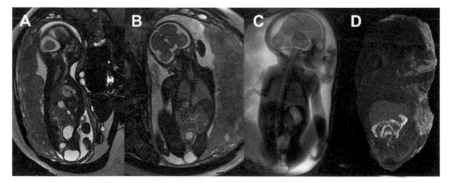

**Fig. 1.** 28 + 3 gestational weeks sagittal (*A*) and coronal (*B*) steady-state free precession sequence. Coronal thick-slab T2-weighted sequence (*C*), and T1 weighted sagittal z-projec-tion (*D*): sacrococcygeal teratoma with extra- and intracorporal cystic part. T1 weighted hy-perintensity of the meconium-filled rectum shows compression and displacement of this part of the large bowels.

As a small number of animal studies have suggested a possibility of teratogenic effects,[8,9] the safety of higher field strengths (more than 1.5 T) at earlier stages of pregnancy is not clear. Still, when MRI has been used as diagnostic imaging tool after 18 GWs, no ill effects have been reported so far. For example, it has been reported that MRI does not demonstrate effects on fetal heart rate patterns,[10] an important marker of fetal health close to term. In short, most human studies assessing the risk of MRI suggest that there are no ill effects to the mother or fetus.

A PubMed literature search of "magnetic resonance imaging fetus" limited to human studies in core clinical journals in the last 10 years, reveals subtle trends in cohorts and in the fetal MRI studies performed. For example, fetal MRI cohort sizes have been growing (**Fig. 2**), ostensibly in response to the need for reliable MRI standards, especially compared with the massive numbers of ultrasound studies that form the basis of ultrasound morphometric and clinical reference standards. Also of note is the increase in organ systems studied during the same period. Imaging studies of the fetal central nervous system (CNS) always have comprised a significant part of fetal MRI, but in the last 10 years, other fetal organs and organ systems, such as the lung and abdomen, and most recently the heart, have grown in prominence in publications. These trends reflect the growing number of indications for fetal MRI.

## RECENT ADVANCES IN FETAL CENTRAL NERVOUS SYSTEM MRI

Cerebral anomalies account for approximately 9% of all isolated anomalies and manifest in 15.9% of multiple malformations,[11] constituting a major impetus for prenatal diagnosis. Of all organ systems in the developing fetus, studies of the developing CNS have benefited most from the image quality and detail that MRI provides. The high resolution of imaging in MRI can identify the critical but extremely small and subtle changes in CNS landmarks, especially at early gestational ages (GA). These changes can manifest in gross MRI morphology, the brain microarchitecture, or the activity of the fetus when assessed in a dynamic sequence. Therefore, MRI has been useful in three regards: (1) the quantification of brain growth and structural

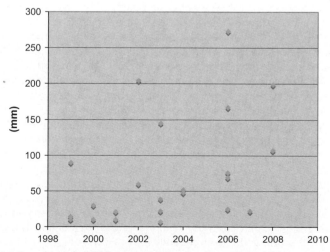

**Fig. 2.** Increases in cohort size of fetal magnetic resonance central nervous system studies as a function of date.

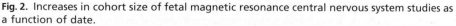

abnormalities using biometry, (2) the qualitative evaluation of CNS microstructure, and (3) the qualitative assessment of dynamic fetal movements in utero.

### Quantification of Brain Growth and Brain Pathology

As an objective method of assessing fetal growth, the clinical implications of morphometric evaluation cannot be underestimated. Willocks and colleagues[12,13] can be regarded as the pioneers in the field of fetal cephalometry. They introduced the quantification of fetal brain growth by standardized parameters, such as the commonly used biparietal diameter.[14] Since then and to this end, ultrasound parameters were re-evaluated repeatedly, and have been used clinically for decades to evaluate fetal brain or skull structures. They remain the standard screen for normal morphology.

Existing postmortem histologic measurements can help validate standardized measurements of fetal brain parameters for MRI, but with some significant limitations. Correlative studies are subject to postmortem changes in the tissue architecture, both microscopic (eg, autolysis) and macroscopic (eg, collapse of ventricular spaces). Dying fetuses tend to bleed in the germinal zone, and thereby provide a dimension of error. The postnatal environment can collapse or distort cerebrospinal fluid (CSF) spaces. Edema makes initial measurements inaccurate and technically challenging. When the brain is fixed postmortem, shrinkage of the tissue is quite pronounced. Because of the high water content of the immature brain, volumetric measurements may be reduced to as much as 70% of their prefixed state,[15] affecting linear dimensions. Despite these setbacks, however, MRI has made a significant impact on the morphometry of structures in the fetal CNS in recent years. This is supported by multiple studies, as detailed next. One study[16] examined the effect of MRI on changes in diagnosis and clinical management of fetuses suspected of having CNS anomalies with ultrasound. In 31.7% (46 of 145) of fetuses with abnormal ultrasound findings, MRI findings changed the diagnosis. Additionally, they found their results were GA-dependent. The mean GA of the 46 fetuses with changes in diagnosis (26.3 weeks) was significantly greater than that of the 99 fetuses with no major change in diagnosis (23.3 weeks, $P<.01$). This finding may suggest that the pathology becomes more apparent with age in both ultrasound and MRI, but does not refute that MRI is a powerful diagnostic adjunct to ultrasound, particularly in earlier weeks, when it would appear that ultrasound is less sensitive. Further contribution of MRI to prenatal CNS assessment is reflected in its diagnostic utility in the evaluation of ventriculomegaly in utero. A large university study[17] examined 167 cases of isolated mild ventriculomegaly (IMV) (ie, unilateral or bilateral ventriculomegaly with no associated anomaly at time of diagnosis). In this study, IMV was diagnosed around 26.5 GWs. In addition to associated anomalies, MRI studies identified three criteria that were associated with an unfavorable outcome: atrial width greater than 12 mm, progressive ventricular enlargement, and asymmetrical and bilateral ventriculomegaly (**Fig. 3**).

Extensive MR templates of gyration and sulcation of the developing fetal brain have been researched, best seen in an extensive 2004 study of both normal and pathologic fetal brains in utero.[17] This study assessed data only after GW 22. Additionally, the standard parameters in 22 to 25 GWs in the previous literature were derived from a very small number of cases.[11] As aforementioned, standardized measurements of brain parameters in fetuses less than 25 GWs previously were extrapolated from ultrasound and histologic measurements. Thus, the MRI morphometry in less than 24 weeks had been significantly lacking until further exploration of fetal brain parameters from 18 to 25 GWs was undertaken recently.[18]

Measurements of fetal brain parameters before 24 GWs present some specific imaging difficulties. The structures themselves are very small. For example, between

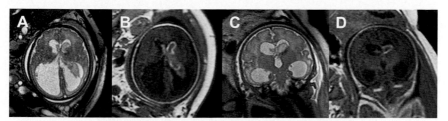

**Fig. 3.** 36 + 6 gestational weeks: axial (A) steady-state free precession sequence, correspond-ing axial T1 weighted sequence (B), and coronal T2 weighted (C) and T1 weighted (D) sequences depicting blood degradation products in a fetus with an intraventricular hemor-rhage. In this case, the etiology of bilateral ventriculomegaly could be explained by obstruc-tions of the Foramen of Monro and at the level of the aqueduct.

18 and 24 GWs, the width of the third ventricle can range from 2 to 3 mm, and the length of the corpus callosum can range between 12 and 18 mm. Additionally, the plane of acquisition can be very sensitive to rotation, and certain structures, because of their size, may be subject to high error due to changes in the plane alone.

As technology has enabled thinner and thinner slices (2 mm generally is considered the lower end of slice thickness range), reassessment of the definition of the parame-ters is important. The fronto-occipital diameter (FOD) used to be a standard measure-ment in the sagittal midline of the fetal brain that measured the longest distance between the occipital and frontal lobe poles. As the slices have become thinner, a perfectly midline sagittal slice can avoid the frontal and occipital lobes completely, remaining instead mostly within the interhemispheric fissure (**Fig. 4**). Therefore, this study suggested that FOD—an important parameter to assess fetal CNS health—might be measured axially, in a plane perpendicular to the brain stem that reflects the longest length between frontal and occipital poles (**Fig. 5**).

This study[18] evaluated the same brain parameters as Garel's study,[17] but focused on GA between 18 and 25 GWs with a much larger study sample. Additionally, it

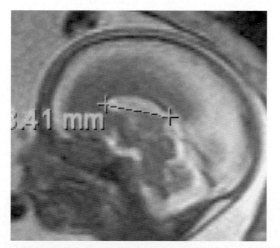

**Fig. 4.** 24 + 3 gestational weeks; sagittal T2 weighted midline plane exhibiting measurement of corpus callosum in oligohydramnios. Note that a midline sagittal slice does not capture the frontal and occipital poles completely.

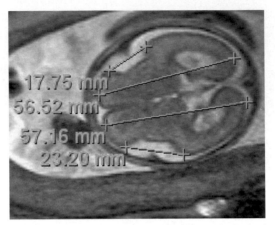

**Fig. 5.** 22 + 4 gestational weeks; T2 weighted axial plane in which the lateral ventricles are largest. Anteroposterior interopercular distance (APIPD) customarily is measured between the most extreme anterior and posterior edges of the Sylvian fissure (measuring 56.52 mm and 57.16 mm). Note that the right APIPD (measuring 23.20 mm) is significantly greater than the left (17.75 mm). In this plane, fronto-occipital diameter also can be measured between the extreme poles of the frontal and occipital lobes.

re-evaluated the morphometric definition of certain brain parameters, such as the aforementioned FOD, to take advantage of recent advances in technology and thinner slices. Many parenchymal brain parameter measurements, such as the length of the corpus callosum (**Fig. 6**), cranial and bone biparietal diameter, and the transverse cerebral diameter, were found to have a linear rate of growth through the period 18 to 25 GWs, a rate of growth consistent with the trends seen in earlier studies.[19] These previous studies corroborated the trends, although they themselves did not attempt to set down standardized measurements for each GW.

Some structures, like the corpus callosum (see **Fig. 4**), are easy to define and measure. Their morphology is such that its measurement is not sensitive to variations

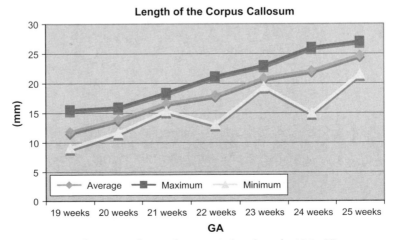

**Fig. 6.** Measurement of corpus callosum from gestational weeks 19 to 25.

in the acquisition plane, and their regular trends reflected this. Generally speaking, the clinical morphometric definition must be easy for practitioners to use, yet also reflect the expected trends in growth for clinical use. Some structures in the CNS, however, can be difficult to define for repeated weekly measurements by clinicians for a few reasons. The structures can change drastically between GWs. For example, the shape and axis of the lateral ventricles change quite dramatically over the course of brain development, from large rounded spaces until approximately 24 GWs, to thin angled slits nearing term.

In the aforementioned study,[18] it was found that certain brain parameters could be assessed better volumetrically. Measurements of brain spaces, such as diameter of the lateral ventricles, diameters of the third and fourth ventricles, and the interhemispheric diameter, were found to show high intrasample variability (**Fig. 7**). This, too, reflected the variability found within earlier studies.[20,21] This variability in nonparenchymal brain measurements could be attributed to two factors. First, the high error of measuring such small structures contributes significantly, being comprised of smaller intrinsic errors. These errors include motion artifacts, error intrinsic to the pulse sequences, slice thickness, and screen pixels (in-plane resolution of 0.7 mm results in an inaccuracy of up to 10% of a structure with a length of 7 mm). But secondly, the variability in measurements may reflect the three-dimensional variability of spaces, and suggest that volumetric measurement may be superior. The lateral ventricles, for example, varied significantly in diameter as slices progressed through the brain in all three orthogonal planes. So although the trend in **Fig. 7** is linear for the average width of the lateral ventricles, high variability also is found to be present.

A parameter that shows this much variability reflects the difficulty in defining the parameter itself, or reflects the variability between fetuses at the exact same location. Difficulties with the lateral ventricles may not be limited to those measurements made earlier than 24 GWs. Another study compared contemporaneous ultrasound and three-dimensional MRI reconstructions in uncomplicated nulliparous term (37 to 40 GWs) pregnancies.[20] This study showed acceptable correlation between both

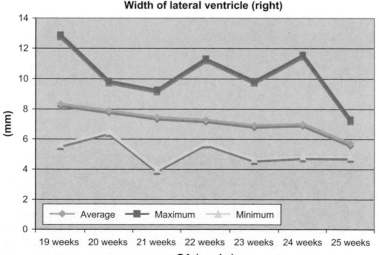

**Fig. 7.** Measurement of width of right lateral ventricles from gestational weeks 19 to 25.

modalities for head circumference, abdominal circumference, and biparietal diameter, but poor correlation with ultrasound for both right and left ventricular atrial diameters.[20] Regardless of the source of error, the data suggest that simple two-dimensional measurements of spaces in the developing fetal brain may not be as reliable as three-dimensional volumetric analysis and that further exploration of three-dimensional volumetrics may prove that it is a more dependable way to achieve nonparenchymal measurements. Fetal brain volumetry has been validated further with a study[21] examining 50 consecutive fetuses at 17 to 37 weeks of GA referred for MRI for ventriculomegaly. As suggested by the previous data, lateral ventricular volumes (and the supratentorial parenchyma) were deemed to be reliably measured with fetal brain volumetry. Inter- and intraobserver variability were low, and the effect of the imaging plane was considered negligible.

Volumetric analysis of the parenchyma also may prove to have clinical applications. Fetal brain volumetry additionally was used to study fetal posterior fossa volume (PFV).[22] The study suggested that fetal PFV could be a measurable parameter for second and third trimester fetuses with anomalies that manifest in the posterior fossa, such as Chiari II and Dandy-Walker. The standard two-dimensional ultrasound transverse cerebellar diameters cannot quantify PFV and are only an indirect measure of the fossa size. In the study, the authors found that the relationship between PFV (in cubic centimeters) and EGA (estimated gestational age in weeks) was described well by a single exponential function (PFV=0.689 exp [EGA/9.10]), and may prove to be another parameter with clinical application.[22]

Volumetric measurements, however, do present some difficulties and inefficiencies that must be overcome to be clinically useful and accessible. Difficulties with partial volume averaging, given the slice thickness at early GAs, add another dimension of error.[22] Additionally, volumetric measurements take longer to process than a normal two-dimensional measurement, a single plane taking as long as 19 minutes in this study.[22] Although this time may be adequately short for particular cases that require attention, it may not be sufficiently quick to screen fetal health (eg, for ventriculomegaly). Therefore, certain advances in the computer programs may be necessary before fetal brain volumetry can be implemented effectively.

The discussion of fetal brain morphometry should include recent work on hemispheric asymmetry. Aside from the problem of interindividual variability in brain structure and in brain growth dynamics, significant hemispheric asymmetry already exists at early stages of fetal development. The degree of fetal brain asymmetry depends on the actual developmental stage and on the brain region examined. After the initial descriptions of hemispheric asymmetry in the adult brain by Geschwind and Levitsky,[23] postmortem studies of fetal brains reported an asymmetrical development of sulci and gyri most pronounced at the end of the second trimester and in the perisylvian cortex regions.[24] An ultrasound study revealed significant hemispheric differences in ventricular size in a series of fetuses with normal neurodevelopmental outcome.[25] Ongoing analysis of fetal brain asymmetry moreover has revealed size differences between the right and left fetal temporal lobes.[5] This hemispheric asymmetry was corroborated further in the 2008 study of fetal brains between 19 and 25 GWs,[18] as the measured right anteroposterior interopercular distances (APIPD) were consistently larger than the left between 19 and 25 GWs (see **Fig. 5**). Advanced computerized fetal MRI and shape analysis is currently performed to assess and quantify the degree of fetal brain asymmetry in vivo. These data require corroboration but raise intriguing questions; it is likely that the normal and potentially abnormal development of lateralization in the human brain will provide important insights into neurodevelopmental outcome.

## Qualitative Assessment of Fetal Brain Parenchyma and Microstructure

MRI's ability to assess fetal brain microstructure has proven to be a significant diagnostic advantage for cases in which abnormalities of the underlying tissue architecture are important. The underlying architecture of fetal brain tissue does not display enough impedance differences to be identified with ultrasound.[5] Therefore, qualitative assessment of the fetal brain microstructure has depended upon histology, and more recently on MRI.

A review in 2006[26] correlated histologic and MRI findings of the transient cerebral zones that manifest during different GWs. The studies assessed in the review further validate the clinical utility of the visually detailed imaging found in MRI, stating that transient zones in the fetal brain parenchyma can be seen in MRI as early as 10 GWs. In addition, several histologically correlated transient features in earlier studies are possible to detect that previously had gone unnoticed (**Fig. 8**), suggesting that the capabilities of MRI to assess fetal brain microstructure have not been exhausted. Although **Fig. 8** only shows three distinct neuroarchitectural laminae in an in vivo fetus, in vitro MRI studies[26] have shown that it is theoretically possible for MRI to detect the seven neuroarchitectural laminae demonstrated histologically between 17 and 28 GWs.

## Diffusion Tensor Imaging and Tractography

An important and promising development in the field of diagnostic fetal MRI is diffusion tensor imaging (DTI) and tractography. DTI makes use of diffusion weighted imaging (DWI) technology. Anisotropic (hindered) and isotropic (nonhindered) diffusion of protons generate the image contrast in DWI. In addition, DWI has high diagnostic sensitivity for identifying acute hypoxic ischemic fetal brain lesions.[5] The technology used in DWI has been used to evaluate in utero normal and pathologic brain tissue architecture in two dimensions.

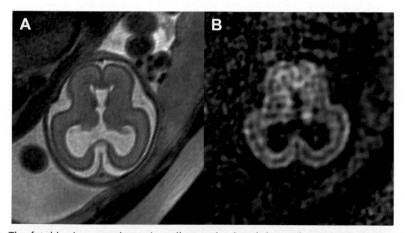

**Fig. 8.** The fetal brain parenchyma is well organized and shows three transient neuroarchitectural zones in (A) axial T2 weighted and (B) diffusion weighted images of a fetus with atypical holoprosencephaly at 24 GW. The outermost layer is the cortical plate, which is hypointense in T2 weighted images, and hyperintense in diffusion weighted images. The subplate is the middle layer, and it has signals opposite from the cortical plate (hyperintense in T2 weighted, hypointense in diffusion weighted). The innermost third layer is the ventricular/subventricular zone with ganglionic eminences, and it has the same signals as the cortical plate.

Taking DWI a step further, DTI uses different electromagnetic field gradients to measure the anisotropy and directionality of Brownian motion in more than six orientations. The degree of anisotropic diffusion depends on the microstructural composition of a certain tissue. Anisotropy is increased when diffusion is hindered by microstructural obstacles, such as cell membranes and organelles, myelin, or axonal elements. This allows a noninvasive characterization of a certain tissue component and the three-dimensional reconstruction of the tissue microstructure such as the architecture of the developing fetal brain. In the postmortem and laboratory setting, high-resolution DTI already has been applied in embryonic and fetal brains. Correlation with histology proved that high-resolution postmortem DTI is able to visualize even subtle structures of the fetal brain.

Currently, the greatest challenge in translating postmortem DTI for use in in vivo fetal MRI is the persistent occurrence of fetal and maternal motion. After sequence optimization (greater slice thickness, lower resolution), however, and by the use of acceleration factors, it is possible to acquire in utero DTI data that can be postprocessed further.[27] As a recent study shows,[28] this technique allows the visualization of corticospinal and callosal pathways in 40% of the examined cases. Especially in situations where fetal motion typically is restricted (cephalic presentation, premature rupture of membranes, advanced GA), these major pathways of the fetal brain may be depicted successfully (**Fig. 9**). This study[28] also provided further evidence for the asymmetrical development of the human brain in utero. Fractional anisotropy (FA) and axial [$\lambda$1] and transverse [$\lambda$2, $\lambda$3] eigenvalues are diffusion parameters used to assess the microstructure and maturity of specific white matter regions. This study reported that higher FA and $\lambda_1$ of the right sensorimotor pathway structures led to significant differences in the length of the right and left corticospinal and thalamocortical connectivity, further supporting asymmetrical maturation of fetal white matter.

Ultrasound does not have the capability to evaluate the evolution and development of fetal white matter. Thus, DTI may further underscore the importance of fetal MRI in the in vivo examination of fetal brain parenchyma and contribute an additional dimension of antenatal imaging. Further technical improvements and a more liberal use of sedation in cases with pending severe brain abnormalities may establish DTI as part

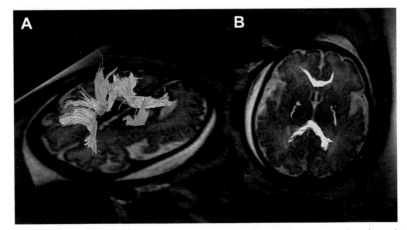

**Fig. 9.** In utero diffusion tensor imaging and tractography at 37 + 6 gestational weeks: two-dimensional projection of the trajectories of the genu and splenium of the corpus callosum (A) and three-dimensional appearance of the bilateral corticospinal tracts and the corpus callosum (B).

of the standard sequence repertoire in the MRI assessment of normal and abnormal fetal brain morphology and function.

## Assessment of Fetal Dynamic States: Function and Movement

Early in the second trimester, cortical folding patterns have not yet emerged in the fetal brain, and quantitative morphometry alone can prove insufficient. MRI dynamic sequences investigate qualitative dimensions of fetal health, namely, the assessment of general movements and movement abnormalities that often are found in cases of brainstem pathologies.

As fetal MRI usually is performed after 17 GWs, earlier patterns of activity such as startles, well documented in ultrasound studies, are seen only rarely.[29] From 18 GWs onwards, general movements and primitive reflexes, as well as small intrinsic movements (eg, those involving the diaphragm, eyes, and tongue) and details of general movements (eg, those involving the hands and fingers) may be observed.[30] Seizures may be identified during the study. Dynamic studies presenting repeatedly abnormal movement patterns can be correlated with structural morphologic findings to confirm a suspected diagnosis. A 2006 study using cine MRI (this study's term for dynamic studies) and two-dimensional fast imaging employing steady-state acquisition (FIESTA) MRI[31] reached the following conclusions. The implementation of parallel imaging with two-dimensional FIESTA has obviated fetal motion as a limitation for prenatal imaging, and cine MRI can illustrate fetal motion with high clinical reliability. The information provided by cine MRI can give critical information for postnatal prognosis, especially in the case of severe CNS abnormalities.

Currently, it is not clear whether fetal behavioral patterns result from the expression of certain genes, or if epigenetic factors (eg, the intrauterine environment) influence fetal activity and lead to individual postnatal variations of movement patterns.[31] Of note, a complete absence of movement during the 30- to 45-minute MRI examination does not assure fetal pathology. Only in the case of abnormally fixed fetal posture (usually characterized by carpopedal positioning of the hands and clubfeet) can a diagnosis of akinesia be made.[32]

In short, dynamic sequences manage to give three-dimensional information about the fetus by displaying two-dimensional images in real time. Watching a fetus move in utero provides much information regarding the neurologic and musculoskeletal function of the fetus, and thereby supplies prognostic information.

## ADVANCES IN MRI ASSESSMENT OF PLACENTAL STRUCTURE

Given the dependence on normal placental transfer of oxygen and energy substrate, the ability to assess placental structure and function using MRI would constitute a major advance. The placenta is vascularized heavily, and utero-placental infarction is a significant risk factor for interuterine growth restriction. Determination of an intact placenta and sufficient utero-placental circulation is an essential component of every antenatal examination. The placenta goes through morphologic changes during gestation, well documented with ultrasound imaging and Doppler ultrasound. Ultrasound studies remain the primary imaging modality for macroscopic abnormalities, but MRI can serve as an adjunct modality for antenatal examinations that are difficult to visualize secondary to disorders or disadvantageous anatomic structures or alignment of the mother or fetus.[33]

One study of 100 normal singleton pregnancies examined the placentas to determine an MRI standard of reference, and was able to confirm the clear morphologic changes (**Fig. 10**) documented by ultrasound.[33] That said, adverse fetal positions

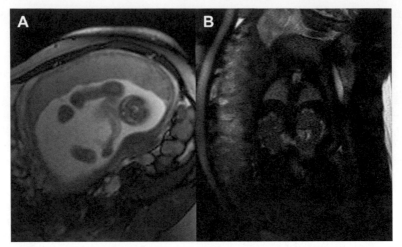

Fig. 10. Steady-state free precession sequence of a placenta at 20 + 1 gestational weeks (GWs) with regular homogenous signals (*A*). At 33 GWs (*B*), the signal characteristics are physiological rather inhomogeneous, showing delineable placentomes.

and certain antepartum pathologies (eg, oligohydramnios and obesity) can limit ultrasound image resolution of the placenta. In cases like these, where ultrasound cannot give a clear diagnosis, MRI is an excellent adjunct imaging modality. In addition, MRI findings have been correlated well with histology. A retrospective study[34] examined 45 singleton pregnancies from 19 to 35 GWs with placental pathologies on MRI scans. Placental hemorrhages (retroplacental hematoma, intervillous thrombi, subchorionic hematoma) and ischemic lesions were visualized with fetal MRI (**Fig. 11**).

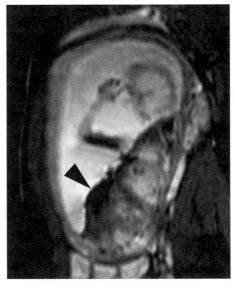

Fig. 11. Echoplanar sequence of a placenta with subchorionic hematoma (*black arrowhead*, hypointense signals on the placental surface) at 19 gestational weeks.

Chorioamnionitis and perivillous fibrin deposition, however, showed few signal changes, which likely reflected small changes in the placenta. The study concluded that fetal MRI could be a promising tool for assessing placental insufficiency.

## SUMMARY: THE FUTURE

Relative to other imaging modalities, fetal MRI remains in the early stages of evolution. Certain anatomically defined parameters that have been established for decades in ultrasound and postmortem histology are still being defined to satisfaction in MRI, even as advances in technology (increases in field strength, new pulse sequences) continue. The advantages of MRI include its notable soft tissue detail, high spatial resolution, planar capabilities, and large field of view. Evidence accumulates from in vivo human studies that MRI does not contribute to fetal anomalies and disorders, but fetal MRI still is used sparingly. As MRI becomes less costly, and the acquisition time of images decreases, expanding the use of fetal MRI clinically may be appropriate. Three categories in fetal MRI warrant further exploration to expand on current fetal assessment: volumetric measurement, DTI and tractography, and motion degradation technology.

### Volumetric Measurements

Currently, volumetric measurements have proven too expensive and time-intensive for everyday screening and diagnostic measurements. Regarding the CNS, two-dimensional ventricular space measurements in early GWs are unreliable diagnostic parameters because of their highly variable nature and inherent error. Further research is warranted to verify three-dimensional and volumetric measurements and to further streamline the process, because early diagnosis of ventricular pathology (eg, hydrocephalus) has such significant clinical implications that two-dimensional measurements in both ultrasound and MRI do not suffice. Three-dimensional reconstruction of fetal brains may not be feasible as everyday clinical adjuncts today, but as the algorithms advance, this method likely will prove an exceptional means of morphometric analysis.

### Diffusion Tensor Imaging and Tractography

Although in its very early stages, DTI and tractography deserve further exploration. The noninvasive characterization of CNS tissue and the three-dimensional reconstruction of the tissue architecture may lead to identification of the most subtle structures and pathologies of the fetal brain. DTI and tractography currently are used only in postmortem and laboratory settings, but their application in fetal brain pathology has been corroborated by histology. This imaging technique will benefit from technological advances that reduce fetal motion in MRI.

### Motion Degradation Technology

High-quality MRI depends on a minimization of motion. One study[35] has evaluated the use of snapshot MRI with volume reconstruction and reported a higher signal-to-noise ratio. This technology images the target volume repeatedly and uses a slice-to-volume registration method that achieves alignment of each slice within 0.3 mm. Fetal MRI has a particular interest in this minimization, as sedation of fetuses currently is avoided.

Follow-up studies in these areas will contribute to prenatal diagnosis, in hopes of further discerning postnatal neurodevelopmental consequences. In doing so, one can elucidate further the complex interactions between nature and nurture in shaping the human brain, mind, and behavior.

**REFERENCES**

1. Miller E, Ben-Sira L, Constantini S, et al. Impact of prenatal magnetic resonance imaging on postnatal neurosurgical treatment. J Neurosurg 2006;105(Suppl 3): 203–9.
2. Danzer E, Hubbard AM, Hedrick HL, et al. Diagnosis and characterization of fetal sacrococcygeal teratoma with prenatal MRI. AJR Am J Roentgenol 2006;187(4): W350–6.
3. Kubik-Huch RA, Huisman TA, Wisser J, et al. Ultrafast MR imaging of the fetus. AJR Am J Roentgenol 2000;174(6):1599–606.
4. Guidelines for diagnostic imaging during pregnancy. ACOG Committee Opinion No. 299. American College of Obstetricians and Gynecologists. Obstet Gynecol 2004;104:647–51.
5. Prayer D, Kasprian G, Krampl E, et al. MRI of normal fetal brain development. Eur J Radiol 2006;57:199–216.
6. Roe v Wade, 410 US Reports 113 (1973).
7. Kaempf JW, Tomlinson M, Arduza C, et al. Medical staff guidelines for periviability pregnancy counseling and medical treatment of extremely premature infants. Pediatrics 2006;117(1):22–9.
8. Carnes KI, Magin RL. Effects of in utero exposure to 4.7 T MR imaging conditions on fetal growth and testicular development in the mouse. Magn Reson Imaging 1996;14(3):263–74.
9. Magin RL, Lee JK, Klintsova A, et al. Biological effects of long-duration, high-field (4 T) MRI on growth and development in the mouse. J Magn Reson Imaging 2000; 12(1):140–9.
10. Vadeyar SH, Moore RJ, Strachan BK, et al. Effect of fetal magnetic resonance imaging on fetal heart rate patterns. Am J Obstet Gynecol 2000;182(3):666–9.
11. Ouahba J, Luton D, Vuillard E, et al. Prenatal isolated mild ventriculomegaly: outcome in 167 cases. BJOG 2006;113(9):1072–9.
12. Willocks J, Donald I, Duggan TC, et al. Foetal cephalometry by ultrasound. J Obstet Gynaecol Br Commonw 1964;71:11–20.
13. Willocks J, Donald I, Campbell S, et al. Intrauterine growth assessed by ultrasonic foetal cephalometry. J Obstet Gynaecol Br Commonw 1967;74(5):639–47.
14. Campbell S. An improved method of fetal cephalometry by ultrasound. J Obstet Gynaecol Br Commonw 1968;75:568–76.
15. Kretschmann H-J. Brain growth. Bibliotheca Anatomica Number 28. Basel (Switzerland): Karger Publishers; 1986.
16. Levine D, Barnes PD, Robertson RR, et al. Fast MR imaging of fetal central nervous system abnormalities. Radiology 2004;232(1):306–7.
17. Garel C. MRI of the fetal brain: normal development and cerebral pathologies. New York: Springer-Verlag; 2004.
18. Chung R, Kasprian G, Brugger P, et al. Oral presentation, "Normal MRI fetal brain parameters: 19–24 weeks". American Society of Neuroradiology conference. New Orleans, Los Angeles, May 31–June 5, 2008.
19. Reichel TF, Ramus RM, Caire JT, et al. Fetal central nervous system biometry on MR imaging. AJR Am J Roentgenol 2003;180(4):1155–8.
20. Hatab MR, Zaretsky MV, Alexander JM, et al. Comparison of fetal biometric values with sonographic and 3D reconstruction MRI in term gestations. AJR Am J Roentgenol 2008;191(2):340–5.
21. Kazan-Tannus JF, Dialani V, Kataoka ML, et al. MR volumetry of brain and CSF in fetuses referred for ventriculomegaly. AJR Am J Roentgenol 2007;189(1):145–51.

22. Chen SC, Simon EM, Haselgrove JC, et al. Fetal posterior fossa volume: assessment with MR imaging. Radiology 2006;238(3):997–1003.
23. Geschwind N, Levitsky W. Human brain: left–right asymmetries in temporal speech region. Science 1968;161:186–7.
24. Chi JG, Dooling EC, Gilles FH. Gyral development of the human brain. Ann Neurol 1977;1:86–93.
25. Achiron R, Yagel S, Rotstein Z, et al. Cerebral lateral ventricular asymmetry: is this a normal ultrasonographic finding in the fetal brain? Obstet Gynecol 1997;89: 233–7.
26. Rados M, Judas M, Kostović I. In vitro MRI of brain development. Eur J Radiol 2006;57(2):187–98.
27. Bui T, Daire JL, Chalard F, et al. Microstructural development of human brain assessed in utero by diffusion tensor imaging. Pediatr Radiol 2006;36(11): 1133–40.
28. Kasprian G, Brugger PC, Weber M, et al. In utero tractography of fetal white matter development. Neuroimage 2008;43(2):213–24.
29. Nijhuis JG. Fetal behavior. Neurobiol aging 2003;24(Suppl 1):S41–6 [discussion: S47–9, S51–2].
30. Prayer D. Oral presentation. "Behavioural Patterns in utero" Neurogenomics and Neuroimaging of Developmental Disorders symposium and workshops. Dubrovnik, Croatia, April 30–May 5 2009.
31. Guo WY, Ono S, Oi S, et al. Dynamic motion analysis of fetuses with central nervous system disorders by cine magnetic resonance imaging using fast imaging employing steady-state acquisition and parallel imaging: a preliminary result. J Neurosurg 2006;105(Suppl 2):94–100.
32. de Vries JI, Fong BF. Changes in fetal motility as a result of congenital disorders: an overview. Ultrasound Obstet Gynecol 2007;29(5):590–9.
33. Blaicher W, Brugger PC, Mittermayer C, et al. Magnetic resonance imaging of the normal placenta. Eur J Radiol 2006;57:256–60.
34. Linduska N, Dekan S, Messerschmidt A, et al. Placental pathologies in fetal MRI with pathohistological correlation. Placenta 2009;30(6):555–9.
35. Jiang S, Xue H, Glover A, et al. MRI of moving subjects using multislice snapshot images with volume reconstruction (SVR): application to fetal, neonatal, and adult brain studies. IEEE Trans Med Imaging 2007;26(7):967–80.

# Fetal Neurological Assessment Using Noninvasive Magnetoencephalography

Curtis L. Lowery, MD[a,b,*], Rathinaswamy B. Govindan, PhD[b],
Hubert Preissl, PhD[b], Pam Murphy, BSN, RN[a,b], Hari Eswaran, PhD[b]

**KEYWORDS**
- Magnetoencephalography • Fetus • Neonates • Brain activity
- Evoked responses • Maturation

The maturational process of the developing brain is reflected by changes in fetal behavior patterns, both spontaneous and induced, which can be observed over gestation. Herschkowitz[1] tabulates the time line for the development of these prenatal activities in terms of weeks of gestational age (GA). Some important features include reflex response elicited by touch (7 GA), limb movements (10 GA), coordinated movements (16 GA), slow (16 GA) and rapid (23 GA) eye movements, cyclic motor activity (21 GA), startle response to vibroacoustic stimulation (24 GA), response to light (28 GA), sleep cycles (34 GA), regular breathing movements (35 GA), and habituation to repeated vibrotactile stimulation (38 GA).

It is clear that to track functional development in the fetal brain we must be able to reliably monitor its biophysical signals during gestation. Fetal brain activity was first recorded noninvasively by Lindsey[2] in 1942 using abdominal electrodes; however, technological limitations of the time yielded poor-quality signals. Advances in technology over the past decade have enabled researchers to investigate directly the functional development of the fetal brain through two emerging techniques: functional magnetic resonance imaging (fMRI)[3,4] and fetal magnetoencephalography (MEG).[5] There are several advantages and disadvantages to both techniques. fMRI has inherent limitations and safety issues, but delivers both functional and anatomical information. In contrast, fetal MEG is a noninvasive method with superior temporal resolution, but does not provide any direct anatomical information. The technique of

[a] Division of Maternal-Fetal Medicine, Department of Obstetrics and Gynecology, University of Arkansas for Medical Sciences, 4301 West Markham Street, #518, Little Rock, AR 72205, USA
[b] Department of Obstetrics and Gynecology, University of Arkansas for Medical Sciences, 4301 West Markham Street, #518, Little Rock, AR 72205, USA
* Corresponding author. Department of Obstetrics and Gynecology, University of Arkansas for Medical Sciences, 4301 West Markham Street, #518, Little Rock, AR 72205.
*E-mail address:* lowerycurtisl@uams.edu (C.L. Lowery).

Clin Perinatol 36 (2009) 701–709
doi:10.1016/j.clp.2009.07.003
0095-5108/09/$ – see front matter. Published by Elsevier Inc.

perinatology.theclinics.com

fetal MEG stems from that of adult MEG, which is a well-established investigational tool.[6,7] MEG records magnetic signals generated by electrical currents in biological tissue.[8] In contrast to electric currents, magnetic signals are not distorted by the different layers of biological tissue.[9] Because MEG has the capacity to record nondistorted magnetic signals directly in a noninvasive manner, it is uniquely suited to the study of the magnetic fields generated in the fetal brain.

## NONINVASIVE DEVICE FOR RECORDING FETAL BRAIN ACTIVITY

SARA (SQUID Array for Reproductive Assessment) is a unique MEG device designed for the noninvasive recording of fetal brain activity. Funding was obtained in 1998 for its construction at the University of Arkansas for Medical Sciences, where it has been in successful operation since 2000. SARA was designed to fill a great need in current fetal evaluation techniques: the need for direct assessment and monitoring of the neurological status of the fetus. These measurements are of significant clinical benefit because they provide a method to assess those fetuses at risk for brain damage in utero, and are especially important in the management of high-risk maternal conditions. Conditions that increase the risk for organ damage in the fetus and particularly the risk of hypoxia to the developing brain include maternal diabetes, hypertension, and other diseases, or maternal activities (eg, smoking) that cause fetal growth restriction. Because SARA can record signals within the mother's abdomen related to changes in electrical flow, applications that are possible include measurement of fetal heart activity, uterine contractile activity, and fetal body movement. A cradle that fits the SARA sensor array has been designed to enable MEG studies in the newborn that can then be correlated with previous fetal studies. In this review, we provide a general overview of the technology and its potential application to fetal medicine. A large number of studies that have been conducted and published describing this device since it was brought into operation are referenced throughout the article.[5,10–20]

## RECORDING METHODS

The SARA system's array of 151 primary sensors is curved to fit the shape of the maternal abdomen (**Fig. 1**). In addition, 29 reference SQUID sensors are located at a distance away from the mother and fetus and are used to detect and attenuate the ambient environmental magnetic noise and vibration signals. To monitor the neurological status of the fetus, we have performed serial studies (starting at 28 weeks of gestation) of the fetal auditory evoked response (AER),[10–13] visual evoked response (VER),[14,15] and spontaneous brain activity.[16,17] Current clinical studies are aimed at improving the monitoring methods of maternal-fetal health and assisting physicians in better management of pregnancy and labor.

All studies performed using SARA were approved by the University of Arkansas for Medical Sciences–Human Research Advisory Committee, and consent was obtained from all subjects. The routine recording sessions range from 6 to 12 minutes in a continuous mode at a sampling rate of 312.5 Hz and a bandpass of dc to 100 Hz. The position and orientation of the mother's abdomen, relative to the sensor array, are determined using three localization coils placed at fiduciary points on the mother's right and left sides, and spine at the level of the umbilicus. These coils do not interfere with the MEG recordings. Fetal head position is defined using a portable ultrasound scanner when the patient sits in front of the array. The ultrasound probe is placed on the surface of the maternal abdomen exactly over the fetal head. A fourth localization coil is then attached to the maternal abdomen to provide additional positional

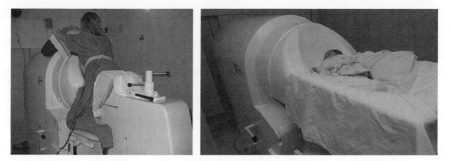

**Fig. 1.** The left panel shows a pregnant subject seated on the SARA system. The right panels shows a neonate positioned in the cradle for a study.

information related to sensor coordinates. The ultrasound examination to evaluate fetal head position is repeated at the end of the study.

## AUDITORY EVOKED RESPONSES

The AER is the neuroelectric response of the auditory system in the brainstem, midbrain, and the cortex to sound stimulation. A large number of components have been described in the human averaged auditory evoked potential. These components can be divided into brainstem (first 10 milliseconds), middle latency (40 milliseconds), and long latency (50 to 250 milliseconds). Several authors[21–23] have reviewed the utility of evoked responses in predicting neurological outcome in neonates. It is generally agreed that AERs are useful in diagnosing hearing loss[24] and are associated with neuromotor impairment, but produce a high rate of false negative results. Some of these negative results may be a consequence of the sensitivity of evoked responses to time elapsed following injury,[25] arguing for the earliest possible measurements (eg, fetus in utero). Tharp[26] associated fetal brain injury with the development of abnormal evoked response in the newborn and also suggested that hydrocephalus can produce severe changes in the brainstem auditory evoked response.[27,28] Several studies show that the auditory evoked response is a useful predictor of brain death.[29,30]

Hepper and Shahidullah[31] reported that as early as the 19th week of gestation, fetuses showed motor responses to pure tone stimuli in the low frequency range of human hearing (500 Hz). They demonstrated that by the 27th week of gestational age, 96% of fetuses in their study responded to 250-Hz and 500-Hz tones. Furthermore, 100% of fetuses responded to tones with frequencies of 1000 Hz and 3000 Hz at 33 and 35 weeks of gestational age, respectively.

Based on these early studies, the standard auditory stimulus used by fetal MEG researchers is a tone burst. The experimental protocols we have tested include the following parameters: Frequency—500 Hz to 1 kHz, Duration—100 ms to 1 s, Interstimulus Interval—1 to 2 s, and Intensity (measured outside in the air)—100 to 120 dB. The auditory stimuli were generated using STIM software (Neurosoft, El Paso, TX). The sound stimulation was delivered to the maternal abdomen overlying the fetal head from a speaker mounted outside the magnetically shielded room, through plastic tubing with an inflated balloon at the distal end.[18] The sound intensity was measured in the air, both at the air-filled bag (120 dB) and in the shielded room (100 dB). For the newborn studies, the balloon was suspended in the midline over the cradle above the newborn's head.[12] Each ear was stimulated separately by turning the baby appropriately with one ear exposed to the direction of the sound. The auditory evoked potentials were sampled at a frequency of 312.5 Hz from 151 magnetic sensors for 6 epochs lasting 1 minute each.

The general approach of most fetal AER studies is to search for an evoked component around 200 ms, which is interpreted as a delayed component corresponding to the adult N100. Various fetal MEG investigators (including our group) have recorded peak AER amplitude ranging from approximately 30 to 175 fT and the latency of the primary response component from 125 to over 200 ms. **Fig. 2** shows a representative response with 500-ms tone duration obtained from a 33-week fetus.

## VISUAL EVOKED RESPONSES

Woods and Plessinger[32] recorded VERs in fetal lambs using implanted scalp electrodes. Their studies demonstrated that the visual system develops progressively during fetal life and is functional before birth. Also, the few studies conducted on human fetuses have observed changes in fetal behavioral states, including heart rate pattern, body movements, and eye movements, in response to visual stimulation.[33,34] Based on the fact that light stimulus has been successfully used to measure the visual functional development of preterm and term newborns,[35–37] we investigated the response to light generated by fetal visual cortical areas. We developed a flash visual stimulus system, based on stimulus parameters used for observing fetal behavioral patterns, to elicit the VER. The light source, located outside the shielded room, uses a light emitting diode (LED) array (Opto Technology model OTL630A-5-10-66-E, wavelength 625 nm). A 7.7 m long fiber-optic cable channels the light flash from the LED array (outside the shielded room) to the maternal abdomen. One end of the light guide is attached to a light source and the other end to an 18-in, plastic, multifiber dispersing device. The light delivered to the maternal abdomen is very safe and similar to the level used in other studies.[33] The

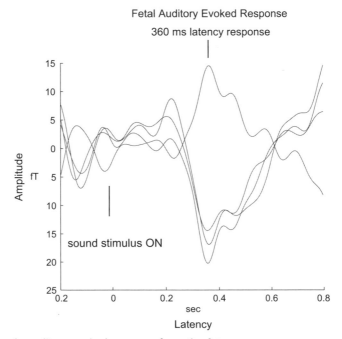

Fetal Auditory Evoked Response

360 ms latency response

**Fig. 2.** A sample auditory evoked response from the fetus.

LED array emits light at wavelength of 629 nm, which is in the visible range (red light). The peak illuminance at the exit of the fiber-optic cable, measured over 33 ms duration light pulse, was 8800 lux. This light pulse was considered safe for the fetus because it is of short duration, contains no short wavelength radiation, and has intensity much lower than sunlight on a bright day (approximately 100,000 lux). Also, the radiant power was 2.79 microwatt/sq-cm in a 33-ms pulse, which is less than a continuous source, eg, a 60-W light bulb; therefore, the issue of thermal damage to tissues does not arise. Preliminary feasibility studies[14] were done with 33-ms flash stimuli, and more recent studies[15] were performed using 100- and 500-ms duration stimuli with an interstimulus interval of 2 seconds. **Fig. 3** shows an averaged VER observed at a latency of 350 ms from 180 light flashes presented to a fetus.

The results of our light studies have shown a decrease in latency over gestation in low-risk fetuses. These results are similar to newborn studies that have shown the shortening of latencies of evoked responses[35–38] with increasing age, suggesting the ongoing maturation of the visual system. These latencies provide information about the maturation of the visual pathway. Increased myelination results in faster conduction along the nerve fibers, resulting in decreased latency values.

## FETAL STUDIES IN HIGH-RISK PREGNANCIES

Evoked responses and the spectral power of the spontaneous activity have been analyzed in 170 high-risk pregnancies. High-risk and low-risk fetuses have been compared.[19]

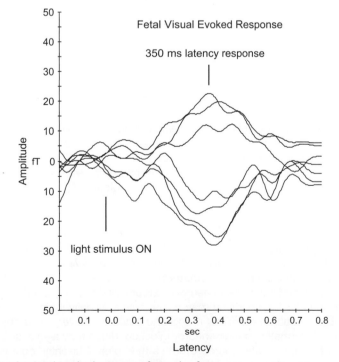

**Fig. 3.** A sample visual evoked response from the fetus.

AERs were investigated in growth-restricted fetuses compared with fetuses of adequate growth. AER latencies of the controls were consistent with existing literature. This study was based on 73 recordings starting at 27 weeks of gestation on 29 pregnant mothers carrying singleton fetuses. Subjects with known chromosomal abnormalities, fetal infections, and stillbirths were excluded. Of the 29 mothers, 15 had uncomplicated pregnancies of adequately growing fetuses and were recruited as control subjects. The remaining 14 women had fetuses with estimated weights below the 10th percentile for gestational age (GA) by ultrasound measurement according to the method of Hadlock and colleagues.[39] After birth, the prenatally classified growth-restricted group was sub-classified as asymmetric and symmetric fetal growth, depending on their growth pattern by ponderal index (PI). Overall, growth-restricted fetuses showed a delay in maturation of auditory-evoked responses[20] as compared with longitudinal studies on low-risk pregnancies. Further, symmetrically growth-retarded fetuses (SGF) had the longest latencies after adjusting for gestational age. When compared with that of normal fetuses, the latency delay for SGF was significantly longer, as was the latency delay for SGF pooled with asymmetrically growth-retarded fetuses (AGF). The latency delay for AGF alone was not statistically significant.

Spontaneous activity powers were estimated in the four frequency bands (delta, theta, alpha, and beta) and compared between the high-risk and low-risk groups using Student $t$ test; a $P$ value less than .10 was considered to be statistically significant. There was a significant difference between the groups in at least one of the spectral bands. The 12 spontaneous recordings in this group were from fetuses that were determined to be growth restricted (IUGR) by ultrasound measurements of estimated fetal weight below the 10th percentile for gestational age, which ranged from 29 to 39 weeks' gestation. Normalized spectral power for each of the spontaneous recordings was computed. Further, fetal spectral power was plotted in each of the four bands in relation to the neonatal outcome, based on standard birth weight classification of newborns. Of the four bands, the normalized spectral power of the theta band showed a significant difference between the two groups. The mean of theta band after birth in the SGA group was 0.063 (SD 0.007), whereas the mean of the appropriate for gestational age (AGA; >10th percentile for gestational age) group was 0.050 (SD 0.004). In summary, although ultrasound showed that 12 fetuses had evidence of growth restriction, this was confirmed in only five infants at birth, all of whom had higher spectral power in the theta band on their MEG recordings. The high false positive rate of projected IUGR based solely on ultrasound measurements is well known. However, in this group of 12 fetuses, the SARA system was able to differentiate those who were truly growth restricted from those who had normal growth at birth. The addition of this kind of physiological assessment to standard morphometric testing would be of great benefit in the effort to reliably diagnose the physiologically affected fetus.

## SUMMARY

Should the diagnostic accuracy of spontaneous fetal MEG be validated in pregnancies at risk for fetal neurological impairment, this technique will prove highly useful in managing complications such as prematurity, in utero asphyxia, preeclampsia, fetal growth restriction, and exposure to neurodevelopmental toxins. Specifically, information on fetal neurological condition may assist timing of delivery in cases of chronic fetal stress by selecting the optimal mode and place of delivery for a compromised fetus. In future, information on fetal neurological condition may also assist the development of potential perinatal neuroprotective therapies. Currently, cost is a limiting factor for its routine clinical use. However, the benefit of this technology lies in the assessment of high-risk pregnancies because current antepartum fetal assessment tests suffer from a high false positive rate (50% to 75%). It is anticipated that MEG will develop as a secondary test after positive initial screening tests to reduce the high false positive rate in high-risk pregnancies that are currently referred to larger centers for follow-up assessment, thereby reducing the rate of unnecessary premature deliveries.

## ACKNOWLEDGMENTS

This study was supported by National Institutes of Health (NIH) grants NINDS/R01NS036277-08A1 and NIBIB/R01EB07826-01A1, USA.

## REFERENCES

1. Herschkowitz N. Brain development in the fetus, neonate and infant. Biol Neonate 1988;54:1–19.
2. Lindsey DB. Head and brain potentials of human fetuses in utero. Am J Psychol 1942;55:412–7.
3. Fulford J, Vadeyar SH, Dodampahala SH, et al. Fetal brain activity in response to a visual stimulus. Hum Brain Mapp 2003;20:239–45.
4. Fulford J, Vadeyar SH, Dodampahala SH, et al. Fetal brain activity and hemodynamic response to a vibroacoustic stimulus. Hum Brain Mapp 2004;22:116–21.
5. Lowery CL, Eswaran H, Murphy P, et al. Fetal magnetoencephalography. Semin Fetal Neonatal Med 2006;11(6):430–6.
6. Lounasmaa OV, Hamalainen M, Hari R, et al. Information processing in the human brain: magnetoencephalographic approach. Proc Natl Acad Sci U S A 1996;93:8809–15.
7. Baillet S, Mosher JC, Leahy RM. Electromagnetic brain mapping. IEEE Signal Process Mag 2001;18(6):14–30.
8. Murakami S, Zhang T, Hirose A, et al. Physiological origins of evoked magnetic fields and extracellular field potentials produced by guinea-pig CA3 hippocampal slices. J Physiol 2002;544:237–51.
9. Malmivuo J, Plonsey R. Bioelectromagnetism. Oxford: Oxford University Press; 1995.
10. Preissl H, Lowery CL, Eswaran H. Fetal magnetoencephalography: current progress and trends. Exp Neurol 2004;190:S37–43.
11. Preissl H, Lowery CL, Eswaran H. Fetal magnetoencephalography: viewing the developing brain in utero. Int Rev Neurobiol 2005;68:1–23.
12. Holst M, Eswaran H, Lowery CL, et al. Development of auditory evoked fields in human fetuses and newborns: a longitudinal MEG study. Clin Neurophysiol 2005;116(8):1949–55.
13. Eswaran H, Lowery CL, Wilson JD, et al. Fetal magnetoencephalography—a multimodal approach. Dev Brain Res 2005;154:57–62.
14. Eswaran H, Wilson JD, Preissl H, et al. Magnetoencephalographic recordings of visual evoked brain activity in the human fetus. Lancet 2002;360(9335):779–80.
15. Eswaran H, Lowery CL, Wilson JD, et al. Functional development of the visual system in human fetus using magnetoencephalography. Exp Neurol 2004;190:S52–8.
16. Rose DF, Eswaran H. Spontaneous neuronal activity in fetuses and newborns. Exp Neurol 2004;190:S28–36.

17. Eswaran H, Haddad N, Shihabuddin BS, et al. Non invasive detection and identification of brain activity patterns in the developing fetus. Clin Neurophysiol 2007;118(9):1940–6.
18. Eswaran H, Wilson JD, Preissl H, et al. Short-term serial magnetoencephalographic recordings of fetal auditory evoked responses. Neurosci Lett 2002; 331(2):128–32.
19. Lowery CL, Govindan R, Murphy P, et al. Assessing cardiac and neurological maturation during the intrauterine period. Semin Perinatol 2008;32(4):263–8.
20. Kiefer I, Siegel ER, Preissl H, et al. Delayed maturation of auditory-evoked responses in growth-restricted fetuses revealed by magnetoencephalographic recordings. Am J Obstet Gynecol 2008;199(5):503.e1–7.
21. De Vries LS. Neurological assessment of the preterm infant. Acta Paediatr 1996; 85(7):765–71.
22. Majnemer A, Rosenblatt B. Evoked-potentials as predictors of outcome in neonatal intensive-care unit survivors: review of the literature. Pediatr Neurol 1996;14(3):189–95.
23. Taylor MJ, McCulloch DL. Visual evoked potentials in infants and children. J Clin Neurophysiol 1992;9(3):357–72.
24. Guerit JM. Applications of surface-recorded auditory evoked potentials for the early diagnosis of hearing loss in neonates and premature infants. Acta Otolaryngol 1985;421:68–76.
25. Beverely DW, Smith IS, Beesley P, et al. Relationship of cranial ultrasonography, visual and auditory evoked responses with neurodevelopmental outcome. Dev Med Child Neurol 1990;32(2):210–22.
26. Tharp B. Neonatal and pediatric electroencephalography. In: Aminoff M, editor. Electrodiagnosis in clinical neurology. New York: Churchill Livingstone; 1986. p. 77.
27. Tharp B. The electroencephalographic aspects of ischemic hypoxic encephalopathy and intraventricular hemorrhage. In: Yabuuchi H, Watanabe K, Okada S, editors. Neonatal brain and behavior. Nagoya (Japan): University of Nagoya Press; 1981. p. 71–8.
28. Tharp B, Scher MS, Clancy RR. Serial EEG's in normal and abnormal infants with birth weights less than 1200 grams—a prospective study with long term follow up. Neuropediatrics 1989;20(2):64–72.
29. Starr A. Auditory brainstem responses in brain death. Brain 1976;99:543–54.
30. Zubick HH, Fried MP, Epstein MF, et al. Normal neonatal brainstem auditory evoked potentials. Ann Otol Rhinol Laryngol 1982;91:485–8.
31. Hepper PG, Shahidullah BS. Development of fetal hearing. Arch Dis Child 1994; 71(2):F81–7.
32. Woods JR, Plessinger MA Jr. The fetal visual evoked potential. Pediatr Res 1986; 20:351–5.
33. Kiuchi M, Nagata N, Ikeno S, et al. The relationship between the response to external light stimulation and behavioral states in the human fetus: how it differs from vibroacoustic stimulation. Early Hum Dev 2000;58:153–65.
34. Peleg D, Goldman JA. Fetal heart rate acceleration in response to light stimulation as a clinical measure of fetal well-being. A preliminary report. J Perinat Med 1980;8:38–41.
35. Hrbek A, Mares P. Cortical evoked responses to visual stimulation in full-term and premature newborns. Electroencephalogr Clin Neurophysiol 1964;16:575–81.
36. Birch EE, O'Connor AR. Preterm birth and visual development. Semin Neonatol 2001;6:487–97.

37. Shepherd AJ, Saunders KJ, McCulloch DL, et al. Prognostic value of flash visual evoked potentials in preterm infants. Dev Med Child Neurol 1999;41(1):9–15.
38. Scherjon SA, Ongerboer de Visser BW, et al. Fetal brain sparing associated with accelerated shortening of visual evoked potential latencies during early infancy. Am J Obstet Gynecol 1996;175(6):1569–75.
39. Hadlock FP, Harrist RB, Martinez-Poyer J. In utero analysis of fetal growth: a sonographic weight standard. Radiology 1991;181(1):129–33.

# Index

*Note:* Page numbers of article titles are in **boldface** type.

## A

Abruptio placenta, 552
Adrenoleukodystrophy, 631–632
Akinesia/hypokinesia, in inborn errors of metabolism, 625
Amphetamines, fetal effects of, 599–600
Anaerobic glycolysis, in cerebral metabolism, 538
Anemia, in infections, 643
Antidepressants, fetal effects of, 600–607
Asphyxia, brain injury in, 581–582
Association of dysplastic and disruptive lesions, in inborn errors of metabolism, 625
ATP synthase defects, 628–630
Atrophy, cerebral, in inborn errors of metabolism, 625
Auditory evoked responses, in magnetoencephalography, 703–704
Autism, vermal malformations in, 519

## B

Basal ganglia, hypoxic injury of, 583–586
Basic helix-loop-helix proteins, in neocortex development, 506–507
Behavior, selective serotonin reuptake inhibitor effects on, 600–607
Biogenic amine transporters, fetal effects of, 607–608
Blindness, cortical, 509
Blood flow, cerebral. *See* Cerebral blood flow and metabolism.
Brain, fetal. *See* Fetal brain.

## C

Calcification, cerebral
    in inborn errors of metabolism, 625
    in infections, 644–646
Cardiac signal monitoring, **683–684**. *See also* Heart rate monitoring.
    electrocardiography in, 679–680
    evolution of, 674–675
    new methods for, 677–679
    spectral analysis of, 676
    standard of care for, 675–676
Cardiovascular collapse, hypoxic injury in, 583–586
Catecholamines
    fetal effects of, 607–608
    methamphetamine effects on, 599–600, 607–608
Cell membrane defects, 623
Cerebellar hypoplasia, in infections, 649

Clin Perinatol 36 (2009) 711–722
doi:10.1016/S0095-5108(09)00084-0
0095-5108/09/$ – see front matter © 2009 Elsevier Inc. All rights reserved.

perinatology.theclinics.com

# Moving?

## Make sure your subscription moves with you!

To notify us of your new address, find your **Clinics Account Number** (located on your mailing label above your name), and contact customer service at:

**Email: journalscustomerservice-usa@elsevier.com**

**800-654-2452** (subscribers in the U.S. & Canada)
**314-447-8871** (subscribers outside of the U.S. & Canada)

**Fax number: 314-447-8029**

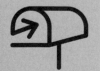

**Elsevier Health Sciences Division**
**Subscription Customer Service**
**3251 Riverport Lane**
**Maryland Heights, MO 63043**

\*To ensure uninterrupted delivery of your subscription, please notify us at least 4 weeks in advance of move.